Veterinary
Epidemiology

Veterinary Epidemiology

PRINCIPLES AND METHODS

S. WAYNE MARTIN

ALAN H. MEEK

PREBEN WILLEBERG

IOWA STATE UNIVERSITY PRESS / AMES

To our families

S. Wayne Martin, D.V.M., Ph.D., is professor in the Department of Veterinary Microbiology and Immunology, Ontario Veterinary College, University of Guelph, Ontario, Canada.

Alan H. Meek, D.V.M., Ph.D., is chairman of the Department of Veterinary Microbiology and Immunology, Ontario Veterinary College, University of Guelph, Canada.

Preben Willeberg, D.V.M., Ph.D., D.V.Sc., is professor in the Department of Forensic and State Veterinary Medicine, Royal Veterinary and Agricultural University, Copenhagen, Denmark.

© 1987 Iowa State University Press, Ames, Iowa, 50014

Orders: 1-800-862-6657   Fax: 1-515-292-3348
Office: 1-515-292-0140   Web site: www.isupress.edu

⊖ Printed on acid-free paper in the United States of America

Authorization to photocopy items for internal or personal use, or the internal or the personal use of specific clients, is granted by Iowa State University Press, provided that the base fee of $.10 per copy is paid directly to the Copyright Clearance Center, 222 Rosewood Drive, Danvers, MA 01923. For those organizations that have been granted a photocopy license by CCC, a separate system of payments has been arranged. The fee code for users of the Transactional Reporting Service is 0-8138-1856-7/87 $.10.

First edition, 1987

Library of Congress Cataloging-in-Publication Data

Martin, S. Wayne
  Veterinary epidemiology.

  Bibliography: p.
  Includes index.
  1. Veterinary epidemiology. I. Meek, Alan H.
II. Willeberg, Preben. III. Title.
SF780.9.M37 1987   636.089′44   87-3169
ISBN 0-8138-1856-7

Last digit is the print number: 9 8 7

C O N T E N T S

P R E F A C E

THE PURPOSE of this textbook is to provide an introductory, yet comprehensive, source of information on epidemiology for veterinary students, researchers, and practitioners. There has not been a textbook that presents analytic epidemiology as a science, basic to veterinary medicine's efforts in health management (herd health) as well as in clinical medicine.

In domestic animal industries the emphasis is on aggregates rather than individuals, and epidemiology has become closely integrated with the formulation and implementation of health maintenance programs. As such, epidemiology will increase in importance as population-oriented health programs become more widely integrated into livestock production systems. It is hoped that the approaches and methods described will assist private practitioners in becoming more involved in formal health management programs, both individually and in conjunction with an epidemiology unit. At the same time, there is a need for those focusing on companion animals to develop a population approach to disease control. Knowledge of the natural history of disease in these populations is of great value for preventive programs, whether these programs are implemented at the population or individual animal level. In addition, structured methods of problem solving and the design and interpretation of clinical trials, when integrated with concepts of sensitivity, specificity, predictive value, and agreement beyond chance levels should enable clinicians to more adequately assess and improve their effectiveness in terms of diagnostic strategies, selecting and interpreting diagnostic tests, and in prognostic and therapeutic activities.

Modern epidemiology overlaps many areas of biometrics; however, we have attempted to minimize statistical techniques. Numerical methods are provided in the chapters on sampling methods, measurement of productivity and disease frequency, and disease causation, since an understanding and working knowledge of these are prerequisites to applying epidemiology in the field. An introductory course in biostatistics would be a useful, but not essential, prerequisite to enhance understanding of this text, since we assume a familiarity with basic statistical notation and operations. This text also contains a chapter on descriptive epidemiologic methods with examples, plus two chapters devoted to features of study design. The chapters on theoretical epidemiology and economics are intended as introductions to these areas of veterinary activity. The last three chapters provide many example applications of the concepts and methods presented earlier in the book. Chapter 12 is particularly pertinent to present and future practitioners.

Throughout the text, we have used examples from the literature to illustrate principles, concepts, and methods. These examples relate to a wide variety of veterinary activities, and we offer no apologies for frequently citing our own work in this regard.

Early drafts of this book were written such that it would be suitable, in size and content, to support a course for veterinary students of 25–30 hours duration. However, with the increasing emphasis on epidemiology at both the professional undergraduate and post-graduate levels, the scope and detail of the text were increased to provide the basis for a 60–80 hour course. Earlier versions have been used for course notes and extension education purposes. The feedback from these students has been invaluable in guiding the book's current structure and content. A recurrent finding in using earlier versions of the book has been that students become much more critical readers of the literature, regardless of their affinity for epidemiology. We see this as a positive result and hope this trend continues.

For those instructors with only 20–30 hours of lecture time in which to teach epidemiology, we suggest that the core ideas of sampling design, measuring disease frequency, statistical evaluation, and epidemiologic measures of association can be presented in a few hours without stressing the associated calculations. Similarly, the major features of observational study design (representativeness of study subjects, valid definitions of exposure and disease, and ensuring comparability of study groups) as well as the additional features of field trials (random assignment, blindness, compliance, and equality of follow up) can be summarized to fit within these time constraints. The book can then serve as a future reference for the details on these subjects.

Only recently have significant numbers of veterinarians attempted to formally link epidemiologic principles with their daily activities. Needless to say this will be an iterative process, but the ultimate goal of serving society, and especially the domestic animal industries, in an optimal manner demands that we continue on this path. We hope this book is of benefit to the veterinary profession and welcome comments or suggestions for its improvement.

Finally, we owe a debt of gratitude to many who have assisted us in preparing this book. In particular, Ian Dohoo, University of Prince Edward

Island, for his assistance with Chapter 12; Mats Rudemo, Royal Veterinary and Agricultural University, Copenhagen, who read an early version for statistical correctness; Tim Carpenter, University of California, Davis, who critiqued Chapters 8 and 9; and David Hird who, with his students, performed a general review of the manuscript. Others to whom we owe a special debt include Nicole Gorman for her patient typing and Margaret Montgomery and Ann Hollings for their proofreading of the manuscript.

A NOTE ON EPIDEMIOLOGY TEXTS

A NUMBER of introductory texts in epidemiology, most of which relate to human health, are available to supplement the material in this book. Some of these texts are: *Epidemiology: Principles and Methods* (MacMahon and Pugh 1970); *Primer of Epidemiology* (Friedman 1973); and *Foundations of Epidemiology* (Lilienfeld and Lilienfeld 1980). More advanced texts include *Epidemiologic Research: Principles and Quantitative Methods* (Kleinbaum, Kupper, and Morgenstern 1982) and *Causal Thinking in the Health Sciences: Concepts and Strategies* (Susser 1973). An excellent text which describes the relationship between epidemiology and infectious diseases is entitled *Natural History of Infectious Diseases* (Burnet and White 1972). In veterinary medicine, the benchmark textbook has been *Epidemiology in Veterinary Practice* (Schwabe, Riemann, and Franti 1977); unfortunately, this text is now out of print. A useful set of notes has been collated into a book form called *Introductory Veterinary Epidemiology* (Blackmore and Harris 1979), and a text emphasizing biometrics in veterinary epidemiology entitled *Statistical Epidemiology in Veterinary Science* (Leech and Sellers 1979) is available. *Patterns of Animal Disease* (Halperin 1975) contains many useful and interesting epidemiologic examples. Although not written as an epidemiology text, a recently published guide, *Interpreting the Medical Literature* (Gehlbach 1982), is an excellent primer in epidemiology.

In practice, epidemiologic principles are closely allied with the economics of health and disease. In order to foster the growth and application of epidemiologic and econometric skills in veterinary medicine, an organization called the International Society for Veterinary Epidemiology and Economics was formed and held its inaugural meeting in 1976. This association has held four symposia to date: the first in Reading, England, 1976; the second in Canberra, Australia, 1979; the third in Arlington, Virginia, 1982; and the fourth in Singapore, 1985. The proceedings of these symposia contain much useful information (see reference list).

Finally, an international journal, *Preventive Veterinary Medicine,* was initiated in 1982, under the editorship of H. Riemann. This journal contains a variety of articles on methodology as well as on the application of epidemiologic and econometric techniques to prevent and control disease in animal populations.

References

Association of Teachers of Veterinary Public Health and Preventive Medicine. 1983. Proc. 3rd Int. Symp. Vet. Epidemiol. Econ. Sept. 1982, Arlington, Va.

Blackmore, D. K., and R. E. Harris. 1979. Introductory Veterinary Epidemiology. Palmerston North, N.Z.: Massey Univ.

Burnet, M., and D. O. White. 1972. Natural History of Infectious Disease. Cambridge, England: Cambridge Univ. Press.

Ellis, P. R., A. P. M. Shaw, and A. J. Stephens, eds. 1976. New techniques in veterinary epidemiology and economics. Proc. 1st Int. Symp. Vet. Epidemiol. Econ., July 1976, Reading, England.

Friedman, G. D. Primer of Epidemiology. 1973. Toronto, Canada: McGraw-Hill.

Geering, W. A., R. T. Roe, and L. A. Chapman, eds. 1980. Proc. 2nd Int. Symp. Vet. Epidemiol. Econ., May 1979, Canberra, Australia.

Gehlbach, S. H. 1982. Interpreting the medical literature: A clinician's guide. Lexington, Mass.: Collamore Press, Heath.

Halperin, B. 1975. Patterns of Animal Disease. Baltimore, Md.: Williams & Wilkins.

Kleinbaum, D. G., L. L. Kupper, and H. Morgenstern. 1982. Epidemiologic Research: Principles and Quantitative Methods. Belmont, Calif.: Wadsworth.

Leech, F. B., and F. C. Sellers. 1979. Statistical Epidemiology in Veterinary Science. New York, N. Y.: Macmillan Co.

Lilienfeld, A. M., and D. E. Lilienfeld. 1980. Foundations of Epidemiology. 2nd ed. New York, N. Y.: Oxford Univ. Press.

MacMahon, B., and T. F. Pugh. 1970. Epidemiology: Principles and Methods. Boston, Mass.: Little, Brown.

Riemann, H. P., ed. 1982/83. Preventive Veterinary Medicine. Amsterdam, The Netherlands: Elsevier.

Schwabe, C. W., H. P. Riemann, and C. E. Franti. 1977. Epidemiology in Veterinary Practice. Philadelphia, Penn.: Lea & Febiger.

Susser, M. 1973. Causal Thinking in the Health Sciences: Concepts and Strategies in Epidemiology. Toronto, Canada: Oxford Univ. Press.

PART **I**

Basic
Principles

CHAPTER 1

Epidemiologic Concepts

1.1 Meaning and Scope of Epidemiology

Epidemiology is a very old science, yet it did not flourish until after the "germ theory" of disease causation became established in the 1800s. Since that time, and until approximately 1960, epidemiology has been closely allied with microbiology in the battle against disease. Subsequent to 1960, epidemiology has become a more holistic discipline, and many factors in addition to the specific agent are investigated to determine their role as potential causes of disease (Schwabe 1982). Concurrently, the use of quantitative methods has become more widespread in epidemiologic research. In veterinary medicine the latter trend has been most pronounced in the last decade. As the emphasis both in veterinary education and practice shifts from the individual animal toward the population, the need for the veterinarian to have skills in quantitative methods will be accentuated. This text has been written in an attempt to assist veterinary students and veterinarians in developing quantitative epidemiologic skills that can be applied to population medicine. It contains a number of introductory epidemiological methods and examples of their application.

Epidemiology may be defined as the study of the patterns of disease that exist under field conditions. More specifically, epidemiology is the study of the frequency, distribution, and determinants of health and disease in populations. Thus, the epidemiology of a disease is the population analogue to the pathogenesis of disease in individuals, and in this context epidemiology is a fundamental science for medicine in populations.

To some, epidemiology is merely a set of methods; however, the use of these methods frequently leads the practitioner to a holistic, population-oriented way of thinking about health and disease that is quite different from the individual patient-oriented approach of clinical medicine. In many instances, the unit of concern in epidemiologic studies is not the individual but rather groups or categories of individuals such as the pen,

3

herd, or flock. Despite this difference in unit of concern, epidemiology requires the same attention to detail and observer skills as clinical medicine and the other biologic sciences.

One method of exploring and understanding epidemiology is by elaborating the previous definition. First, it is noted that epidemiology is the study of the frequency and distribution of disease. Initial clues about the etiology of a disease are often provided by its distribution. That is, information about what animals are affected and where and when a disease occurs often is suggestive of the causes of disease. Subsequently, it will be necessary to formally identify some of the determinants (causes) of the disease, (i.e., to explain why the disease occurs with the objective being to reduce its severity or frequency of occurrence). These details may be obtained by formally contrasting the characteristics of healthy versus diseased individuals, or by contrasting the characteristics of groups having a relatively high frequency of the disease versus groups having either none or a low frequency of the disease of interest. (Studies of the latter type are called case-control studies, and along with other types of analytic observational studies, they are introduced in Chapter 2 and elaborated in Chapter 6.)

Determinants, those factors that influence health and disease, are commonly called causes of disease. In epidemiology the word determinant is used to describe any factor that when altered produces a change in the frequency or characteristics of disease. Therefore, as will be stressed throughout this text, few diseases have a single cause. Host factors (such as age, breed, and sex) frequently are determinants of disease. Many determinants are external to the individual animal, as opposed to the internal factors that relate to the pathogenesis of disease. Putative causes of disease may be referred to as exposure or risk factors (or as independent, predictor, or explanatory variables) because they are suspected of producing the outcome of interest. The presumed effect, usually either health (as measured by productivity) or disease occurrence, is called the outcome, response, or dependent variable. (Variable refers to a property, factor, or characteristic of an individual or group being measured, rather than meaning "changeable.") For example, in a study of the association between immune status (e.g., level of serum antibodies) and the occurrence of disease, immune status is the independent and health status the dependent variable. If the impact of disease on the level of production were being studied, production would be the dependent variable and the presence or absence of disease the independent variable.

Disease and health are not redundant in the above definition, since in all epidemiologic studies both "diseased" and "healthy" animals should be present. As one example of their dual value, contrasting the characteristics of diseased versus healthy animals can provide valuable clues about the causes of disease. Nonetheless, health and disease are relative terms and their definitions usually depend on the circumstances in which they are applied. Hence some working definitions are in order.

Disease may affect individuals in either a subclinical or clinical form. Clinical disease represents the state of dysfunction of the body detectable by one or more of a person's senses. In contrast, subclinical disease represents a functional and/or anatomical abnormality of the body detectable only by selected laboratory tests or diagnostic aids. Although subclinical disease usually is less serious for the individual than clinical disease, it may be more important for the population because of its frequency. As a general rule, regardless of the primary cause(s) of the disease, the number of animals subclinically diseased will be much larger than the number clinically diseased. In this regard, it is particularly important to make a distinction between infection and disease. Infection with most agents (including microorganisms and parasites) of so-called infectious diseases does not lead to clinical disease in the majority of infected animals. In many cases the infected animals appear to be healthy. For present purposes, an animal that is neither clinically nor subclinically diseased is by definition healthy. Most populations comprise varying proportions of healthy, subclinically diseased, and clinically diseased individuals, with the proportions being subject to change over time.

Although health in humans has been defined as a state of complete physical, mental, and spiritual well being, in veterinary medicine, productivity is often used as a surrogate measure of health. In domestic animal populations, whether a disease is present or not is usually less important than the frequency with which the disease occurs and its subsequent impact on productivity. In this context, whereas disease may limit productivity, disease per se may not be the most important limiting factor of production. Other factors (such as management decisions, improper housing, or inadequate feeding practices) may have a greater impact on production in many situations (Williamson 1980). The association of these factors with health status may be investigated in a manner similar to studying the impact of disease on production using the techniques described in this text.

Due partly to the premise that the herd or flock is more important than the individual, the unit of concern for the epidemiologist frequently is an aggregate or population of animals, not an individual (e.g., it is more important that the feedlot is healthy than that a particular animal is healthy). Even when the individual is the unit of concern (e.g., in a study of the effect of vaccination on the health status of individuals), epidemiologic techniques are limited to groups (categories of individuals) rather than to an individual. Epidemiologists do observe individuals within the groups, but the conclusions are based on the experience of the group. Despite this limitation, inferences derived from groups may be extrapolated under certain circumstances to individuals (see 1.5). ("Population" is used throughout this text in two senses — first, to describe the total number of animals in a group being studied who are biologically at risk of the event under study, and second, to refer to the larger number of individuals of a particular type or species about which inferences are being made, based on information from a sample.)

One dimension for conceptualizing the structure of populations is that they are composed of a number of levels of organization. For example, the levels of organization from smallest to largest may be conceptualized in the following manner: cells of similar structure or function form organs, organs form body systems, and individuals are composed of body systems. Litters, pens, or herds are composed of a number of individuals; a collection of herds in one geographic area would form a local industry; and the local industries together would make up a larger animal industry, such as the swine or dairy industry. Each higher level of organization has characteristics beyond those of the lower levels. Individuals have more properties or characteristics than the sum of all the body systems; likewise, herds of animals have more properties than the individuals that compose them.

The level of organization selected for a specific study (the sampling unit in observational studies and the experimental unit in field trials) is the unit of analysis for that study. The unit of analysis often is not the individual animal; for example, if pens of pigs are the sampling units in an observational study, the unit of analysis would be the pen. Recognition of the correct unit of analysis is important for a number of reasons in addition to those already described. The unit of analysis may constrain the causal inferences about individuals that can be drawn from a sample (see 5.6.1) and, in addition, the unit of analysis is the basis for determining the degrees of freedom used in statistical testing.

It should be obvious from the definition and the preceding discussion that the setting for most epidemiologic work is the field (farm, animal clinic, city, nation, etc.) rather than the laboratory. Thus, epidemiologic observations relate to and are derived from field situations, although the analysis of data based on these observations may be conducted in a laboratory environment. Suitably stored and analyzed data will give the epidemiologic laboratory the same essential role in population medicine as the clinical pathology or microbiologic laboratory in individual animal medicine. In another sense, epidemiology is the diagnostic tool for populations, analogous to the role of clinical medicine as the diagnostic tool for individuals.

Finally, all animals, including humans, are possible subjects for epidemiologic study. Historically, epizootiology has been used to describe studies of disease in animal populations, and epidemiology for similar studies in human populations. Since a literal translation of "epidemiology" is the study (logos) of what is upon (epi) the population (demos) and because of the many similarities between human and animal medicine, there is little need to continue to use the term epizootiology. For those wishing to retain the distinction between studies of disease in animals and humans, the linguistic problems associated with this carried to the extreme would result in terms such as epiornithology, epiicthyology, and epiphytology to describe the study of diseases in populations of birds, fish, and plants respectively.

1.2 Purposes of Epidemiology

The major purpose of epidemiology is a pragmatic one; namely, to provide data on which a rational decision for the prevention and/or control of disease in animal populations can be based. In domestic animals this involves optimizing health (productivity) and not necessarily minimizing the occurrence of disease. Many medical disciplines have a similar general purpose. The special contribution of epidemiology is providing information describing the frequency and distribution of health and disease, identifying factors influencing the occurrence and severity of disease in the population of concern (in its natural setting), and quantitating the interrelationships between health and disease.

To fulfill these purposes, an epidemiologic study might be carried out to estimate the frequency of disease (e.g., the rate of infertility in dairy cows) or to identify factors that might cause the disease of concern (e.g., whether the type of ration is associated with the rate of respiratory disease in feedlot cattle). The former activity is known as descriptive epidemiology because its primary purpose is to describe what the syndrome is, who is affected, where the disease occurs, and when it occurs. The latter activity is called analytic epidemiology because the primary emphasis is on the collection and analysis of data to test a hypothesis; that is, to provide answers to why the disease occurred.

The relationship between development of disease and the operational purposes of epidemiology is shown in Figure 1.1. These operational purposes include primary, secondary, and tertiary prevention of disease. (This ordering not only represents a convenient way of differentiating among these purposes, but also reflects their inherent utility in the health care of populations. That is, society should emphasize primary rather than tertiary prevention as a means of improving health status. Health will improve only marginally by killing weeds and treating disease.) Primary prevention includes those activities directed toward preventing exposure to causal factors, particularly the complexes of factors that are sufficient to produce disease. Quarantine and vaccination are examples of primary prevention. Vaccination does not prevent exposure to the agent but can prevent a sufficient cause from forming by rendering the animal immune to the level of challenge by the agent under field conditions.

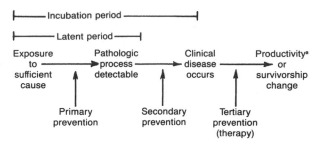

1.1. Relationship between development of disease and operational purposes of
epidemiology.

Secondary prevention includes those activities designed to detect disease processes as early as possible before clinical disease occurs. The underlying and biologically reasonable principle is that early detection will allow
treatment and hence increase the probability of restoring the individual to
full health and reducing production losses. Despite the reasonableness of
this argument, its basis should be formally evaluated whenever possible.
Screening tests to detect brucellosis and tuberculosis, somatic cell counts to
detect mastitis, regular examinations of the postpartum cow, and metabolic
profiles are examples of tests used in secondary prevention.

Tertiary prevention is more commonly known as therapeutics. It has
been noted that for economic reasons tertiary prevention, especially in domestic animals, is somewhat of a salvage operation. However, despite the
best efforts to prevent disease, it will occur (it is hoped much less frequently), and many veterinarians will continue to be employed primarily in
the therapeutic role. At present, much of the time spent during a veterinarian's education is devoted to understanding the pathogenesis of disease,
diagnosing disease, and instituting an adequate therapeutic (including sur-
gical) regime. Yet, epidemiologic skills can increase the clinician's abilities
at tertiary prevention. The concepts of field trials (Chapter 7) are applicable to clinical trials and the evaluation of therapeutic regimes. In terms of
diagnosing disease, various forms of decision analysis (see Chapter 9) are
becoming more widely used as an aid to understanding the process of differential diagnosis as well as for evaluation of alternative therapeutic strategies. Epidemiologic studies are used infrequently to study the pathogenesis
of disease; nonetheless, the results of epidemiologic studies often provide

indirect but useful clues about the nature of the disease process.

As shown in Figure 1.1, the period between exposure to an agent (infection) and the occurrence of clinical disease is referred to as the incubation period. Infectious agents often have different incubation periods, and this knowledge can be of value when investigating or predicting disease outbreaks. The latent period for infectious diseases refers to the period between infection and shedding of the organism and is usually shorter than the incubation period. For noninfectious diseases, it is the period between exposure to the agent and the occurrence of detectable pathologic changes.

As previously mentioned, high production can be a cause of disease as well as being affected, usually adversely, by the occurrence of disease (Figure 1.1). Monitoring productivity at the herd and the individual animal level often provides the first clue that something is wrong biologically. Hence production monitoring should be an integral component of a health management program, a feature that will be elaborated in subsequent chapters. A simplified concept of production monitoring is shown in Figure 1.2. By monitoring production, disease may be detected at an early stage; hence production monitoring is a form of secondary prevention. For instance in Figure 1.2 production decreases could have been used to predict the subsequent occurrence of calfhood diseases and/or those occurring at the second calving. The diagram also implies that level of production could be used to detect subclinical diseases (e.g., mild metritis at the first calving) as well as the occurrence of other events such as estrus.

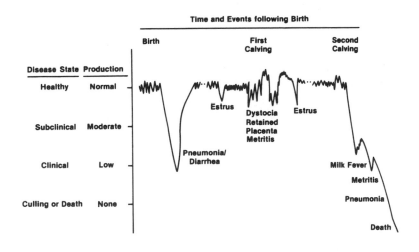

1.2. Hypothetical relationship between production monitoring and disease states and other events. Production level can be measured in calves by weight gain or feed efficiency and after first calving in milk production per day.

1.3 Basic Concepts

Most epidemiologic work is based on four principles or concepts about health and disease (see MacMahon and Pugh 1970, Chapter 1). The first and perhaps oldest concept is that disease occurrence is related to the environment of the species being studied. Here environment includes the physical, biological, and sociological (ethological) milieu of an individual. The origin of this concept is usually attributed to the Hippocratic writings in "On Airs Waters and Places," although the factual basis for this belief has been disputed (Roth 1976). To identify the specific environmental factors leading to disease occurrence, epidemiologists frequently compare environments where disease is prevalent to those where it is infrequent or absent.

Weather is a major component of the environment, and its role as a determinant of many parasitic diseases and vectorborne infections is well documented. For example, warm, wet weather provides optimal environment for most helminth parasites to survive outside the host. Dryness is usually harmful to their survival, while most survive cold weather quite well. Similarly, warm, wet conditions provide a very suitable environment for the survival and multiplication of insects that can serve as vectors of disease. However, less obvious effects (such as the impact of weather on morbidity and mortality) are poorly documented and understood. In a study designed to investigate the association between weather and survivorship of dairy calves in California, the results indicated that the number of births each day, the risk of death for calves born each day, and the day of death were all influenced by weather extremes (Martin et al. 1975).

Weather also could exert its effects on calf health in indirect ways. In hot climates, cows kept in an open paddock will seek shade during the day to reduce heat stress. However, most cows prefer to calve in more isolated, quiet areas and will usually leave the shaded areas and deliver their calf near the periphery of the paddock. Subsequent to parturition, the cow is torn between her mothering instincts such as licking and drying her calf and assisting it to nurse and her desire to return to the shaded area. Many cows choose the latter, and the calf is deserted and left in the hot sun. This can severely compromise the calf since the temperature regulating mechanisms of the newborn are subject to extremes in temperature, and the calf can lose large amounts of body fluids attempting to maintain its body temperature within reasonable limits. Thus lack of mothering, failure to obtain adequate amounts of colostrum, and stress of maintaining its body temperature can singly and jointly greatly increase the susceptibility of a calf to a number of infectious agents. Because of this, many calves succumb to enteritis, septicemia, and pneumonia, greatly reducing the likelihood of surviving the early postpartum period. Nonclimatic components of the environment, such as management and housing, also appear to exert a great effect on calf health in particular and on disease occurrence and productivity in general. Most of the evidence on this matter, however, is based largely on clinical impressions, and relatively few formal studies on the role of these factors have been conducted.

Although conceptually some prefer to have a separate category for agents in the host-environment-agent triad (see Fig. 1.3a), the preference here is to treat agents as a component of the environment (see Fig. 1.3b) and to evaluate their importance in perspective, relative to other environmental factors that influence the health status of animals. It may be noteworthy that host and agent factors receive much emphasis in veterinary education, most schools having departments formally structured to study these factors. Few medical or veterinary schools have departments whose faculty are devoted to the study of the environment or the relationship between the environment and host. This may lead to a failure to appreciate the multiple ways environmental factors exert their effects. It also may narrow the concepts of disease causation and methods of disease control. Knowledge of the involvement of specific infectious and/or toxic agents in a disease has been extremely helpful in controlling many diseases. At the

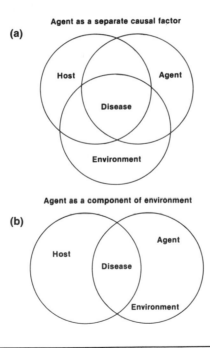

1.3. Relationship among host characteristics, environmental factors, agents, and disease.

same time, however, it has tended to lead to the overreliance on antimicrobials and vaccines as the primary means of disease control. In discussing this subject, White (1974) stresses the need for a more holistic ecological view of health and disease.

The second principle of epidemiologic work is to count the occurrence of natural events such as births, disease and death. Quantification per se is perhaps the most obvious aspect of modern day epidemiology and points out the need for veterinarians to have knowledge of basic demographic and statistical techniques. Using this approach, and despite the incompleteness and inaccuracies of the available data (the Bills of Mortality), it was demonstrated in the mid-1600s that many biological phenomena when taken in mass were quite predictable. John Graunt, who is credited with this observation, is often viewed as the father of demography and as such contributed greatly to both statistics and epidemiology. "It may be of interest . . . that the father of demography was not a trained statistician, nor a trained epidemiologist, but (a draper) a careful and original thinker who reasoned that if disease was more common in one area, in one sex, in one population, there had to be a reason which required exploration and which, upon identification, could lead to a reduction of illness. This, after all, is still the basic goal of the epidemiologist" (Wynder 1975).

This predictability of mass events is used implicitly and explicitly by veterinarians and is a cornerstone of epidemiologic field studies. Clinicians implicitly make use of this feature as an aid to diagnosis (e.g., by knowing that certain diseases—milk fever, left displaced abomasum, and reticuloperitonitis—occur much more frequently at or near parturition than at other times in a cow's life). Epidemiologists explicitly use this feature (e.g., castrated cats fed dry cat food and housed only indoors are much more likely to develop feline urologic syndrome than noncastrated cats fed moist foods and allowed exercise outdoors, or as another example, the morbidity curve in recently transported feedlot animals is much more predictable than which individual will develop disease). Implicitly, this feature stimulates the inquiring mind to seek reasons to explain why a disease occurs in certain circumstances and not others (e.g., why wildlife rabies appears to be more common in relatively urbanized areas than in more isolated rural areas).

It may be worthwhile to note that a medical or veterinary degree is not essential for a person to an epidemiologist (White 1974). Certainly, both historically and presently, many people not specifically trained in medicine contribute greatly to the field of disease prevention and control, if not specifically to epidemiology. The exact training and educational requirements to become a "card-carrying" epidemiologist have been the subject of much debate, mainly in response to the formation of a professional college to certify epidemiologists (Lilienfeld 1980; Stallones 1980). Veterinarians, because of their excellent biological training, have made great contributions to health maintenance and disease prevention. To an extent the statement that "every veterinarian is an epidemiologist" is true, yet this should not detract from the additional benefits to be obtained by formal training in epidemiology.

The third concept of epidemiologic work is to utilize nature's experiments whenever possible. Because the epidemiologist usually is involved in nature's experiments only as an observer, such studies are termed observational studies. As an example, in a study to assess the effect of different ventilation systems on pneumonia in swine, one could identify sufficient numbers of swine—some raised in barns ventilated by one system, some raised in barns ventilated by other systems, and some raised in barns with no formal system for exchange of air—and note the extent of pneumonia in pigs raised under these specific ventilation systems. If carefully planned and analyzed, field observations such as these can provide much useful information on the effectiveness of various types of ventilation systems, as well as the relationship of other factors to health and disease. In many such instances experimental studies are too impractical, and thus observational studies provide the only remaining scientific avenue of investigation. Yet, despite the practical utility and scientific validity of observational studies, many medical scientists dismiss or play down the results of such nonexperimental work. The logical basis for their dismissal is often unclear or nonexistent, and a detailed discussion concerning observational and experimental studies will be provided in subsequent chapters.

Sometimes it is possible to observe natural situations that simulate manipulative experimental conditions quite closely. A classic example of such a study is Dr. John Snow's investigation of cholera epidemics in England during the 1800s, some 30 years prior to the identification of the cholera bacillus (MacMahon and Pugh 1970; Susser 1973).

Dr. Snow noted the nature of the disease, a profuse diarrhea, and observed that although most members of a household became infected, the doctors and nurses who cared for them usually remained healthy. On this basis, he believed the disease was not directly contagious, but that contamination of the water supply by feces was a major method of disease transmission. (He had difficulty convincing his colleagues of this because miasma—bad air—was the major explanation of disease causation at that time.)

To test his hypothesis, Snow analyzed data from Bills of Mortality and was able to show a close association between the company supplying water and the level of cholera in different areas of London. The Southwark and Vauxhall and the Lambeth companies both obtained water downstream from the sewage outlet in the Thames River, and people in the areas served by these companies experienced higher mortality rates than people in other areas of London. After the 1849 epidemic, Lambeth moved its inlet upstream. Subsequently, in the 1853 cholera epidemic, people receiving water from this company had much lower levels of mortality from cholera than people in the same area who received water from Southwark and Vauxhall. Snow used this change of inlet location to study the occurrence of cholera in households. In one area of London this change resulted in the two companies supplying water to houses on the same streets, the residents in the area often not recognizing this fact. He cleverly developed a screening test to determine which company supplied water to each house when the occupants, relatives, or previous owners were unsure of the source of their water (downstream water had a high salt content). By doing this, Snow was able to show that people in houses supplied with water from Southwark and Vauxhall had a much higher rate of cholera than those supplied by Lambeth. By carefully documenting the water supply, the number of deaths, number of cholera cases, and number of people at risk in each household, Snow was able to convince the authorities that a clean water supply was indeed the key to preventing cholera epidemics. (Using households as the sampling unit rather than larger units defined by water supply was a significant improvement in Snow's ability to identify the cause of cholera in individuals. It is in fact a general principle that if the unit of concern is individuals, then individuals should be the sampling unit if one hopes to detect a direct cause of disease.)

The history of contagious bovine pleuropneumonia (CBPP) and its eradication from North America provide further insight into the usefulness of field observations, when attempting to understand and/or control disease (Law 1887; Jasper 1967; Schwabe 1984). CBPP (lung fever) was probably present in Asia for hundreds of years before the nineteenth century. It was probably spread throughout Europe by the movement of cattle as a sequel to the Napoleonic wars and was introduced into North America, Australia, and probably Africa by shipments of infected cattle.

The first recorded case of lung fever introduced into the United States was in a cow purchased from an English ship in 1843. Later shipments of cattle from Holland to America (1859) were also known to be infected. The disease had a long incubation period, approximately 4–7 weeks, and was usually progressive, with severe debility or death within a few weeks to months subsequent to clinical onset. Field observations suggested that animal to animal contact was the major route of transmission, although spread by fomites (human clothes or boots, infected barns, feed, and manure) was known to have occurred. Effective transmission usually required close and prolonged animal-to-animal contact, although numerous examples of its spread after brief contact are cited (Law 1887). (Interpretation of the historical information on this subject is difficult because other respiratory diseases may have been confused with CBPP.)

Initially, much debate centered on "spontaneous generation" versus "contagion" as an explanation for the pattern of disease occurrence. However, with careful documentation of cases and outbreaks (descriptive epidemiology), it became clear that imported or purchased cattle were the most logical source of the disease in almost every instance. Experiments were also conducted to demonstrate conclusively that the disease was contagious and did not arise spontaneously. It was noted, however, that the disease spread more rapidly and tended to be more severe during the summer than during the winter; this feature may have been of help in the eradication program. (The disease was more difficult to control in warmer climates such as Australia, a country that only recently became CBPP-free.) Early uncoordinated control efforts by individual veterinarians and farmers proved unsuccessful at slowing the spread of the disease, and by 1886 it had spread to Illinois, Kentucky, and Missouri. Consequently, the export of meat and meat products to England from the United States was terminated; the embargo lasting for almost 35 years, long after CBPP had been eradicated.

In 1856 the Bureau of Animal Industry was formed in the United States under the direction of Daniel Elmer Salmon, and in 1887 Congress provided sufficient funds to begin a large-scale organized eradication program. These activities included case-finding, slaughter of infected animals and/or herds, disinfection with lime and/or sulphur as well as fodder and manure disposal on infected farms, and quarantine, both for cattle entering the United States and for cattle movement within the continent. Through these activities CBPP was eradicated by 1892, at least 6 years before Nocard, a French veterinarian, cultured and identified the direct cause of the disease, a mycoplasma agent. This successful campaign was the first major triumph of organized veterinary medicine in North America. Today, the eradication of CBPP and the work of Snow on cholera serve to remind epidemiologists that control of disease is possible without a complete understanding of its etiology or pathogenesis provided that a sufficient amount of its natural history is known. Knowing the natural history of a disease often suggests weak links in the causal chain, that if broken can prevent the spread and/or persistence of the disease.

The fourth basic concept of epidemiology is that controlled field experiments should be performed whenever possible. However, they should be performed in the species of interest and in its natural environment. Such experiments, often called field trials, are analogous to laboratory experiments requiring the same design and performance rigor. In field trials the type, timing, and level of challenge are left to nature; the possible modifying effects of the natural environment are incorporated in the trial such that the results are directly applicable to practical situations. Thus, although a major part of epidemiologists' work involves observational studies, the necessity to conduct experiments under field conditions can not be overemphasized. For example, Snow's ultimate evidence incriminating contaminated water as the major factor in the cholera outbreaks was obtained from an experiment; his experiment involved removing the handle of the Broad Street pump at a major contaminated water source in this area of the city. This forced the people to walk to a more distant but clean water source. Subsequently, a dramatic decline in morbidity and mortality from cholera occurred in this area of London, while people in other areas supplied with contaminated water continued to experience high levels of sickness and death.

A number of new drugs, vaccines, and feed additives have been marketed for prophylactic and therapeutic purposes. At the same time, many programs, including the construction of new buildings, have been proposed to prevent or control disease. If these products or programs were as effective as originally claimed, there would be little need for the continuous supply of new programs and products. Changes in resistance patterns, emergence of new agents, and new demands from industry and society (e.g., protection against residues) may place demands on the biologic industries to supply better products. However, many biologics and disease control programs are not adequately tested to ensure that they are efficacious under field conditions at the time of marketing. Often, officials in charge of licensing biologics do not believe that field trials are practical or valid; hence most governmental licensing agencies do not require formal randomized field trials to be conducted prior to licensure. It is an unfortunate truism that efficacy under controlled laboratory conditions is often not validated under actual field conditions. A review of bovine respiratory disease vaccines discusses and highlights some of these problems (Martin 1983).

Today most progressive medical schools stress the need for controlled trials to ensure that medical practitioners do more good than harm when they administer biologics to their clients. As mentioned, some veterinarians and medical doctors advance the argument that testing biologics or disease prevention programs under "real-world" conditions is inappropriate because of the lack of control over challenge; others believe that any experimentation with clients' animals is unethical. In general, the epidemiologic stance on this matter is that it is necessary to evaluate biologics and disease control programs under the conditions that will be used in the field and to alter the management systems and/or develop new biologics as required. Field-trial design can make allowance for the probability of challenge, the likely effectiveness of the product being evaluated, etc. Failure to experiment may allow the widespread use of ineffective programs or potentially dangerous biologics, which might prove more costly biologically and economically than the original disease.

1.4 Nature of Epidemiologic Studies

Epidemiologic studies follow the general scientific method. Hypotheses are derived from clinical observations and descriptive studies (descriptive epidemiology and case reports) in combination with existing knowledge about the disease. (Recall that Snow's original hypothesis was based on his clinical observations, and his initial descriptive studies provided results consistent with his hypothesis.) These theories are then tested by a formal study, the results of which either validate or modify current knowledge. The process is repeated, each iteration of this cycle bringing the investigators closer to the solution of the problem.

At any point different disciplines may be at very different stages of this cycle (e.g., there may be much knowledge about the pathogenesis of a disease yet little knowledge about the natural history of that disease), and given the current burgeoning of knowledge, today's facts will probably change in the near future. It is partially for this reason that this text stresses concepts (organizing principles) and methods whose rate of change is much slower than that of facts. In this regard, Schwabe (1982) has summarized five scientific revolutions in veterinary medicine (the profession's response to the recognition by researchers and practitioners that the prevailing concepts were inadequate to solve prevailing problems) and the new developments these revolutions produced. In terms of disease causation, the concepts have evolved from supernatural forces, to natural forces (miasma), humoral imbalances, and man-created filth (sanitary awakening) to specific etiologic agents. Today most medical professionals accept the concept of multiple determinants (i.e., host, agent, and environmental factors).

The formal evaluation of hypotheses is central to the advancement of medicine. The three distinctly different approaches to hypothesis testing are observational studies, controlled experiments, and theoretical studies.

In observational studies, the epidemiologist observes but does not attempt to influence or directly control the independent or dependent variables under study. That is, the epidemiologist has no control over which animals are exposed to a specific factor (e.g., vaccination) and no control over the challenge of that factor (e.g., the presence or absence of specific organisms). (The presence of the investigator may indirectly influence the factors under study, however. This is true when studying management factors, particularly when the study is conducted over a prolonged period. Revealing initial results can similarly induce owners to change their management practices before the study is completed. These unintentional effects need to be considered when performing and interpreting the results of observational studies.)

Experiments may be laboratory- or field-centered and may be classified as true experiments if formal random allocation to treatment is used and quasi experiments if formal random allocation is not used. As previously mentioned, it is an epidemiologic tenet that field trials (controlled experiments) may be required to assess how well products and programs work under field conditions (e.g., how well a vaccination regime works under field conditions). In laboratory experiments the investigator exerts direct control over the treatment (e.g., vaccination) and challenge (exposure) of the animals under study. This control can greatly enhance the precision of the results obtained relative to observational methods and field experiments, but the conditions of the experiment may differ sufficiently from actual field conditions so as to greatly restrict the extrapolation of the results beyond the actual experimental setting. The more natural the experimental setting, the less likely this is to be a problem. Regardless of where the experiment is performed, in true experiments the investigator exerts control over the actual allocation of treatment to individuals using a formal random process. In quasi experiments the investigator personally assigns the treatment rather than using formal random allocation. True experiments are much more likely to yield valid results than quasi experiments, particularly if the investigator is seeking to prove a point rather than trying to solve a biologic problem.

For a variety of reasons there are few examples of well-conducted field trials in the veterinary medical literature. Many veterinarians understand basic principles of experimentation, but laboratory experiments often utilizing germ-free animals, single-agent disease models, or highly controlled trials in atypical environments have dominated research interest. Although the latter experiments provide much useful basic scientific information, they are not substitutes for well-performed field trials. It is hoped that the use of experimentation under field conditions will become more widespread.

An example may help to clarify the difference between observational studies and experiments. There has been renewed interest in assessing the efficacy of vaccines against respiratory disease in feedlot calves, particularly when vaccination is conducted 3–4 weeks prior to shipment of calves to feedlots (preimmunization or prevaccination). In a field trial of these vaccines, individual calves were randomly (a formal, not haphazard, process) assigned to receive or not receive specific vaccines. The calves were identified by ear tag and followed to the purchasing feedlot; the subsequent rates of treatment for respiratory disease were noted (Martin et al. 1983). At the same time, an observational study was conducted based on the extent of respiratory disease in prevaccinated calves sold as part of a program to encourage preconditioning (weaning, creep feeding, and vaccination) and prevaccination (vaccination only). The owners of the prevaccinated calves had decided to vaccinate their calves; the decision was not influenced by the investigator. Nonprevaccinated calves in the same feedlots, many from the same saleyard, served as controls (Church et al.

1981). What then is the key difference between these two studies? The main difference is the control offered by the process of randomization. In the field trial, randomization ensured that the vaccinated and unvaccinated groups were comparable and thus prevented other factors, known and unknown, from biasing the results. (Technically, randomization allows one to calculate the probability of dissimilarities in the groups after assignment; it does not guarantee that the groups will be similar.) In the observational study a large number of differences may have existed between the vaccinated and unvaccinated calves, and these could magnify or reduce the true effect of the vaccine(s). Thus the evidence from one observational study is much less convincing than evidence from one field experiment, but the observational study is much easier to perform. In this instance both the experimental and observational study results suggested little if any benefit from prevaccination. (Note in this analytic observational study that the unit of analysis was a group of calves, not an individual calf. The importance of this difference will be elaborated in Chapters 2 and 7.)

The theoretical approach to hypothesis testing has expanded with the advent of modern computers and represents a major new and expanding activity for epidemiologists. In studies of this type, some form of model is used in an attempt to mimic reality. If the model can simulate field conditions closely, it may be used to test a large number of hypotheses without having to do expensive and time-consuming field studies. Although the use of this approach has only recently gained attention and credence in veterinary medicine, appropriate models can greatly enhance our ability to test multiple theories in a short period. For example, a model of mastitis in dairy herds (Morris 1976) can be used to investigate biologic and economic results from various control strategies. Similarly, a model of *Fasciola hepatica* in sheep (Meek and Morris 1981) can be used to assess alternative treatment strategies for sheep under various stocking densities and paddock conditions. Even much simpler mathematical models, such as the Reed-Frost model of disease transmission in populations, are illustrative of the principles that underlie the spread of infectious diseases (Schwabe et al. 1977). This approach to the study of disease will be described later (Chapter 8), and although still in its infancy, computer modelling will likely become an integral part of decision making in veterinary medicine.

1.5 Sequence of Causal Reasoning

Since observational studies are central to epidemiologic work and their use is only now becoming widespread in veterinary medicine, it may be instructive to review the reasoning process associated with these studies. In observational studies the sequence of causal reasoning might be described as a three-stage process. First, it is necessary to ascertain whether the independent variable (the exposure factor) is statistically associated with the dependent variable (the outcome). Second, if the variables are associated statistically, there is a set of accepted criteria to assess whether the variables are likely to be causally associated. Finally, the nature and consequences of the causal association may be elaborated, using for example, path models, simulation models, or actual experimentation.

Thus the study of associations is central to observational studies. The way in which epidemiologists use "association", in contrast to its general use by veterinarians and biologists, is perhaps best explained with an example. Suppose *Haemophilus somnus* is isolated from 30% of lungs of cattle with pneumonia. Does this mean that isolating the organism and having pneumonia are associated? In common usage, the word association describes two events occurring together (physically, functionally, or temporally) in the same individual. Thus in everyday parlance they would appear to be associated. However, epidemiologically speaking, there is insufficient information to reach such a conclusion. For two events to be associated epidemiologically, they must occur together more or less frequently than would be expected from chance alone. For an epidemiologic association, *H. somnus* must be present more or less frequently in cattle with pneumonia than in cattle without pneumonia. Notice that a formal comparison group is always required to measure association. That is, non-diseased animals are compared to diseased animals, and unexposed animals serve as a comparison for exposed animals. Statistical tests to evaluate the likelihood that the observed association (i.e., the difference in frequency of the factor or disease) is due to sampling error (i.e., chance variation) will be described in subsequent chapters.

Associations describe the relationship for categories of individuals rather than for a particular individual. As an example, there is a valid association between castration and feline urologic syndrome, the categories being castration status and urologic disease status. The association does not say that a particular cat developed urologic syndrome because it was castrated, nor does it say that a particular cat did not develop urologic disease because it was not castrated. It could happen in an individual cat that castration prevented the disease, although the general tendency was in the opposite direction. However, the stronger the association (the group experience), the more likely it is that the association based on categories of individuals may apply to individual cats. Thus if 90% of agammaglobulinemic calves die within 28 days of birth and only 2% of calves with normal levels of gammaglobulin die in that period, it would very likely be true to say that an individual agammaglobulinemic calf died because of the lack of globulins. Arguments such as this that move from the general (the study result) to the specific (the individual) are termed deductive. Arguments that move from the specific (the study) to the general (the reference population) are called inductive. For either type of argument to be of value, the study results must be valid; hence this text stresses methods of design likely to enhance the validity of results.

The above scenario also illustrates the difficulty in establishing the cause(s) of an event in individual animals. If an aborted fetus is infected with bovine virus diarrhea virus (a putative cause of abortion), what is the likelihood that the fetus was aborted because of this viral infection? In other words, what is the probability that bovine virus diarrhea virus was the cause of abortion in this fetus? Further study of this text should provide the reader with a basis for attempting to answer this and similar questions.

References

Church, T., R. Williams, D. Karen, and G. Bradshaw. 1981. Alberta certified feeder program, 1980–81. Edmonton, Canada: Alberta Dep. Agric.

Jasper, D. E. 1967. Mycoplasmas, their role in bovine disease. J. Am. Vet. Med. Assoc. 151:1650–55.

Law, J. 1887. The Lung Plague of Cattle, Contagious Pleuro-pneumonia. *In* The Farmers Veterinary Advisor. Ithaca, N. Y.: Cornell Univ.

Lilienfeld, A. M. 1980. The American College of Epidemiology. Am. J. Epidemiol. 111:380–382.

MacMahon, B., and T. F. Pugh. 1970. Epidemiology: Principles and Methods. Boston, Mass.: Little, Brown.

Martin, S. W. 1983. Vaccination: Is it effective in preventing respiratory disease or influencing weight gains in feedlot calves? Can. Vet. J. 24:10–19.

Martin, S. W., C. W. Schwabe, and C. E. Franti. 1975. Dairy calf mortality rate: The association of daily meteorological factors and calf mortality. Can. J. Comp. Med. 39:377–88.

Martin, W., P. Willson, R. Curtis, B. Allen, and S. Acres. 1983. A field trial of preshipment vaccination, with intranasal infectious bovine rhinotracheitis-parainfluenza-3 vaccines. Can. J. Comp. Med. 47:245–49.

Meek, A. H., and R. S. Morris. 1981. A computer simulation model of ovine fascioliasis. Agric. Syst. 7:49–77.

Morris, R. S. 1976. The use of computer modelling in epidemiological and economic studies of animal disease. Ph.D. thesis, Univ. of Reading, Reading, Eng.

Roth, D. 1976. The scientific basis of epidemiology: An historical and philosphical enquiry. Ph.D. thesis, Univ. of Calif., Berkeley.

Schwabe, C. 1982. The current epidemiologic revolution in veterinary medicine, pt 1. Prev. Vet. Med. 1:5–15.

Schwabe, C. W. 1984. Veterinary Medicine and Human Health. 3rd ed. Baltimore, Md.: Williams & Wilkins.

Schwabe, C. W., H. P. Riemann, and C. E. Franti. 1977. Epidemiology in Veterinary Practice. Philadelphia, Penn.: Lea & Febiger.

Stallones, R. A. 1980. Letter to the editor. Re: The proposed American College of Epidemiology. Am. J. Epidemiol. 111:460.

Susser, M. 1973. Causal Thinking in the Health Sciences: Concepts and Strategies in Epidemiology. Toronto, Canada: Oxford Univ. Press.

White, K. 1974. Contemporary epidemiology. Int. J. Epidemiol. 3:295–303.

Williamson, N. B. 1980. The economic efficacy of a veterinary preventive medicine and management program in Victoria dairy herds. Aust. Vet. J. 56:1–9.

Wynder, E. 1975. A corner of history: John Graunt, 1620–1674, the father of demography. Prev. Med. 4:85–88.

C H A P T E R *2*

Sampling Methods

Good sample design is an essential component of surveys and analytic studies. Hence, this chapter contains methods for obtaining data from a representative subset (sample) of a population and makes inferences about the characteristics of the population. Other aspects of data collection (e.g., questionnaire design) are discussed in 6.1.

Sometimes data from a census are available to describe events in a population; no sampling is required and hence no information is lost, as can occur when selecting only a subset of the population. More frequently, data are available from only a subset of the population, and that subset may or may not have been selected by formal sampling methods. For example, data from outbreak investigations or routinely collected data from hospitals or client records (e.g., case reports) may be viewed as arising from a sample of the population, although no formal sampling is used. As will become apparent, there are fewer problems in extrapolating from data obtained by formal planned sampling than from data whose collection was unplanned.

There are two reasons why an epidemiologist would take a planned sample of a population. One is to describe the characteristics (i.e., frequency and/or distribution of disease or production levels) of a population. Examples might include selecting a sample of dairy cows to estimate the extent of subclinical mastitis in a population and selecting a sample of the dog population to estimate the percentage vaccinated against diseases such as rabies. Descriptive studies such as these are called surveys. The process of collating and reporting information from planned surveys, routinely collected data, or outbreak investigations is termed descriptive epidemiology (see Chapter 4).

The second reason for taking a planned sample is to assess specific associations (e.g., test hypotheses) between events and/or factors in the population. Examples would be a sample designed to look for associations between the type of milking equipment and milking procedures and the level of mastitis in the herd, or a study designed to test the hypothesis that certain phenotypes of dogs are more susceptible to bone cancer than others. Studies such as these are analytic studies, and the process of collating, analyzing, and interpreting the information is termed analytical epidemiology (see Chapter 6). In practice, the differences between these types of observational studies often become nebulous. For example, it is not uncommon to do some hypothesis testing using data from surveys. Nonetheless, since the main emphasis of surveys differs from hypothesis testing, the distinction is maintained to simplify and add order to the description of the underlying sampling strategies.

Whether the study is a survey or an analytic study, how the study members are obtained from the population (i.e., the method of sampling) will determine the precision and nature of extrapolations from the sample to the population. Planning the sampling strategy is a major component of survey design. Although sampling per se is only a small part of the design of an analytic study, its central importance is indicated by the fact that the three common types of analytic studies are named on the basis of the sample selection strategy.

Further details on sampling are available in a number of texts (Snedecor and Cochran 1980; Cochran 1977; Levy and Lemeshow 1980; Leech and Sellers 1979; Schwabe et al. 1977). An excellent manual on sampling in livestock disease surveys is provided by Cannon and Roe (1982).

2.1 General Considerations

State the objectives clearly and concisely. The statement should include the parameters being estimated and the unit of concern. Usually, it is best to limit the number of objectives, otherwise the sampling strategy and study design can become quite complex.

The investigator usually will have a reference or target population in mind. This population is the aggregate of individuals whose characteristics will be elucidated by the study. The population actually sampled is often more restricted than this target population, and it is important that the sampled population be representative of the target population. It would be inappropriate to attempt to make inferences about the occurrence of disease in the swine population of an entire country (the target population) based on a sample of swine from one abattoir or samples obtained from a few large farms (the sampled population). As another example, data from diagnostic laboratories usually are not representative of problems in the source population and hence would not be appropriate for estimating disease prevalence.

In planning a sample, note the type and amount of data to be collected. If the objectives are straightforward and few in number, this aspect of planning is easy. At this stage of planning, explicit definitions of the outcome must be considered. That is, in a study to estimate the frequency of metritis in dairy cows, the outcome (metritis), must be clearly defined. This increases the scientific validity of the study and allows other workers to compare their results (similarities and differences) to those of the survey. Related to this matter is the data collection method (e.g., personal interview, mailed questionnaire, special screening tests). Identifying the validity and accuracy of data collection methods are discussed in Chapter 3.

Because the results of samples are subject to some uncertainty due to sampling variation, it is important to consider how precise (quantitatively) the answer needs to be. The results of different samples will, in general, not be equal; the greater the precision required (the smaller the sample to sample variation), the larger the sample must be. Factors that influence the number of sampling units required in surveys are discussed in 2.2.8, analytic studies in 2.4.4.

Prior to selecting the sample, the sampled population must be divided into sampling units. The size of the unit can vary from an individual to an aggregate of individuals, such as litters, pens, or herds. The list of all sampling units in the sampled population is called the sampling frame. Often because of practical considerations, although the unit of concern may be individuals, aggregates of individuals are used as the initial sampling unit. For example, although the objective might be to estimate the prevalence of brucella antibodies in cattle (the unit of concern), the initial sampling unit might be the herd, since a list of all cattle in the population would be difficult to construct. In other instances, to estimate the average somatic cell count of milk in dairy herds, the unit of concern is the herd and it also could be the sampling unit (e.g., a convenient way of obtaining a representative sample of milk from the herd would be to take an aliquot portion of milk from the bulk milk tank).

Finally, before proceeding with the full study it is important to pretest the procedures to be used. Such pretesting should be sufficiently rigorous to detect deficiencies in the study design. This would include the sample selection, clarity of questionnaires, and acceptability and performance of screening tests. This pretest should also be used to evaluate whether the data to be collected in the actual study are appropriate to answer the original objectives.

2.2 Estimating Population Characteristics in Surveys

To provide a practical illustration of the different methods of survey sampling, assume that the investigator wishes to estimate the percentage of adult cows (beef and dairy) in a large geographic area that have antibodies to enzootic bovine leukosis virus. The unit of concern is the cow, and the true but unknown percentage of reactor cows in the target population is the parameter to be estimated. N represents the number of cows in the population and n the number of cows in the sample.

2.2.1 Nonprobability Sampling

Nonprobability sampling is a collection of methods that do not rely on formal random techniques to identify the units to be included in the sample. Some nonprobability methods include judgment sampling, convenience sampling, and purposive sampling.

In judgment sampling representative units of the population are selected by the investigator. In convenience sampling, the sample is selected because it is easy to obtain; for example, local herds, kennels, or volunteers may be used. Using convenience or judgment sampling often produces biased results, although some people believe they can select representative samples. This drawback and the inability to quantitatively predict the sample's expected performance suggest these methods rarely should be used for survey purposes. In purposive sampling, the selection of units is based on known exposure or disease status. Purposive sampling is often used to select units for analytic observational studies, but it is inadequate for obtaining data to estimate population parameters.

Examples of the application of nonprobability sampling to estimate the prevalence of enzootic bovine leukosis virus include the selection of cows from what the investigator thinks are representative herds and the selection of cows from herds owned by historically cooperative or nearby farmers.

The following sampling methods belong to a class known as probability samples. The discussion assumes that sampling is performed without replacement; hence an individual element can only be chosen once.

2.2.2 Simple Random Sampling

In simple random sampling, one selects a fixed percentage of the population using a formal random process; as for example, flipping a coin or die, drawing numbers from a hat, using random number generators or random number tables. ("Random" is often used to describe a variety of haphazard, convenience and/or purposive sampling methods, but here it refers to the formal statistical procedure.) Strictly speaking, a formal random selection procedure is required for the investigator to calculate the precision of the sample estimate, as measured by the standard error of the mean. In practice, formal random sampling provides the investigator with assurance that the sample should be representative of the population being investigated, and for the parameter being estimated, confidence intervals are calculated on this premise. Despite mathematical and theoretical advantages, simple random sampling is often more difficult to use in the field than systematic sampling (described in 2.2.3). Consider the procedure for selecting a sample of 10% of feedlot steers as they pass through a handling facility. In simple random sampling, a list of randomly obtained numbers—representing, for example, the animals' identification (i.e., ear tags) or the order of the animals through a handling facility—would be prepared beforehand to identify the animals for the sample. The practicalities of using such a list in a field situation (e.g., losing count of animals and/or continuously having to refer to a list of numbers) may make this type of sampling inappropriate.

To obtain a simple random sample of cows for the prevalence of enzootic bovine leukosis antibodies one would obtain a list of n random numbers between 1 and N, each number identifying a cow in the sampling frame. Thus the cows selected would be distributed randomly throughout the sampled population.

2.2.3 Systematic Random Sampling

In systematic sampling the n sampling units are selected from the sampling frame at regular intervals (e.g., every fifth farm or every third animal), thus the interval k is 5 or 3 respectively. If k is fixed initially, n will vary with N; whereas if n is fixed initially, k becomes the integer nearest to N/n. When systematic methods are used, the starting point in the first interval is selected on a formal random basis.

Systematic sampling is a practical way to obtain a representative sample, and it ensures that the sampling units are distributed evenly over the entire population. There are two major disadvantages of this method. First, it is possible that the characteristic being estimated is related to the interval itself. For example, in estimating the prevalence of respiratory disease in swine at slaughter, one might systematically select a day of the week (e.g., Wednesday) to examine lungs. If swine slaughtered on Wednesdays were not representative of swine slaughtered on the other days of the week (e.g., because of local market customs), a biased result would be obtained. The second disadvantage is the difficulty of quantitatively assessing the variability of estimates obtained by systematic random sampling. In practice, one uses methods appropriate for simple random sampling to obtain these estimates.

If N/k is not an integer, some bias will result in the sample estimate because some animals (elements) will have more impact on the mean than others. This is of little concern if N is large and k is small relative to N. To prevent this bias, select the desired k and draw a random number (RN) between 1 and N; then divide RN by k and note the remainder. This remainder identifies the starting point between 1 and k (i.e., a remainder of 0 means the starting point is the kth individual, a remainder of 2 the second individual, and so forth) (Levy and Lemeshow 1980, p 76).

In sampling to estimate the prevalence of antibodies to enzootic bovine leukosis virus, using a list of all N cows in the area in question (the sampling frame), the initial animal to be tested would be selected from the first N/n animals randomly. Subsequently, every kth cow would be tested. In selecting 10% of steers, one could randomly select a number between 1 and 10 (say 6) and then the 6th, 16th, 26th, etc. animal through the facility would be included in the sample.

2.2.4 Stratified Random Sampling

In stratified sampling, prior to selection, the sampling frame is divided into strata based on factors likely to influence the level of the characteristic (e.g., prevalence of antibodies) being estimated. Then a simple random or systematic random sample is selected within each stratum.

Stratified sampling is more flexible than simple random sampling because a different sampling percentage can be used in the various strata (e.g., 2% in one stratum and 5% in another). Also, the precision of the sample estimate may be improved, because only the within-stratum variation contributes to the variation (standard error) of the mean in stratified sampling; whereas in simple random sampling both the within-stratum and the between-stratum variation are present. A graphic illustration of this feature is shown in Figure 2.1.

In simple random sampling, the variability of the estimate of prevalence has components related to both within-herd type and between-herd type variation in prevalence. In stratified random sampling, the variability of the estimate has components related to only the within-herd type variation in prevalence; hence its variability is expected to be less than that

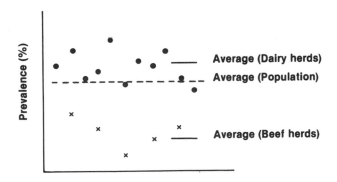

2.1. Prevalence of disease X in population of dairy and beef cattle herds: relationship of sampling design to variability of sample means.

obtained in simple random sampling. For example in Figure 2.1 the variability of the prevalence in beef herds, about the mean for beef herds, and the variation of the prevalence in dairy herds, about the mean for dairy herds, are much smaller than if type of herd is ignored and the variation of herd disease prevalence about the overall mean is calculated. Variation (see Table 2.1) of the mean (estimate of prevalence) is calculated using standard formula for the variance or its square root, the standard deviation. The standard deviation of a mean is referred to as a standard error.

The obvious disadvantage of stratified sampling is that the status of all sampling units, with respect to the factors forming the strata, must be known prior to drawing the sample. In general, the number of factors used for stratification should be limited to those likely to have a major impact on the value of the characteristic (e.g., prevalence of antibodies) being estimated.

As an example of this method and given that dairy cows are likely to have a higher rate of enzootic bovine leukosis antibodies than beef cows, one should obtain a more precise estimate of the population mean (prevalence) if strata were formed based on type of cow. Also, if 60% of the cow population N comprised dairy cows, 60% of the sample n should be dairy cows. This is called proportional weighting, and it keeps the arithmetic involved in calculating the sample statistic simple. Cows would be selected within each stratum by using simple random or systematic random sampling methods.

In the sampling methods discussed, the sampling unit and the unit of concern are the same (i.e., a cow). These methods are well suited for sampling from laboratory files or from relatively small groups of identifiable animals. However, the practical difficulty of obtaining a list (the sampling frame) of all cows in a large geographic area such as a province or state is a drawback. Additionally, with stratified sampling, the appropriate characteristics of each sampling unit must be identified (e.g., as dairy or beef in the previous example). To overcome these problems, allow flexibility in sampling strategy, and decrease the cost of the sampling, it is often easier to initially sample herds or other natural aggregates of animals within the area, although individual animals are the units of concern. Two of the more common sampling methods used for this purpose are cluster and multistage sampling.

2.2.5 Cluster Sampling

In cluster sampling, the initial sampling unit is larger than the unit of concern (e.g., usually the individual). Clusters of individuals often arise naturally (e.g., litters, pens, or herds) or they may be formed artificially (e.g., geographic clusters). Administrative units such as counties may also be used as artificial clusters for sampling purposes. The clusters (sampling units) can be selected by systematic, simple, or stratified random methods;

all individuals within the sampling units are tested.

Sometimes the group, be it a herd, pen, or litter, is the unit of concern, and therefore is not considered to be a cluster. Some examples of this situation are investigations to classify herds as to whether they are infected with enzootic bovine leukosis; estimation of the mean somatic cell count for dairy herds using bulk tank milk samples; and estimation of the mean herd milk production or days to conception.

In the bovine leukosis example, a cluster sample could be obtained by taking a simple random sample of all herds in the sampled population and testing all cows within the selected herds. From the formula in Table 2.1, note that the variability of the mean of the cluster sample is a function of

Table 2.1. Formulas for estimating simple characteristics of populations

Type of random sample	Estimates of mean	Estimates of precision (standard error of mean)
Simple	$\bar{y} = \Sigma y_i/n$	$se(\bar{y}) = (s^2/n)^{1/2}$ where $s^2 = \Sigma (y_i - \bar{y})^2/(n-1)$ $s^2 = \bar{p}\bar{q}$ for attributes

y_i = value of variable y in ith individual. If an attribute (e.g., disease) is being measured, $y_i = 1$ if present and 0 if absent; hence $\bar{p} = \Sigma y_i/n$ and $\bar{q} = 1 - \bar{p}$

n = sample size and N = population size

If $n/N > 0.1$, then s^2 is adjusted by multiplication by $1 - n/N$

Stratified	$\bar{y}_{st} = \Sigma W_j\bar{y}_j$ or $\bar{y}_{st} = \Sigma y_{ij}/n$	$se(\bar{y}_{st}) = [\Sigma (W_j^2 s_j^2/n_j)]^{1/2}$ where $W_j = N_j/N$ and $s_j^2 = \Sigma (y_{ij} - \bar{y}_j)^2/(n_j - 1)$ $s_j^2 = \bar{p}_j\bar{q}_j$ for attributes

The subscript j indicates the stratum

W_j = population weighting factor: the proportion of the population in the jth stratum, i.e., N_j/N. Second formula for the mean assumes proportional weighting, i.e., $w_j = W_j$

Y_{ij} = value of variable y in ith individual in jth stratum. If an attribute is being measured, $Y_{ij} = 1$ if present and 0 if absent

$\bar{y}_j$ = mean of jth stratum
n_j = number of individuals in jth stratum in sample
N_j = number in jth stratum in population

If $n_j/N_j > 0.1$, each s_j^2 may be adjusted by multiplying by $1 - n_j/N_j$

Cluster (*equal sized clusters only*)	$\bar{y}_{cs} = \Sigma \bar{y}_c/m$ $= \Sigma y_{ic}/mn$	$se(\bar{y}_{cs}) = (s^2/m)^{1/2}$ where $s^2 = \Sigma (\bar{y}_c - \bar{y}_{cs})^2/(m-1)$

$\bar{y}_c$ = mean of variable y in cth cluster; it is $\bar{p}_c$ for attribute variables, but treat these as continuous variables
y_{ic} = value of ith individual in cth cluster. If an attribute is being measured, $y_{ic} = 1$ if present and 0 if absent
m = number of clusters in sample (M is number of clusters in population) each containing n individuals
Adjust s^2 if $m/M > 0.1$ using multiplication by $1 - m/M$

the between-herd variance and the number of clusters m in the sample, not the number of animals in the sample.

2.2.6 Multistage Sampling

This method is similar to cluster sampling except that sampling takes place at all stages. As an example of two-stage sampling, one would begin as in cluster sampling by selecting a sample of the primary units (e.g., herds) listed in the sampling frame. Then within each primary unit, a sample of secondary units (e.g., animals) would be selected. Thus the difference between cluster and two-stage sampling is that subsampling within the primary units is conducted in the latter method.

Multistage sampling is used because of its practical advantages and flexibility. The number of primary (n_1) and secondary units (n_2) may be varied to account for different costs of sampling primary versus secondary units as well as the variability of the characteristic being estimated between primary units and between secondary units within primary units (see 2.2.9).

To continue with the bovine leukosis example, one could proceed in the same manner as cluster sampling, but after selection of the herds (the primary units), a simple or systematic random sample of cows within each herd (the secondary units) would be selected. This process could be extended to three-stage sampling by selecting small geographic areas as the primary units, selecting herds within these areas as secondary units, and finally selecting animals within the herds as tertiary units. Whenever possible, one should select each stage's sampling units with probability proportional to the number of individuals they contain. This minimizes the error of estimate and stabilizes the sample size. The main disadvantage of cluster and multistage samples is that more individuals may be required in the sample to obtain the same precision as would be expected if individuals could be selected with simple random sampling.

As an illustration of multistage sampling, suppose that in the bovine leukosis example there are M farms (say 120) and N animals (say 8000) in the population. The objective is to estimate the proportion of animals having enzootic bovine leukosis antibodies using a sample size of 800 ($n = 800$). The sampling frame would have the format shown in Table 2.2.

Suppose the number of primary sampling units (farms) to be selected is 40(n_1) and, on average, 20(n_2) secondary units (animals) will be selected from within each primary unit. (Note that $n_1 \times n_2 = n$.) If the number of animals in each herd was unknown, one could take a simple or systematic random sample of 40 herds and randomly select a fixed percentage (i.e., 30% $= Mn/mN$) of the animals in each herd for testing. When the number of animals in each herd is known, a more optimal procedure is to sample the primary units with probability proportional to their size, and then to select a fixed number of animals from each herd. In this example, the initial step is to randomly select 40 numbers within the range of 1 to 8000. Each of

Table 2.2.   Format for a sampling frame for two-stage sampling

Farm number	Number of animals	Cumulative number of animals
1	62	1–62
2	48	63–110
3	74	111–184
4	36	185–220
.	.	.
.	.	.
.	.	.
119	42	7900–7941
120	59	7942–8000

the random numbers will identify a farm according to the cumulative number column. Subsequently, 20 animals may be randomly selected from each farm. Both of these procedures give each individual the same probability of being selected. Since it is assumed that sampling is without replacement, if a farm is identified twice, another should be selected randomly. (Technically it would be better to randomly select twice the number of animals from that herd.) If fewer than 20 animals are present in a specified herd, the practical solution is to test all available animals.

A modification of this method to ensure that each farm may be selected only once is the use of systematic random techniques. For example, the selection interval k is found by dividing the total number of animals N by n_1 (in this case, $k = 8000/40 = 200$). A number is then selected randomly from the range 1 to k (e.g., 151). The remaining 39 numbers (351, 551, etc.) would identify the farms to include in the sample. This process will select a farm only once, providing the interval k is greater than the number of animals on the largest farm.

2.2.7   Calculating the Estimate

The point estimate of the prevalence of reactors in the population, the parameter $P(T+)$, is the test-positive proportion in the sample, the statistic $p(T+)$ or $\bar{p}$. To calculate this statistic the number of test positives are added together and divided by the sample size. (This assumes a proportionally weighted sample when stratified sampling is used, which is self-weighting in terms of the mean. The same approach is also used for estimates obtained from cluster or multistage samples. See Snedecor and Cochran 1980 for details.) Calculating the estimate of a population mean (say average milk production) is performed in an analogous manner (see 3.6).

EXAMPLE CALCULATIONS   In the enzootic bovine leukosis example, if 125 of 2000 cows were test-positive, the estimate of the prevalence of reactors in the population would be $\bar{p} = 125/2000 = 0.063$ or 6.3%. If a simple random sample or systematic random sample were used to obtain the sample, the variability of the point estimate would be:

$$\text{Variance } (\bar{p}) = \bar{p}(1 - \bar{p})/n = 0.063 \times 0.937/2000$$
$$V(\bar{p}) = 0.295 \times 10^{-4}$$
$$\text{Standard Error } (\bar{p}) = V(\bar{p})^{1/2}$$
$$SE(\bar{p}) = 0.0054 \ (0.54\%)$$

These estimates could be written as 6.3% ± 0.5% (*SE*). With moderately large sample sizes, 65% of all possible sample means will be within 1 standard error of the true mean, 95% within 1.96 standard errors, and 99% within 2.6 standard errors. The calculation of a confidence interval as an extension of the above facts is described in 3.6. More complex calculations are required to determine the variability of means obtained from cluster or two-stage samples (see Table 2.1). Since the clusters are rarely of equal size, the reader can use the formula shown in Table 2.1 for the initial calculations, but should consult one of the reference texts for details of more accurate methods.

2.2.8   Sample Size Considerations

Accurate determinations of the sample size required for a survey can be quite detailed, and most complex surveys will require the assistance of a statistician. For less complex surveys one of the following formulas should provide suitable estimates.

To determine the sample size n necessary to estimate the prevalence of reactors $P(T+)$ in a population (the mean of a qualitative variable, morbidity rates or mortality rates, see 3.2 and 3.3), the investigator must provide an educated guess of the probable level of reactors $\hat{P}$ (read "P hat"), and must specify how close to $P(T+)$ the estimate should be.

EXAMPLE CALCULATIONS   Suppose the available evidence suggests that approximately 30% ($\hat{P} = 0.3$) of the cow population will have antibodies to enzootic bovine leukosis. Also, assume the investigator wishes the survey estimate to be within 6% of the true level 95% of the time. (6% is termed the allowable error, or required precision, and is represented in the following formula by L.) Then the required sample size is:

$$n = 4\hat{P}\hat{Q}/L^2 \qquad \text{where } \hat{Q} = 1 - \hat{P}$$
$$= 4 \times 0.3 \times 0.7/0.06^2 = 0.84/0.0036 = 233$$

Thus approximately 230 cows would be needed for the survey.

In general, the number of animals in the population has little influence on the required sample size except when n is greater than $0.1N$. For example, if the herd contained only 200 cows ($N = 200$), the required number of cows is found using the reciprocal of $1/n^* + 1/N$ where n^* is the above sample size estimate. In this instance, the number required to obtain the same precision is the reciprocal of $1/233 + 1/200 = 1/108$; thus the required sample is approximately 108 animals (Cannon and Roe 1982).

When determining the sample size necessary to estimate the mean of a quantitative variable (e.g., production parameters, see 3.6), the investigator needs to supply an estimate of the standard deviation or variance of that variable in the target population and specify how close to the mean the sample estimate should be. Suppose reproductive efficiency as measured by the calving-to-conception interval is the event of interest. Assume that the available evidence suggests that the standard deviation of this interval is 20 days, and the investigator wishes the sample to provide an estimate within 5 days of the true average 95% of the time. Then $\hat{S} = 20$ and $L = 5$, and the required sample size is:

$$n = 4\hat{S}^2/L^2 = 4 \times 20^2/5^2 = 1600/25 = 64$$

Thus approximately 64 cows are required for the survey.

The number 4 in the previous formulas is the approximate square of $Z = 1.96$, which provides a 95% confidence level. If the investigator wished to be 99% certain that the results would be within $\pm L$ of the true level, 6.6 (the approximate square of $Z = 2.56$) should be substituted for 4. The reader is encouraged to experiment with different values in each of the above formulas to assist in understanding the consequences of these changes.

In using the above formulas, it is assumed that the sampling unit is the same as the unit of concern. When using cluster or multistage sampling, an upward adjustment in the sample size may be required to obtain the desired precision in the estimate. If the disease is not very contagious and/or the within-primary-unit correlation coefficient is small, a two to three times increase in the sample size should be appropriate. For very contagious diseases, the necessary sample size may have to be increased five to seven times (Leech and Sellers 1979). These increases are based on rule-of-thumb, and more accurate formulas as described in 2.2.9 should be used when the appropriate information on the within- and between-herd variances is available.

2.2.9 Cost considerations in survey design

Frequently, the investigator must perform the sampling under monetary as well as practical and biologic constraints. Thus, rather than only specifying the precision of the estimate, the investigator may seek to obtain the highest precision for a specified cost or, conversely, the least cost for a specified precision.

Simple probability sampling procedures are not particularly flexible in terms of meeting monetary constraints, other than altering (usually reducing) the total number of sampling units studied. However, stratified sampling allows the investigator to select different numbers of units from different strata, depending on the relative costs associated with sampling in each stratum. The basic rule is to reduce the number of samples in strata with high sampling costs and to increase the number with lower sampling costs. The optimal stratified sample will have stratum weights proportional to $N_j S_j / C_j^{1/2}$ where N_j is the number in the population in stratum j, S_j is the standard deviation of the parameter being measured in stratum j, and C_j is the cost of sampling in stratum j. If the resulting sample is not proportionally weighted according to the population structure, the calculation of the sample mean should be done using the weighting formula in Table 2.1.

Cluster sampling is often used because of practical difficulties in obtaining a sampling frame in which the individual is the sampling unit. Thus circumventing these "practical difficulties" by using cluster sampling is really a reaction to economic constraints. For example, it may cost less to sample 4000 swine using cluster sampling than to sample 1000 using random sampling, although the precision of the estimate obtained by the latter may be greater than that obtained using cluster sampling with more individuals.

The most flexible sampling method to take account of cost factors is multistage sampling. In two-stage sampling one may vary the number of primary and secondary units selected according to the costs of sampling primary units (e.g., herds) as well as the costs of sampling secondary units (e.g., animals within a herd). In the enzootic bovine leukosis example, the cost of traveling to a herd to obtain samples may be large relative to the cost of obtaining a sample from an individual cow once on the farm. This would suggest an increase in the number of secondary units (cows) and a decrease in the number of primary units (herds) to reduce the total cost of sampling. The balance between primary and secondary sampling units can be investigated formally. If c is the total monies available for sampling, c_1 the cost of sampling primary units, and c_2 the cost of sampling secondary units, the relationship between these costs and the numbers of primary and secondary units is:

$$c = c_1 n_1 + c_2 n_1 n_2$$

The appropriate number of secondary units n_2 to select, minimizing costs for a given precision, or vice-versa (Snedecor and Cochran 1980), is found using:

$$n_2 = (c_1 s_2^2 / c_2 s_1^2)^{1/2}$$

The number of primary units n_1 may then be found using the previous formula, since c, c_1, c_2 and n_2 are known. If $c_1 = c_2$, then n_2 is merely a function of the respective variances; namely, $n_2 = (s_2^2 / s_1^2)^{1/2}$.

EXAMPLE CALCULATIONS   Suppose a person wished to estimate the blood globulin level in mature dairy cows. Assume that the total money available for the project (c) is $10,000, that it will cost an average of $100 per farm ($c_1$) to sample each herd (this includes travel costs), and that the cost per cow (c_2) is $10 once at the herd (this includes the cost of blood vials, needles, technician time, and laboratory analysis). Assume also that the between-herd variability (s_1) in globulin concentration is 8g/l and the within-herd (cow-to-cow) variability (s_2) is 4 g/l. On this basis,

$$n_2 = (100 \times 4^2 / 10 \times 8^2)^{1/2} = 2.5^{1/2} = 1.6$$

Since n_2 should be an integer, round 1.6 to 2 cows per herd. Now, solve the initial cost equation for n_1.

$$10,000 = 100 n_1 + 10 \times 2 n_1 = 120 n_1$$
$$n_1 = 83$$

Thus, approximately 80–85 herds would be used, taking 2 cows per herd.

Despite the high cost per herd, the relatively large between-herd variability dictates that a large number of herds are required. In this instance, if $c_1 = c_2$, the ratio $(s_2^2 / s_1^2)^{1/2}$ indicates that one animal (the minimum number) per herd should be selected.

2.3   Sampling to Detect Disease

As part of many disease control or eradication programs, entire herds or flocks are tested to ascertain if the specified disease is present or, conversely, to ensure that the disease is absent. However, testing entire herds or flocks is expensive, and the veterinarian may have to accept the results of testing only a portion of the animals.

When sampling is used for this purpose, a frequently asked question is, What sample size is required so that the veterinarian can be 95% or 99% confident that the herd or flock is disease-free if no animals or birds in the sample give a positive test result? To actually prove (i.e., be 100% certain) that a disease is absent from a population requires testing almost every individual. For example, to prove that atrophic rhinitis was not present in a

5000 pig feeder operation would require the examination of the snout of virtually every pig.

Despite these limitations, sampling can provide valid insight into the health status of the population, because it is rare for only one animal in a herd to have the disease of interest. Infectious diseases tend to spread, and even infrequent noninfectious diseases would be expected to cluster somewhat within a herd, assuming environmental determinants of the disease are present. Thus for many diseases, if the disease is present at all, the herd will be likely to contain more than one diseased individual. This knowledge may be utilized when sampling to detect disease. The sampling strategy is designed to detect disease if more than a specified number or percentage (>0) of animals have the disease. The actual number or percentage of diseased animals to specify when making the sample size calculations should be based on knowledge of the biology of the disease. Often, the results of previous testing campaigns will supply useful information. For example, available data might indicate that the percentage of cattle with bovine tuberculosis in infected herds averages between 5 and 10%. These could be used as starting points to determine the possible range of sample sizes required to detect bovine tuberculosis when it is present.

Table 2.3 contains the sample size required to be 95% or 99% certain that at least one animal in the sample would be diseased if the disease were present at or above the specified level. The minimum number of diseased animals assumed to be present in a herd is one, and for populations of greater than 100 individuals, the number of diseased animals is based on assumed prevalences ranging from 1–50%. Note that a formal random sampling method, with individuals as the sampling units, is required if the desired confidence level shown is to be attained. If no formal random selection is used, the confidence one can have in the result is unknown, at least quantitatively. This circumstance may arise when animals are examined at slaughter for the presence of disease (e.g., in slaughter checks of pigs for respiratory disease). The pigs examined may not be representative of the source population; for example, the disease of interest may have a high case fatality rate and hence only disease-free animals survive to market age and weight. Although sample size requirements may be calculated to assist in evaluating the potential workload, one should be cautious and assign only a judgmental level of confidence if no diseased animals are observed in an informal sample such as this. Sometimes it may be assumed with a high degree of certainty that the level of disease in culled animals is much higher than in the source population; these diseases influencing the withdrawal of the animal in the first instance. If a sufficient number of these animals are examined and are found to be disease-free, the source herd or flock may be deemed disease-free, although no formal sampling was used in selecting the culled animals to be examined. (In fact, if a high

Table 2.3. Sample sizes required to be 95/99% confident disease is present at/or below specified prevalence D/N, if no diseased animals are observed

Population size	Prevalence of disease[a]: (D/N) × 100			
	1%	5%	10%	50%
30	29/30	23/27	19/23	5/7
60	57/60	38/47	23/31	5/7
100	95/99	45/59	25/36	5/7
300	189/235	54/78	28/41	5/7
500	225/300	56/83	28/42	5/7
1,000	258/367	58/86	29/43	5/7
10,000	294/448	59/90	29/44	5/7

[a]The minimum number of diseased animals is one, at 1% and 5% prevalence in populations of size 30 and 60 respectively.

The above sample size requirements were derived using the following formula from Cannon and Roe (1982):

$$n = [1 - (1 - a)^{1/D}] [N - (D - 1)/2]$$

where n is the required sample size
a = probability (confidence level) of observing at least one diseased animal in sample when the disease affects at least D/N in population
D = number of diseased animals in population
N = population size
Note: If the column heading D/N is read as the proportion of animals in a population that is tested (n/N), the body of the table provides the expected maximum number of cases in the population.

percentage of culled animals are tested at slaughter, the tested animals essentially are a census of all culled animals. The problem in this case is not so much concerned with sampling, but with the amount of information about the population of interest provided by testing the culled animals.)

EXAMPLE CALCULATIONS Assume that in a population of 1000 (N) swine, there will be at least 10 (D) pigs with atrophic rhinitis, if it is present at all. The sample size required to be 95% ($a = 0.95$) sure of detecting at least one pig with rhinitis is:

$$n = [1 - (1 - 0.95)^{0.1}] [1000 - (9/2)] = 0.259 \times 995.5 = 258$$

To be 99% certain of detecting at least one pig with rhinitis under the conditions in this example, the required sample size is:

$$n = 0.369 \times 995.5 = 367$$

The previous formula may be solved for D, rather than n, and the following formula results:

$$D = [1 - (1 - a)^{1/n}] \ (N - [(n - 1)/2])$$

This formula is useful to provide the maximum number of diseased animals (D) expected in a population, with confidence a, when n individuals are examined and found to be free of disease.

EXAMPLE CALCULATIONS   If 20 randomly selected layer hens from a flock of 5000 are examined and found to be free of pullorum disease, the maximum expected number of infected birds in that flock would be:

$$D = [1 - (1 - 0.95)^{0.05}][5000 - (19/2)]$$
$$= 0.139 \times 4990.5 = 694$$

giving a maximum percentage with pullorum disease of 13.9%. If 200 randomly selected hens were all negative, the maximum expected number infected in the flock would be 73, or a maximum prevalence of 1.5%.

As noted, Table 2.3 can be used to obtain the maximum number diseased by changing the column header D/N to n/N where n/N represents the percentage of the population examined and found disease-free. The body of the table will provide the maximum number of diseased individuals expected in a population of size N.

2.4 Hypothesis Testing in Analytic Observational Studies

The three sampling methods — each denoting a type of analytic study — described in this section differ in the amount of information they provide with respect to the population. Cross-sectional studies are based on a single sample of the population, whereas, in principle, cohort and case-control studies are based on two separate often purposive samples (Fleiss 1973).

To assist the description of these sampling methods, the basic population structure with respect to one exposure factor (often called the independent variable) and one disease (often called the dependent variable) both with two levels, present or absent, is shown below. The letters A, B, C, and D, represent the number of individuals (sampling units) in each factor-disease category in the population.

		Diseased ($D+$)	Not diseased ($D-$)	
Exposed	($F+$)	A	B	$A+B$
Not exposed	($F-$)	C	D	$C+D$
		$A+C$	$B+D$	$N=A+B+C+D$

A variety of rates and proportion can be calculated if the numbers in each of the four cells (factor-disease combination) are known. The objective of analytic studies is to estimate these rates, although not all may be estimated from each study design. See Table 2.4.

For purposes of nomenclature, lowercase characters indicate that the values are derived from a sample, whereas uppercase characters indicate population values. Thus p indicates an estimate, that is a statistic, from a sample, whereas P indicates the corresponding population value or parameter. In discussing numbers of individuals as opposed to proportions, n will be substituted for p. For example, $n(F+)$ is the number of exposed units in the sample which may also be indicated as $(a + b)$.

Table 2.4. Method of calculating major population parameters

Parameter (rate or proportion)	Notation	Calculated using
Exposed	$P(F+)$	$(A + B)/N$
Diseased	$P(D+)$	$(A + C)/N$
Diseased and exposed	$P(F+ \text{ and } D+)$	A/N
Diseased in exposed group	$P(D+/F+)$	$A/(A + B)$
Diseased in nonexposed group	$P(D+/F-)$	$C/(C + D)$
Exposed in diseased group	$P(F+/D+)$	$A/(A + C)$
Exposed in nondiseased group	$P(F+/D-)$	$B/(B + D)$

To clarify the sampling strategy in each of the three analytic study methods, assume the investigator wishes to test if vaccination against selected viruses alters the risk of pneumonia in feedlot cattle. Although it is rare that the structure of the population to be sampled is known, a numerical example is given in Table 2.5. Although based on fictitious data, the example demonstrates the information that would be provided by each of the sampling methods, in comparison to the information that would be available if the population structure was known. With a few modifications, the same approaches to sampling could be used if disease was the independent variable and production the dependent variable (e.g., if the intention were to test the hypothesis that the presence of a disease alters the level of production).

2.4.1 Cross-Sectional Sampling

A sample, usually obtained by one of the previous probability sampling methods, is selected from the population, and each member (sampling unit) is classified according to its current status for the factor and the disease. All of the disease rates in the population may be estimated, based on the results of a cross-sectional sample. Thus this method allows the investigator to learn about the population structure, as well as to test the null hypothesis that the factor (vaccination) and disease (pneumonia) are

Table 2.5.   Demonstration of the anticipated results of sampling a population using cross-sectional, cohort, and case-control methods

Suppose the factor is vaccination and the disease is pneumonia. Further, assume the population has the following structure:

		Pneumonia $D+$	No pneumonia $D-$	Total
Vaccinated	$F+$	12,000	48,000	60,000
Not vaccinated	$F-$	18,000	22,000	40,000
		30,000	70,000	100,000

If 1000 animals were sampled from this population using *cross-sectional* methods, the anticipated results, ignoring sampling error, would be:

		$D+$	$D-$	$p(D+/F)$	
Vaccinated	$F+$	120	480	600	(20%)
Not vaccinated	$F-$	180	220	400	(45%)
		300	700	1000	
	$p(F+/D)$	(40%)	(69%)		

All the population characteristics including those shown in parentheses may be estimated from these data.

If *cohort* sampling were used with 500 individuals per group the results would be:

		$D+$	$D-$	$p(D+/F)$	
Vaccinated	$F+$	100	400	500	(20%)
Not vaccinated	$F-$	225	275	500	(45%)

Only the two characteristics (shown in parentheses) of the population may be estimated from these data.

Finally, if *case-control* sampling were used with 500 individuals per group, the results would be:

		$D+$	$D-$
Vaccinated	$F+$	200	343
Not vaccinated	$F-$	300	157
		500	500
	$p(F+/D)$	(40%)	(69%)

Again, only the two population characteristics (shown in parentheses) may be estimated from these data.

independent events in the population. However, this method of sampling may be impractical when disease frequency is low, because large sample sizes would be required to obtain a sufficient number of cases. In the example in Table 2.5, 120 vaccinated cattle with pneumonia were observed; whereas 180 would be expected if vaccination and pneumonia were independent events. The expected number is derived by multiplying the first row total by the first column total, and dividing by n (i.e., 600 × 300/1000). This calculation is based on statistical theory regarding probabilities of independent events and is the basis of the chi-square test, see 5.2. Since there are fewer observed vaccinated animals with pneumonia than expected, it appears that vaccination may protect against pneumonia.

An example of a cross-sectional study is presented in Table 2.6. This northern California study was designed to estimate the frequency of acute bovine pulmonary emphysema and to identify factors associated with this disease (Heron and Suther 1979). A list of all herds in three counties (the sampling frame) was obtained from the California Bureau of Animal Health. Then a stratified random sample was used—each county constituted a separate stratum—and a 10% random sample of herds (the sampling unit and the unit of concern) was selected within each county.

Farm owners were interviewed about their husbandry methods, particularly forage management practices. Based on the results of this study, it appeared that approximately 10% of the farms experienced an outbreak of acute bovine pulmonary emphysema during the 4-year study, and that approximately 35% of farm managers used pasture rotation but did nothing specific to prevent the problem. Approximately 2.5 farms (24 × 7/68) or 3.6% of farms would be expected to use pasture rotation and experience the disease if these were independent events; whereas 7 (10.3%) actually did. This suggested a strong association between pasture rotation with no preventive measures and the occurrence of pulmonary emphysema. Additional data indicated that about 3% of the cattle at risk on the affected farms developed pulmonary emphysema. The case fatality rate was 53.8%.

A cross-sectional design was used in a study of factors influencing morbidity and mortality in feedlot calves (Martin et al. 1982). However,

Table 2.6.   Results of a cross-sectional study of the relationship between pasture changes and the occurrence of acute bovine pulmonary emphysema (ABPE) during a four-year period

	Number of herds			
	Affected	Non-affected		$p(D+/F)$
Pasture rotated and no preventive measures taken	7	17	24	(29.2%)
Pasture not rotated or preventive measures taken if pasture rotated	0	44	44	(0.0%)
	7	61	68	
$p(F+/D)$	(100.0%)	(27.9%)		

Source: Heron and Suther 1979, with permission.

Note: The prevalence of pasture rotation with no preventive measures taken was 24/68 = 35.3% of farms.

ABPE occurred during at least one of four years in 7/68 = 10.3% of farms.

ABPE and pasture rotation with no preventive measures taken occurred together in 7/68 = 10.3% of farms.

Other estimates of rates applying to the source population are shown in parentheses.

since no formal sampling was used to select collaborators, it is not known how closely the distribution of various risk factors or the prevalence of disease found in the study might be to population values. Thus, although the associations found in the study may be valid, it is difficult to extrapolate certain results beyond the sample (i.e., beyond the groups of cattle under study).

2.4.2 Cohort Sampling

In cohort sampling, a sample of exposed $(F+)$ and a sample of unexposed $(F-)$ sampling units are selected and observed for a period of time, and the rate of disease in each sample is used to estimate the corresponding rates of development of disease in the two populations. Usually when cohort sampling is used, one does not gain information about the frequency of the factor or of the disease in the population. Testing whether the rate of disease in the exposed group is equal to the rate in the unexposed group evaluates the null hypothesis that the factor and disease are independent events in the population. In the example in Table 2.5, a sample of 500 vaccinated animals and a comparison cohort of 500 unvaccinated animals were identified and observed for a specified time to determine the respective rates of pneumonia. In this fictitious data, since only 20% of vaccinated animals and 45% of nonvaccinated animals developed pneumonia, it appears vaccination helped prevent the development of pneumonia.

The two cohorts (i.e., the two exposure groups) are only infrequently selected by a formal random sampling process. Usually they are purposively sampled specifically because of their exposure or nonexposure to the factor of interest. As long as the two groups are comparable in other respects, the effect of the exposure factor can still be evaluated. However, the groups should be demonstratively representative of the exposed and unexposed segments of the population if the results are to be extrapolated beyond the sampling units in the study.

An example of the use of cohort sampling is shown in Table 2.7. The

Table 2.7. Results of a cohort study of the relationship between the place of residence and the extent of pulmonary damage in 7-12-year-old dogs

	Pulmonary tract damage			Rate of lesions $p(D+/F)$
	Severe lesions	No severe lesions	Total	
Urban dogs[a]	224	82	306	(73.3%)
Rural dogs	50	150	200	(25.0%)
	274	232	506	

Source: Reif and Cohen 1970.
[a]This classification was based on known levels of air pollutants in the area, as well as housing density.

objective was to contrast the rate of pulmonary disease in rural $(F-)$ and urban $(F+)$ dogs in an attempt to estimate the impact of living in a relatively unpolluted (rural) versus a polluted (urban) environment (Reif and Cohen 1970). No differences were noted in young dogs. However, significant differences were seen in dogs 7–12 years of age; the highest rates being in urban dogs, suggesting a harmful effect of the polluted environment.

2.4.3 Case-Control Sampling

In case-control sampling, samples of diseased $(D+)$ and nondiseased $(D-)$ individuals are selected, and the proportion of each that has been exposed to the factor of interest is used to estimate the corresponding population proportion. Testing whether these two sample proportions are equal evaluates the null hypothesis that the factor and disease are independent events in the population. In the example in Table 2.5, a group of 500 animals with pneumonia and a sample of 500 animals without pneumonia would be selected, and the proportion vaccinated in each group would be contrasted. If the proportion of cases that were vaccinated (40%) was significantly different than the proportion of controls that were vaccinated (69%), vaccination would be associated with pneumonia. Since the former proportion is smaller, it appears that vaccination protected against the development of pneumonia in this hypothetical example.

Only infrequently are the two groups $(D+$ and $D-)$ obtained by a formal random sampling procedure. Usually the cases are obtained from one or more sources and essentially represent all of the available cases from the purposively selected sources. Often, the comparison group consists of all animals not having the disease of interest from the same source, be that a set of clinic or farm records. Sometimes, however, formal sampling is used. In a study of feline urological syndrome, the cases represented all cats with the disease in the clinic records; whereas the controls were obtained by taking a 10% systematic random sample of cats without the urologic syndrome (Willeberg 1975). In another example, the characteristics of herds with reactors to brucellosis were contrasted with those with no reactors. The data were obtained from the records of a diagnostic laboratory. Since a large number of herd records were available, a 10% random sample of herds having reactors and a 6% random sample of herds not having reactors to bovine brucellosis were selected. (These sampling fractions were selected because initial estimates indicated that they would provide the required number of reactor and nonreactor farms.) (S. W. Martin, pers. comm.)

In a study of factors associated with mastitis in dairy cows (Goodhope and Meek 1980), the case herds were the 550 with the highest milk-gel index in the province of Ontario. Each was matched to the closest herd in the same county with the lowest milk-gel index (i.e., the controls). (The latter selection method helped ensure that the case and control herds were comparable since they were geographically matched.)

An example of case-control sampling is presented in Table 2.8 (Willeberg 1980). Herds with high levels (>5%) of enzootic pneumonia in swine at slaughter (cases) were compared to herds with low levels (<5%) of enzootic pneumonia in their pigs (controls). While a number of characteristics of these herds were contrasted, Table 2.8 demonstrates the association of one factor (herd size) with level of pneumonia. Note that the sampling units are herds, not individual pigs. It is obvious from these data that larger herds (the exposure factor) occur much more frequently among herds with pneumonia problems than in herds with low levels of pneumonia. This suggests a harmful effect of the factor "large herds" on the level of pneumonia.

Table 2.8. Results of a case-control study of the relationship between herd size and pneumonia level in swine herds

	Level of pneumonia	
Herd size	High (>5%)	Low (<5%)
Large (>400 pigs)	67	22
Small (<400 pigs)	49	111
	116	133
$p(F+/D)$	(57.8%)	(16.5%)

Source: Willeberg 1980, with permission.
Note: The unit of concern and of analysis is the herd, not the pig.

2.4.4 Sample Size Considerations

Because of the time and expense required to conduct a valid analytic study, careful consideration should be given to determining the number of animals or sampling units required. The formulas given in Table 2.9 provide a basis for estimating sample sizes when the study is designed to contrast two groups.

EXAMPLE CALCULATIONS Two hypothetical examples will be presented to demonstrate the use of sample size formulas. In the first example, assume that the study is intended to compare the milk production of cows with clinical mastitis to cows not having mastitis (i.e., comparing the means of two quantitative variables). Suppose cows not experiencing clinical mastitis will produce 160 BCM units of milk with a standard deviation of 40 BCM units. (BCM is the breed class average for milk; see 3.6.1.) Further, assume clinical mastitis will reduce milk production by 10% to 144 BCM

Table 2.9.   Formulas for calculating the sample size in observational studies or field trials involving two treatments

If the outcome is measured as a proportion use:

$n = [Z_\alpha(2\bar{P}\bar{Q})^{1/2} - Z_\beta(P_eQ_e + P_cQ_c)^{1/2}]^2 / (P_e - P_c)^2$

If the outcome is expressed as a mean use:

$n = 2[(Z_\alpha - Z_\beta)S/(\bar{X}_e - \bar{X}_c)]^2$

n = estimated sample size for each of the exposed (cases) and unexposed (control) groups. The above formulas are based on large sample size theory; thus, if $n < 10$, double it, and if $n < 25$ increase n by about 1.5 times.

Z_α = value of Z which provides $\alpha/2$ in each tail of normal curve if a two-tailed test is used or α in one tail if a one-tail test is used. If α, the type I error, is 0.05 then the two-tailed Z is 1.96. α specifies the probability of declaring a difference to be statistically significant when no real difference exists in the population.

Z_β = value of Z which provides β in the lower tail of normal curve (Z_β is negative if $\beta < 0.5$). If β, the type II error, is 0.2, the Z value is -0.84. β specifies the probability of declaring a difference to be statistically nonsignificant when there is a real difference in the population.

P_e = estimate of response rate in exposed (or case) group
P_c = estimate of response rate in unexposed (or control) group
$\bar{P} = (P_e + P_c)/2$
$\bar{Q} = 1 - \bar{P}$
S = estimate of standard deviation common to both exposed (cases) and unexposed (control) groups
$\bar{X}_e$ = estimate of mean of outcome in the exposed (or case) group
$\bar{X}_c$ = estimate of mean of outcome in the unexposed (or control) group

Note: Since $P, Q, S,$ and $\bar{X}$ are estimates of population parameters, they should be written with a caret (^); however, the syntax becomes complicated and thus for clarity the caret is omitted.

units. How many cows are required in a cohort study to be 80% (1 - type II error) certain of detecting a difference as large as this, if it exists? Substitution of the above estimates into the second formula for sample size determinations gives:

$$n = 2[(1.96 + 0.84)40/(144 - 160)]^2 = 2(112/ - 16)^2$$
$$= 2(-7)^2 = 2 \times 49 = 98$$

Thus, the investigator should use approximately 100 mastitic and 100 non-mastitic cows for the study.

As a second example, suppose a newly identified organism is present in 40% (P_e) of nasal swabs of feedlot calves with pneumonia, and it is thought to occur in about 15% (P_c) of swabs from feedlot calves without pneumonia. How many calves would have to be examined in a case-control study to be 80% sure of detecting this difference (or greater) if it existed? Note that $\bar{P} = 0.275$ and $\bar{Q} = 0.725$. (This is contrasting the means of two qualitative variables, the means being expressed as rates or proportions.)

$$n = \frac{[1.96(2 \times 0.275 \times 0.725)^{1/2} + 0.84(0.4 \times 0.6 + 0.15 \times 0.85)^{1/2}]^2}{(0.4 - 0.15)^2}$$

$$= (1.24 + 0.51)^2/0.25^2$$
$$= 3.06/0.063$$
$$= 49$$

The investigator should plan to include approximately 50 calves with pneumonia (cases) and 50 calves without pneumonia (controls) in the study.

2.4.5 Cost Considerations in Analytic Studies

Under most practical field conditions, it can be shown that case-control studies require the fewest sampling units of all analytic observational studies to evaluate a specified hypothesis (Fleiss 1973). This and other features of study design make case-control studies a popular choice when selecting a study method (see Chapter 6).

In the previous discussions of sampling for hypothesis testing, equal size groups were used (i.e., the $F+$ and $F-$ groups were of equal size in cohort studies and the $D+$ and $D-$ groups were of equal size in case-control studies). If the costs of obtaining study subjects differ between unexposed and exposed, or cases and controls, the study design can be modified to take this feature into consideration. Although straightforward in principal, the formulas are somewhat complex, and the interested reader should consult the appropriate references for details and examples (Meydrech and Kupper 1978; Pike and Casagrande 1979).

References

Cannon, R. M., and R. T. Roe. 1982. Livestock Disease Surveys: A Field Manual For Veterinarians. Canberra: Australian Bureau of Animal Health.

Cochran, W. G. 1977. Sampling Techniques. Toronto, Canada: John Wiley & Sons.

Fleiss, J. L. 1973. Statistical Methods for Rates and Proportions. Toronto, Canada: John Wiley & Sons.

Goodhope, R. G., and A. H. Meek. 1980. Factors associated with mastitis in Ontario dairy herds: A case-control study. Can. J. Comp. Med. 44:351–57.

Heron, B. R., and D. E. Suther. 1979. A retrospective investigation and a random sample survey of acute bovine pulmonary emphysema in Northern California. Bov. Pract. 14:2–8.

Leech, F. B., and K. C. Sellers. 1979. Statistical Epidemiology in Veterinary Science. New York, N. Y.: Macmillan Co.

Levy, P. S., and S. Lemeshow. 1980. Sampling for Health Professionals. Belmont, Calif.: Wadsworth.

Martin, S. W., A. H. Meek, D. G. Davis, J. A. Johnson, and R. A. Curtis. 1982. Factors associated with mortality and treatment costs in feedlot calves: The Bruce County beef project, years 1978, 1979, 1980. Can. J. Comp. Med. 46:341–49.

Meydrech, E. F., and L. L. Kupper. 1978. Cost considerations and sample size requirements in cohort and case-control studies. Am. J. Epidemiol. 107:201–5.

Pike, M. C., and J. T. Casagrande. 1979. Re: Cost considerations and sample size requirements in cohort and case-control studies. Am. J. Epidemiol. 110:100–2.

Reif, J. S., and D. Cohen. 1970. Canine pulmonary disease. II. Retrospective radiographic analysis of pulmonary disease in rural and urban dogs. Arch. Environ. Health 20:684–89.

Schwabe, C. W., H. P. Riemann, and C. E. Franti. 1977. Epidemiology in Veterinary Practice. Philadelphia, Penn.: Lea & Febiger.

Snedecor, G. W., and W. G. Cochran. 1980. Statistical Methods. 7th ed. Ames: Iowa State Univ. Press.

Willeberg, P. 1975. A case-control study of some fundamental determinants in the epidemiology of the feline urological syndrome. Nord. Vet. Med. 27:1–14.

_____. 1980. The analysis and interpretation of epidemiological data. Proc. 2nd Int. Symp. Vet. Epidemiol. Econ., May 1979, Canberra, Australia.

Measurement of Disease Frequency and Production

3.1 Disease Frequency: General Considerations

Counts of individuals that are infected, diseased, or dead may be used to estimate workload, costs, or the size of facilities required to provide adequate health care for a specific animal population. However, epidemiologists usually wish to estimate the probability of events such as becoming infected, diseased, or dying in populations containing different numbers of individuals. Hence they express these counts as a fraction of the number of animals biologically capable of experiencing the event. The latter group of animals is called the population at risk. Fractions having the general form $a/(a + b)$ (where a is the number of animals with the event of interest, and b is the number of animals at risk of but not experiencing that event) are called either rates or proportions (Elandt-Johnson 1975). In practical terms rates are fractions, but they usually are multiplied by 100 or 1000, etc., so the result is a number greater than 1.

Morbidity and mortality are the two main categories of events for which rates are calculated. However, there are other events of interest to veterinarians and their clients, including culling (the premature removal of animals from a herd or flock), survival to weaning, and pregnancy rate (the probability of becoming pregnant within a specified period). The format for calculating these rates is the same as for morbidity and mortality; hence only the latter will be described in detail in this chapter.

3.1.1 Rates: Specifying the Denominator and Time Components

All rates have an external time component which refers to a period or a point in calendar time (called the study period). This should be specified when reporting results because the rate may change with time, from season to season, or year to year. In addition, a rate is based on an internal time component (ITC), a time period having a duration of less than or equal to the study period. An investigation of the rate of calf mortality might last for a period of three years, but the calculation of the rate could be based on a daily, monthly, yearly, or 3-year basis.

A basic rule in forming a rate is that each animal can only experience the event of interest once during a time period; they cease to be at risk after the event of interest occurs, and for the duration of the internal time period on which the rate is based. Although mastitis can occur more than once during a lactation, if one is calculating the rate of mastitis during a lactation (ITC), only the first occurrence is counted. The easiest way to handle multiple occurrences is to shorten the ITC sufficiently to make the constraints reasonable. That is, several rates of mastitis, one for each 30-day interval postpartum, could be calculated.

In general, there are two different types of rates. The first, called a true rate (in technically precise terms, an incidence density rate), describes the average speed at which the event of interest (i.e., infection, disease occurrence, culling, death) occurs per unit of animal time at risk (Green 1982; Kleinbaum et al. 1982). In human medicine the most common time unit used for the period of risk is a year; however, shorter periods such as days or months are appropriate and often are used in veterinary medicine. The concept of animal time may require elaboration; for example, one animal year of risk may result from one animal being at risk of the event of interest for one year, or 12 animals being at risk for one month (1/12 of a year), or 365 animals being at risk for one day (1/365 of a year). Many other combinations are possible, but the general rule is to multiply the number of animals by their average period at risk to obtain the animal time of risk.

If the data are available, an exact denominator for a true rate is formed by adding each individual time period at risk for all animals in the study. Often, calculating an exact denominator is not practical or necessary. An approximate denominator may be formed by adding the number of animals at risk at the beginning of the time period to the number at risk at the end, dividing the sum by 2 to obtain the average number at risk (NAR), and multiplying the number at risk by the appropriate ITC.

Thus the general formula for a true rate is:

$$\frac{\text{no. animals acquiring event of interest}}{\text{average NAR} \times \text{ITC}}$$

EXAMPLE CALCULATIONS   To illustrate this method of calculating a rate, assume that 3 animals were observed in a study period lasting 1 year.

During the year, 2 develop a disease, 1 at day 120 (0.33 years) and 1 at day 240 (0.67 years). The true rate of disease per animal year using the exact denominator is:

$$2/(1 + 0.33 + 0.67) = 2/2 = 1 \text{ per animal year}$$

The true rate using the approximate denominator is:

$$2/\{[(3 + 1)/2] \times 1\} = 2/2 = 1 \text{ per animal year}$$

The two rates agree because the animals experiencing the event of interest were at risk for an average of exactly 1/2 year. Note that 2 animal years of risk were experienced by these 3 animals during the 1-year study period. Also, the time period on which the rates were based (the ITC) is 1 year, the same as the period of study (the external time component). The ITC of 1 year is represented by $\times$ 1 in the above calculations. If the rate was desired on an animal week basis, the ITC factor $\times$ 52 would be used.

True rates are used when the animal population being studied is very dynamic (with additions and/or withdrawals) during the period representing the ITC. As mentioned, the approximate denominator is used when the exact period of risk of individual animals is unavailable or impractical to obtain. True rates have a minimum value of zero and a maximum value of infinity; true rates apply only to populations and have no interpretation at the individual level. Had both animals developed disease on day 30 (0.08 of a year), the total animal years of risk would have been 1.16 and thus the rate would be 1.72 per animal year, or 172% (172 per 100 animal years). This cannot be sensibly interpreted at the individual animal level.

If a true rate has been calculated based on one internal time period, say x months, and it is desired to determine the rate on the basis of some other time period, say y months, then assuming a constant rate, the rate in the latter period is: true rate in y = true rate in $x(y/x)$.

EXAMPLE CALCULATIONS   In the initial example, the true rate per animal month would be $1 \times 1/12 = 0.08$ per animal month.

The second type of rate, called a risk rate (in technically precise terms, a cumulative incidence rate), provides a direct estimate of the probability as defined in statistics of an animal experiencing the event of interest during the internal time period. (In this text, risk will be used as a synonym for probability and the specific measure of risk will be referred to as a risk rate. The words "at risk" may be used in their usual sense, namely, to denote animals susceptible to that disease.) This method requires that each animal initially at risk be observed for the full duration of the stated time period or until the event of interest occurs. Also, there can be no additions to the number initially at risk. (These constraints are the major reasons that true rates often are used to describe the rapidity with which disease occurrence is changing in natural populations.) If there are withdrawals (losses from the study), for reasons other than the event of interest, the effective denominator is determined by subtracting one half of the number withdrawn from the initial number at risk. (The reason for subtracting one half rather than some other number is more pertinent in biometrics courses.) Risk rates have a minimum value of 0 and a maximum value of 1; risk rates may be interpreted at either the population or individual level.

The general format for a risk rate is:

$$\frac{\text{no. animals acquiring event of interest}}{\text{initial NAR} - \frac{1}{2}\text{ withdrawals}}$$

The risk (probability) form of rate is used whenever possible for analytic purposes (comparing rates statistically), since comparing true rates poses both practical and theoretical problems in terms of testing for statistical significance.

EXAMPLE CALCULATIONS   To illustrate the method for determining a risk rate (the probability of an animal developing disease during a time period of one year) using data from the previous example, is: $2/3 = 0.67$.

The risk form of rate may be multiplied by 100 or 1000 to express it on a per 100 or 1000 animals basis. For example 67% means 67 events per 100 animals initially at risk.

If the risk form of rate has been calculated based on one internal time period (e.g., x months) and it is desired to express the risk rate for a different length of time (e.g., y months), then assuming a constant rate, the risk in the latter period is: risk rate in $y = 1 - (1 - \text{risk rate in } x)^{y/x}$.

EXAMPLE CALCULATIONS   If the risk rate of disease in one year is 0.67, the risk rate in two years is: $1 - (1 - 0.67)^2 = 0.89$.

If a true rate is available and the risk of an animal experiencing the event of interest (in the same time period) is required, the formula to convert a true rate to a risk rate is: risk rate $= 1 - e^{-\text{true rate}}$, where e is the base of natural logarithm. This approximation is extremely good when the true rate is below 0.05 per unit of animal time.

When rates are low (<15%), the technical differences between true rates and the risk form of rates may be ignored primarily because the difference in magnitude between them is of little practical importance. For example, in Table 3.1 the true rate of foot problems is 0.24 per cow year. Using the above formula, the risk rate per year is 0.21, for practical purposes, nearly the same magnitude. On the other hand, there is merit in

Table 3.1. Example calculations: true rates and risk rates

A herd of dairy cows provides the following data for the year 1983: On January 1, there were 60 cows in the herd, 6 of which had foot problems; 42 of the 60 cows calved during the year.

Ten new cows entered the herd during the year, all at the time of calving. Eight of the original cows were culled; 4 of these 8 had calved and subsequently developed left displaced abomasum (LDA) and foot problems (FP); the other 4 cows had no diseases and had not calved.

A total of 8 cows developed left displaced abomasum, 6 of these also developed foot problems. Six other cows acquired foot problems; 32 other cows experienced one or more other diseases.

Two cows died; 1 of these had left displaced abomasum, the other no disease.

What are the morbidity, mortality, culling (crude), and the proportional morbidity rates?

In order to proceed make the following assumptions: The period of risk for left displaced abomasum is short and only cows that calve are at risk; hence, use the initial population at risk — adjusting it for any losses — as the denominator. The period of risk for foot problems is long and cows are affected for their lifetime; hence, use the average population at risk for the denominator.

Morbidity risk rate (LDA) $= 8/[(42 + 10) - 0.5 \times 1 \text{ died}] = 8/51.5 = 0.16$ per year
Mortality risk rate (LDA) $= 1/[(42 + 10) - 0.5 \times (1 \text{ died} + 4 \text{ culls})]$
$\qquad\qquad = 1/49.5 = 0.02$ per year
Case fatality rate (LDA) $= 1/8 = 0.125$. Only deaths shortly after the disease occurrence are of interest, so the 4 culls are not counted as withdrawals.
Proportional morbidity rate (LDA) $= 8/(32 \text{ others} + 6\text{FP} + 8\text{LDA}) = 8/46 = 0.17$
Morbidity true rate (FP) $= 12/\{[(60 - 6) + (54 - 2 \text{ deaths} - 4 \text{ culls} - 12 \text{ cases}$
$\qquad\qquad + 10 \text{ additions})]/2\} \times 1$
$\qquad\qquad = 12/[(54 + 46)/2] \times 1 = 12/50 = 0.24$ per cow year
Crude mortality true rate $= 2/[(60 + 60)/2] \times 1 = 2/60 = 0.03$ per cow year
Proportional morbidity rate (FP) $= 12/46 = 0.26$
Culling true rate $= 8/[(60 + 60)/2] \times 1 = 8/60 = 0.13$ per cow year

noting the differences to avoid confusion when the rates are $> 15\%$.

A practical method of calculating risk rates in dynamic populations circumventing the use of exponentials is:

$$\frac{\text{no. animals acquiring event of interest}}{\text{average NAR}}$$

This formula is very much like the true rate formula given earlier, but in calculating the average NAR the animals developing the event of interest are not subtracted from the NAR at the end of the stated time period. For example, in Table 3.1 the risk rate of foot problems may be calculated using the average of 54 and 58 (46 + 12 cases) as the denominator; namely, $12/56 = 0.21$.

3.2 Morbidity Rates

Morbidity rates describe the level of clinical disease in an animal population and may be crude, cause-specific, attribute-specific (i.e., host characteristic) or a combination of the latter two. Crude rates specify neither disease nor host attributes (e.g., the morbidity rate in feedlot cattle during July was 5%). Such rates may be made more meaningful by specifying the disease (e.g., the morbidity rate due to pneumonia in feedlot cattle during July was 4%) or attributes of the host (e.g., the morbidity rate in feedlot calves less than 8 months of age during July was 9%) or both. The extent to which one should make a rate specific depends on the circumstances involved. Morbidity rates also differ depending on whether new cases (incidence) or only existing cases (prevalence) are of interest. Although it is possible to include the number of new and existing cases in the same rate (called period prevalence), it is usually advisable to keep them separate.

Incidence rates describe the probability, or rapidity, of a new case developing during the stated internal time interval. The general formula for a crude true incidence rate is:

$$\frac{\text{no. animals developing disease during time period}}{\text{average population at risk during time period} \times \text{ITC}}$$

For example, in a study of calf morbidity the formula for the true morbidity rate per animal month would be:

$$\frac{\text{no. calves developing disease during a month}}{\text{no. calf-months at risk during that month}}$$

In most instances, the denominator would be calculated by counting the number of live disease-free calves on the first day of the month, adding this to the number of live disease-free calves on the last day of the month and dividing the sum by 2 (the implied time component being $\times$ 1 month). Calves that developed disease during the month would not be at risk at the end of the month and hence should not be included even if they are alive and disease-free at that time. If detailed calf records were available, the exact denominator could be determined, but often such accuracy is not required.

To directly calculate the probability of disease occurrence in a group of animals (e.g., pigs born in July, cattle entering a feedlot in October, dogs whelping in May), one should use the risk form of incidence rate. For example, the formula for the risk rate of disease in calves born in July would be:

$$\frac{\text{no. calves born in July developing disease}}{\text{no. calves born alive in July}}$$

Note that the disease does not have to occur in July. Usually one specifies a reasonable period of risk for the disease in question, say 28 days for most neonatal diseases.

Host characteristics (attributes) often have a dramatic effect on the probability of disease events (see Chapter 4). Therefore, most rates are restricted to selected ages or breeds of the species in question; the restrictions apply to both the numerator and the denominator of the rate. An example of an attribute specific rate is a neonatal rate, indicating disease or death within 28 days of birth.

The risk form of rate is frequently used when the event(s) of interest is closely related, temporally, to occurrences such as farrowing (birth), entry to a feedlot, or the start of a racing season; the period of follow up begins at the time of the latter events. In these instances, the biologic period of risk usually is short relative to the average duration of observation (study period) of individual animals. For example, since the majority of cases of displaced abomasum (DA) occur within a few weeks of calving, the risk rate formula would be:

$$\frac{\text{no. cows developing DA of those calving in June}}{\text{no. cows calving in June}}$$

In calculating risk rates, the animals in the numerator must belong to the group defined in the denominator. Of course, if individuals cannot be identified readily, or if new animals are added to the at risk group, the true rate formula:

$$\frac{\text{no. cows developing DA in June}}{\text{no. cow months of risk in June}}$$

may be used. Both formulas require that the at risk period for DA be defined. One can convert from the true rate to the risk rate using the formula previously shown. Note that some cows developing DA may not have calved in June and may have contributed little to the denominator. Further, some of those calving in June might develop DA in July, but would not be counted in the numerator although they contributed to the denominator. However, in general and particularly in large, stable populations, these discrepancies cancel each other and the rate remains valid. (See Table 3.1 for illustrative calculations.)

For many infectious diseases, animals previously exposed or vaccinated may not be biologically at risk. Thus the rates can be made more accurate if adjustments are made to the denominator for the number of immune animals in the population, and this information should be used if the circumstances allow. Frequently, however, the number of truly immune animals (as distinct from animals with high-serum titers) is unknown; thus if animals are apparently at risk of the event or disease of interest, they should be counted in the denominator.

In contrast to incidence (a dynamic measure of disease occurrence), the prevalence proportion (also called the point prevalence rate) is a static measure of disease frequency. It is the fraction of the population that is diseased at a point in time. The general formula for a crude prevalence proportion is:

$$\frac{\text{no. animals with disease at a point in time}}{\text{no. animals at risk at that point in time}}$$

Note that for a diseased animal to exist, the animal must first develop the disease (a function of incidence); then the disease must persist and the animal must survive (both a function of duration). Thus, in diseases of short duration or with a high case fatality rate, the incidence rate will likely be greater than the prevalence proportion. Chronic diseases tend to produce prevalence proportions that are greater than the incidence rates. In keeping with common usage, prevalence proportion will be referred to hereafter as prevalence. An approximation that explicitly links incidence rate (IR), prevalence (P) and duration of disease (D) is: $P = IR \times D$. All three quantities must be stated in the same time period (e.g., days).

The terms incidence and prevalence often are used incorrectly, particularly in the reporting of the results of mass serologic or microbiologic testing. By definition, incidence rates require two tests — one at the start of the period of observation to ensure that the animals did not have the disease, and the second to investigate whether the disease developed during the observation period. Rates based on one test or examination are by definition measuring prevalence (existing cases). Quite often, rates derived from clinical diagnostic data are treated as incidence rates, as if they were measuring the relative frequency of new cases. However, these rates most often are based on time of diagnosis, not on time of occurrence of the disease. For diseases that may remain subclinical for months or years before becoming clinically apparent, ignoring this difference could lead to inferential errors. For example, animals born with congenital abnormalities are often thought of as new cases and therefore as incidence cases. However, in order to exist at birth, the abnormality must develop in utero and the fetus must persist (not be resorbed or aborted at an early stage of development). Variation in the severity of the abnormality, with respect to survivability of the fetus, could drastically alter the number of animals with abnormalities observed at or after birth, with no change in the number of new abnormalities. Thus, congenital abnormalities measure prevalence not incidence.

As demonstrated above, it is quite important to differentiate incidence rates from prevalence proportions. First, their magnitude may differ greatly, particularly with chronic diseases. Second, factors associated with acquiring new disease may differ from those associated with having a disease, and only the former are of value for disease prevention. Finally, knowledge of the time period when the disease was acquired assists in demarcating the time period during which causal factors may have operated and, hence, assists in the identification of these factors.

A subtype of an incidence rate is an attack rate. The latter is used when the period of risk is limited, as in simultaneous exposure of a group of animals to noxious gases or contaminated water or food. The general formula for an attack rate (AR) is similar to that for the risk form of rate, namely:

$$\frac{\text{total no. animals that develop disease during specified time period following exposure}}{\text{total no. animals exposed}}$$

Because the biologic period of risk is limited, an attack rate represents the total incidence rate; no new cases would arise from that exposure even if the period of observation were lengthened.

A further modification of morbidity rates, primarily used to study the spread of infectious diseases in defined subgroups (e.g., households) of the population, is the secondary attack rate (SAR), which is calculated as:

$$\frac{\text{total no. animals exposed to first case (proband) that develop disease within range of incubation period}}{\text{total no. animals exposed to proband}}$$

Secondary attack rates are usually applied to natural groupings of animals such as pens or farms. They may also be used to evaluate the communicability of diseases of unknown etiology in an attempt to see if infectious agents might be involved. For infectious diseases, the higher the SAR the more contagious the agent. However, some noninfectious diseases can occur in a manner that may result in a high secondary attack rate. This may occur if there is a variable latent period following a common exposure of individuals within the group, and hence the disease may appear to spread from animal to animal.

3.3 Mortality Rates

Mortality rates describe the quantitative impact of death in an animal population. Two frequently used measures of mortality are the crude and cause-specific mortality rates. The formula for the crude mortality (true) rate is:

$$\frac{\text{total deaths in time period}}{\text{average population at risk in time period} \times \text{ITC}}$$

and the formula for the cause-specific mortality (true) rate is:

$$\frac{\begin{array}{c}\text{total deaths from disease } X \\ \text{in time period}\end{array}}{\text{average population at risk in time period} \times \text{ITC}}$$

The probability (i.e., risk) of dying in a specified time period may be determined by restricting the denominator to those alive at the start of the time period and adjusting this number for any withdrawals, as was described for risk rates. All animals must be observed for the full time period, or until death or withdrawal occurs.

The risk of death in animals with a specific disease may be described using the case fatality rate. The formula for a case fatality rate is:

$$\frac{\begin{array}{c}\text{total deaths from disease } X \text{ within} \\ \text{specified time after diagnosis}\end{array}}{\text{total no. animals acquiring disease } X}$$

Case fatality rates are of greater value in acute than in chronic diseases and are used to describe the virulence of the agent and/or the severity of the disease. (See Table 3.1 for example calculations.)

An approximation that links case fatality rates (CFR), cause-specific mortality rates (CSMTR), and incidence rates (IR) is CFR = CSMTR/IR. Thus under certain assumptions, if any two of these rates are known, the third may be calculated.

3.4 Proportional Rates

Sometimes, (e.g., when summarizing disease occurrence on one farm or in one clinic) an investigator divides the number of animals with a given disease by the total number of diseased animals. In other instances, the number of animals dying from a given disease is divided by the total number of deaths. These are called proportional morbidity or proportional mortality rates respectively. Although they have the form of a rate and often are mistakenly referred to as incidence or prevalence rates, the denominator is only a portion of the actual population at risk. Proportional rates may be affected by independent changes in the numerator, the denominator, or both. Hence proportional rates are potentially misleading, and their use is discouraged in favor of the morbidity or mortality rates described previously.

3.5 Variability of Rates

Risk rates and prevalence proportions are averages subject to variability from sampling error. In calculating this sampling error, the number of animals used to calculate the rate is regarded as if it was a random sample from a larger population. If repeated samples of the same number of individuals n were selected, the calculated rate $\bar{p}$ would vary from sample to sample. The extent of this variability is described by the standard error of the mean and is estimated from the sample to be:

$$SE(\bar{p}) = [\bar{p}(1 - \bar{p})/n]^{1/2}$$

A 95% confidence interval may be constructed using the upper and lower limits of the interval defined by $\bar{p} \pm 1.96 \times SE(\bar{p})$ (see Table 2.1). The interpretation to be placed on the confidence interval is that if many samples were selected and a confidence interval constructed for each, 95% would contain the true population rate. This approximation is quite good provided both $n\bar{p}$ and $n(1-\bar{p})$ are > 5.

EXAMPLE CALCULATIONS   Suppose that in a pen of 100 pigs, 30 develop pneumonia and 5 of these die during the first month on feed. If all pigs were free of pneumonia at the start of the feeding period, the true rate of pneumonia per month is $30/[(100 + 70)/2] = 0.35$ or 35% (i.e., 35 per 100 pig months). The probability of a pig developing pneumonia during the 1-month period (risk rate) is: $30/100 = 0.3$ or 30%.

If the above risk (0.3) remains constant during a 3-month feeding period, the probability of a pig developing pneumonia at least once during the 3-month period is:

$$\text{risk rate (3)} = 1 - [1 - \text{risk rate(1)}]^{3/1}$$
$$= 1 - (1 - 0.3)^3 = 1 - 0.7^3 = 0.66$$

This means that 66% of the pigs (or 100 x 0.66 = 66 pigs) would be expected to develop pneumonia in the 3-month period.

The true rate of mortality is $5/[(100 + 95)/2] = 0.051$ per month, whereas the probability of a pig dying during the first month (risk rate) is $5/100 = 0.050$. (Note that as the true rate decreases, it approximates the risk rate very closely.) If the probability of mortality remained constant for the 3-month feeding period, the probability of a pig dying in the 3-month period is $1 - (1 - 0.05)^{3/1} = 1 - 0.95^3 = 0.14$. This means that 14% of the pigs would be expected to die during the 3-month feeding period.

The probability of a pig dying if it develops pneumonia is found by using the case fatality rate. In this example, the case fatality rate for pneumonia is $5/30 = 0.17$ or 17%. (Note that since the only disease present is pneumonia, the above morbidity and mortality rates are cause-specific.)

If the 100 pigs were viewed as a sample of the feeder-pig population on this farm, one could construct confidence intervals for the average morbidity and mortality risk rates.

For the average morbidity risk rate, the standard error of $\bar{p}$ (0.30) is $SE(\bar{p}) = (0.30 \times 0.70/100)^{1/2} = 0.046$ and hence the 95% confidence limits are 0.21–0.39 (21%–39%).

For the average mortality risk rate, the standard error of $\bar{p}$ (0.05) is $SE(\bar{p}) = (0.05 \times 0.95/100)^{1/2} = 0.022$ and hence the 95% confidence limits are 0.007–0.093 (0.7%–9.3%).

If the 100 animals were obtained by formally sampling a defined population (a herd) with individual pigs being the sampling unit, and if the number studied was greater than 10% of the population, more precise estimates of the standard error may be obtained by adjustment using the finite population correction factor (see Table 2.1). Hence, if there were only 500 pigs in the population, $n/N = 0.2$ and the correction factor for the standard error is $(1 - 0.2)^{1/2} = 0.89$. Thus the best estimate of the standard error of the morbidity rate is $0.046 \times 0.89 = 0.04$, and the best estimate of the standard error of the mortality rate is $0.022 \times 0.89 = 0.02$. The resulting confidence intervals will be slightly narrower; a reflection that 20% of the population was sampled. The reader will now be aware that it is quite difficult to establish standard errors for true rates, hence no discussion of this topic will be presented. If standard errors are desired and the true rate is low (< 10%), one may use the same approach as demonstrated above for risk rates.

3.6 Measuring Production: Basic Statistics

As previously mentioned, the level of production is often used in veterinary medicine as a proxy or surrogate measure for health. As such, production is frequently the outcome of concern (dependent variable) in many veterinary epidemiologic studies. Production, whether it be kilograms of milk per lactation, number of pigs per litter, number of litters per year, weight gain per day, or eggs per bird per year, is considered to be a quantitative variable. The sample distribution of a quantitative variable is best described by the mean ($\bar{y}$) or average, the standard deviation (s), or variance (s^2), and the median. The sampling variability of the mean is described by the standard error of the mean [$SE(\bar{y})$] (see Table 2.1).

The mean is a measure of central tendency and a formula for calculating it is $\bar{y} = \Sigma\, y_i/n$ where y_i is the ith observation, n is the number of observations, and Σ means take the sum of the y_i. The median is another measure of central tendency and is the middle value when the n values are placed in order of magnitude. If n is even, the median is the average of the middle two values of y_i. The median is useful to describe central tendency when the distribution of a variable is not Gaussian (i.e., not bell-shaped or normal), since the median is affected less by extreme values than is the mean. If a distribution has a right skew (long tail to the right) the mean will be greater than the median and vice versa if the distribution has a left skew. Another way of treating skewed data is to transform them (e.g., by taking logarithms of the values) and then taking the mean of the logarithmic values. A common example of this approach is in the description of somatic cell counts in milk.

The standard deviation s is the square root of the variance or mean square s^2 and describes the variability of individual values of y around their mean. Two formulas for calculating s^2 are:

$$s^2 = \Sigma\, (y_i - \bar{y})^2/(n - 1) \quad \text{or} \quad [\Sigma\, (y_i^2) - (\Sigma\, y_i)^2/n]/(n - 1)$$

$$s = (s^2)^{1/2}$$

A number of relatively inexpensive calculators are programmed to calculate $\bar{y}$ and s^2; nonetheless, the above formulas are instructive about the meaning of these statistics.

The n animals on which y and s are based may be viewed as a sample of size n from a much larger population. Repeated samples of the same size would provide other estimates of the average in the population. (One does not actually draw repeated samples but uses the central limit theorem to describe the variability of the sample mean.) The variability among these means is described by the standard error of the mean and this may be calculated as $SE(\bar{y}) = (s^2/n)^{1/2} = s/(n)^{1/2}$.

The standard error may be used to construct a confidence interval for the mean. The upper and lower limits of a 95% confidence interval are calculated using $\bar{y} \pm 1.96 \times SE(\bar{y})$.

When measuring rates of events (e.g., disease) at any aggregate level (e.g., farm level), the rates may be treated as quantitative variables for purposes of description and analysis.

3.6.1   Choosing the Production Parameter

In many studies only a few production parameters are available. However, even if the number of choices is limited, the investigator should try to select parameters that not only measure production, but that may be used as economic indicators, and hence are of value for decision making (Williamson 1980). For example, selecting the number of services per conception as a parameter of reproductive efficiency in dairy health management would probably be unwise; first, many factors including time of first postpartum breeding affect it, and second, this parameter is not a good indicator of important economic aspects of reproduction. The open interval (i.e., the period between parturition and conception) or the percentage pregnant by 100 days postpartum would be more appropriate parameters. A hierarchy of parameters should be used to monitor and/or investigate production decreases in health management programs (see 12.2). Both the mean and the standard deviation are important to note in such instances.

Choosing a suitable measure for milk production in dairy cows will serve as an example of some other considerations that must be taken into account in selecting a parameter. Absolute measures of milk production include the total kilograms of milk produced in a lactation (kg tot) and the kilograms of milk produced in a 305 day period (kg 305). The value of the kg 305 over the kg tot is that differences due to variation in days-in-milk are removed. However, other factors such as the age of cow and the season of calving can also have a major effect on the kg 305 produced. To circumvent these problems, the effects of age and calving season can be removed using an index known as the breed class average for milk production (BCM). In a simple sense, the production of a typical cow is assigned a value of 100 and all other cows are assigned a breed class average score based on their kg 305 adjusted for their age and their season of calving. In general, each BCM unit in a two-year-old cow represents about 45 kg of milk. The BCM allows one to compare the milk production between two groups of cows in the same herd or between two groups of herds without having to worry about the age structure or seasonal distribution of calvings within the groups.

If an investigator wished to compare the milk production of cows with a particular disease to that of cows without that disease, and production data from more than one herd were to be used, the comparison could be biased by differences in the level of production among herds, unless equal numbers of cows with and without the disease were selected from each herd. Another way to obviate this problem is to express each cow's level of production as the deviation (in BCM units) from the average production in her source herd. This parameter is known as the deviation-from-herd-average and is frequently used to remove the herd effect when making cow-level comparisons across many herds.

Although the above example is based on the dairy industry, similar indices for other parameters in other industries are available or can be derived.

3.7   Detecting Subclinical Disease with Screening Tests

The previous sections have been concerned with measuring the frequency and impact of visible events such as clinical disease or death in animal populations. Screening is the application of a test to apparently healthy animals in order to detect infection or subclinical disease. In domestic animals, probably the major economic loss is due to the effects of hidden or subclinical disease. For example, subclinical mastitis is a mild inapparent condition, yet because of its high prevalence, it has a much greater impact on the productivity of dairy herds than the sporadic yet dramatic clinical forms of the disease. In addition, knowledge of the frequency and distribution of infectious and noninfectious agents of disease and of immune responses to these agents can greatly assist our understanding of disease processes and the importance of various agents in manifestationally classified syndromes such as pneumonia or gastroenteritis. Certainly, as mentioned in Chapter 2, the frequency, distribution, and importance of subclinical disease may be very different from that of clinical cases. From an epidemiologic perspective, it may be argued that greater success at preventing disease occurrence can be realized if investigations are concentrated on how infections occur and persist in the absence of disease, rather than using only diseased animals as models of study.

Because the disease process is clinically inapparent, special tests (e.g., the California mastitis test) are required to detect subclinical disease. Also, in addition to what one might consider conventional laboratory tests, epidemiologists include any device or process designed to detect or elicit a sign, substance, tissue change, or response as a test. Thus, examples of tests include common serologic and microbiologic tests for detecting agents or the animal's response to an agent; clinical-pathologic tests designed to measure the number of particular cell types, the levels of tissue enzymes or minerals; as well as questions in personal or mail surveys. Using one or more of our senses during the diagnostic process for the detection of signs or tissue changes (including pregnancy diagnosis and meat inspection findings) could also be included as tests.

Tests are usually considered to be either pathognomonic or surrogate. Pathognomonic tests are those for which the detection of a sign, substance, response, or tissue change is an absolute predictor of the presence of the disease or disease agent. Surrogate tests detect secondary changes, which it is hoped will predict the presence or absence of disease or the disease agent. For example, a positive culture of *Brucella abortus* from a cow's milk sample is pathognomonic for brucella infection. Testing the milk for anti-bodies to *Brucella abortus*, however, is a surrogate test; since it is not measuring the presence of *Brucella abortus* per se, but rather the body's reaction to brucella organisms or cross-reacting antigens. Surrogate tests may produce false-positive results, whereas pathognomonic tests do not. Both types of tests can have false-negative results. Such false results and the question of assessing tests and interpreting the results lead to the subject of sensitivity and specificity (Robertson 1963; Martin 1977; Dodd 1978; Seiler 1979; Martin 1984).

3.7.1 Sensitivity and Specificity

Suppose it is possible to correctly classify animals into two cate-gories — those having disease X and those not having disease X, — using a set of available tests. A new test has been developed, and its ability to differentiate between diseased and nondiseased animals needs to be evalu-ated. (Disease here is used in its broadest sense and includes subclinical disease and/or infection.)

The initial step in the evaluation is to select a sample of animals known to have disease X and a sample known not to have disease X. Atlthough infrequently used in practice, formal random samples of each of these populations will help to ensure that animals to be tested are representative of diseased and nondiseased animals respectively, as this is crucial for ac-curate evaluation of the new test (Ransohoff and Feinstein 1978). It is also important that the new test is biologically independent of the methods initially used to define the true health status of the animals. After appropri-ate animals are selected, they are tested and classified as being positive or negative on the basis of the new test results. The resultant cross classifica-tion of n animals according to their true health status and the results of the screening test may be displayed as follows:

Test result	Actual health status (Disease X)	
	Present ($D+$)	Absent ($D-$)
Positive ($T+$)	a	b
Negative ($T-$)	c	d
	$a+c$	$b+d$

The sensitivity of the test is its ability to detect diseased animals and is defined as the proportion of the diseased animals that test positive, i.e., $a/(a + c)$. The specificity of the test is its ability to detect nondiseased ani-mals and is defined as the proportion of nondiseased animals that test negative, i.e., $d/(b + d)$. (Nondiseased indicates animals that do not have the event of interest; it does not mean 100% healthy.) In combination these two statistics describe how well a test can discriminate between nondiseased and diseased individuals. Note that the epidemiologic usage of "sensitivity" differs from immunologic or pharmacologic usage. In the latter disciplines, a sensitive test is one that detects a small amount of antibody, toxin, enzyme, etc. An immunologically sensitive test may not be epidemiologically sensitive, so one should be careful not to confuse the different meanings. Sensitivity and specificity are calculated in the same manner as risk rates because they are probability statements. To summarize:

$$\text{sensitivity} = a/(a+c) = p(T+/D+)$$
$$\text{specificity} = d/(b+d) = p(T-/D-)$$

In a random sample of the overall population, the true prevalence proportion of disease in the population $P(D+)$ would be estimated by $p(D+)$, i.e., $(a + c)/n$. However, in practice this parameter is almost always unknown; only the test results ($T+$ and $T-$) are available, and hence the estimate of $P(D+)$ is the apparent prevalence proportion $p(T+)$, namely, $(a + b)/n$. Obviously, the true and apparent prevalence proportions are equal only if $b = c$. In general, b tends to be numerically greater than c and thus the apparent prevalence is usually somewhat higher than the actual prevalence, sometimes by a surprising amount.

To summarize, in a random sample of the population,

$$\text{apparent prevalence} = (a + b)/n = p(T+)$$
$$\text{true prevalence}\quad\ = (a + c)/n = p(D+)$$

Note that for most surrogate tests there is an inverse relationship between sensitivity and specificity. That is, if the critical value of the test is altered so that the sensitivity is increased, the specificity will be automatically decreased. This is because the substances being measured may be present in nondiseased as well as diseased animals, although at different levels and with different frequencies, and often their distributions overlap. For example, Figure 3.1 displays the distribution of antibody titers to agent X in a sample of healthy nondiseased (do not have agent X) and a sample of diseased (have agent X) animals. Note that most nondiseased animals do not have a titer to the agent, some have low titers and a very few have high titers. On the other hand, in diseased animals the distribution is somewhat bell-shaped (i.e., a normal or Gaussian distribution). Very few diseased animals have low titers; most have moderate titers, and some have very high titers to the agent. Although the diseased animals have higher titers on average, the two distributions of titers overlap, and this produces an inverse relationship between the sensitivity and the specificity of tests measur-

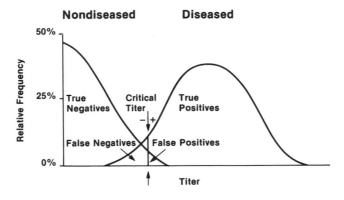

3.1. Distribution of titers to agent X in sample of nondiseased and diseased animals.

ing this antibody response. The resultant sensitivity and specificity will depend on the critical titer selected.

In practice, a critical titer is selected so that animals having titers above that point are considered positive, and those having titers equal to or below that point are considered negative. In terms of the previous 2 x 2 table, diseased animals with titers above the critical titer are the true positives, their number being represented by a; the nondiseased animals with titres below the critical titre are the true negatives, their number being represented by d; the nondiseased animals with titers above the critical titer are false positives, their number being represented by b, and the diseased animals with titers equal to or less than the critical titer are false negatives, their number being represented by c.

If the critical titer is adjusted to increase the sensitivity (i.e., lowered or moved to the left in Fig. 3.1), the number of false-positive animals will increase, hence this decreases the specificity. If the critical titer is altered by moving it to the right to increase the specificity, the sensitivity of the test will decrease, thus there will be a larger number of false negatives. An example of the effect of changing the critical titer when testing for visceral larva migrans using an ELISA test is shown in Table 3.2 (Glickman et al. 1978).

In general, sensitivity and specificity describe the discriminatory power of a test based on a single biologic sample taken at a point in time. They do not describe how well the test would function if applied very late in the disease process as compared to early in the disease process; nor do they

Table 3.2. Sensitivity, specificity, and predictive value of the enzyme-linked immunosorbent assay (ELISA) for the diagnosis of visceral larva migrans

Cut-off log titer of a positive ELISA test	Sensitivity (%)	Specificity (%)	Predictive value	
			Positive (%)	Negative (%)
1	91.3	76.9	70.0	93.8
2	91.3	79.5	72.4	93.9
3	82.6	82.1	73.1	89.2
4	82.6	84.6	76.0	88.9
5	78.3	92.3	85.7	87.8
6	65.2	94.9	88.2	82.2
7	56.5	97.4	92.9	79.2
8	43.5	97.4	90.9	74.5
9	30.4	100.0	100.0	70.9
10	30.4	100.0	100.0	70.9
11	21.7	100.0	100.0	68.4
>12	17.4	100.0	100.0	67.2

Source: Glickman et al. 1978, with permission.

describe how well one could classify the health status of animals based on results from using the test sequentially on the same animals. The same principles apply, however, to the situation where acute and chronic (convalescent) titers are measured, and an animal is declared infected or diseased if there is say a two-fold or four-fold titer rise. Here the question of interest is the ability (i.e., sensitivity and specificity) of a specified increase in titer to discriminate between diseased and nondiseased animals.

3.7.2 Indirect Estimates of Sensitivity and Specificity

Sometimes the test to be evaluated is biologically similar to those available to diagnose the disease, yet estimates of sensitivity and specificity are desired. This is frequently the case with diseases of viral etiology where the virus is difficult to culture, and secondary binding tests are used to detect the presence of antibody to viral antigens. In this instance, the results of the new test can be compared with the results of a bank of standard tests. For this purpose, animals positive to all tests in the bank are assumed to be diseased, and animals negative to all tests in the bank are considered disease-free. Animals with intermediate types of response are excluded from further analyses. The sensitivity and specificity calculations proceed in the usual manner, but the results of the comparisons should be prefixed with "relative" to indicate that the determinations are based on biologically related tests. Usually the results obtained by this method represent maximum values of sensitivity and specificity. The reader should note that comparing the results of one test to the results of a biologically related surrogate test does not allow the establishment of sensitivity or specificity. This procedure can establish which test gives more positive results and the extent of agreement between the tests, but not their ability to differentiate diseased from nondiseased animals.

In other situations, it may prove very difficult to assemble a sufficiently large representative group of nondiseased animals in order to determine the specificity of a test. However, if test results on a relatively large number of representative animals ($n > 1000$) are available, and if it is reasonable to assume that the prevalence of disease is less than 1% and that the test has high sensitivity, an approximation may be used. The approximation is based on the assumptions that all test-positive individuals are false-positives and that disease is rare. Thus specificity can be estimated by $1 -$ (number of test positives)$/n = 1 - (a + b)/n$.

EXAMPLE CALCULATIONS   If 17 of 2000 representative animals have positive tests, then assuming all are false-positive reactions the minimum specificity would be $1 - 17/2000 = 0.9915$ or 99.15%.

Under some circumstances, it may be possible to conduct a detailed follow-up on the test-positive animals and classify them into diseased and nondiseased (false-positive) groups. In this case, assuming a reasonable sensitivity, specificity may be more accurately estimated by:

$$1 - \frac{\text{number of false positives}}{n - \text{number of diseased among test positives}} = 1 - b/(n - a)$$

Finally, if estimates of sensitivity are available, the above estimate may be improved by using a^* instead of a, where $a^* = a/\text{sensitivity}$ (a^* estimates $a + c$).

EXAMPLE CALCULATIONS   If 12 of the above 17 reactors were found to be diseased, the minimum specificity would be $1 - 5/(2000 - 12) = 1 - 0.0025 = 0.9975$ or 99.75%. In addition, if the test was known to be 80% sensitive, an improved estimate of specificity would be $1 - 5/(2000 - 15)$, which to four decimals in this case is also 0.9975 or 99.75%.

3.7.3 Predictive Value of Screening Test Results

The predictive value of a positive test is defined as the proportion of diseased animals among those that test positive; that is, the quantity $p(D+/T+)$ which is calculated using $a/(a + b)$. (Unless otherwise stated, this discussion will be restricted to the predictive value of a positive test result.) Caution is required here because this quantity sounds and looks like $p(T+/D+)$ (i.e., sensitivity), but it is quite different. Predictive value is important because it reflects the way test results are used in the field. Here the question is, Given that an animal has a positive test, what is the likelihood that the animal has the disease or infection under study? This question arises because the true state of health is unknown, hence, the practitioner must argue backward from test results to the likelihood of disease, not from disease status to the likelihood of a specific test result.

The predictive value of a test has been used as a method of test selection. However, the predictive value of any given test is affected by both the sensitivity and the specificity of the test, as well as by the true prevalence of disease in the population. Since the latter usually is unknown, it makes the selection of the "best" test difficult, because the direction of the inequality of predictive values of two tests can be reversed depending on the prevalence of disease. One cannot assume that the test with the highest predictive value is necessarily the most sensitive or specific.

The data in Table 3.3 demonstrate the effect of prevalence of disease on the predictive value of the test result. Note that when the prevalence of disease is 3%, the predictive value of the test is 79.5%. (This is found by dividing 234, the number of test positives, into 186, the number of true positives.) When the prevalence of disease is 0.1% (i.e., one animal per thousand is diseased) the predictive value is 10.7%, and when the prevalence of disease is 0.01% (i.e., one animal per ten thousand) the predictive value of a positive test is 1.2%. Note that the assumed level of sensitivity and specificity, 62% and 99.5% respectively, have not changed except for rounding to obtain whole numbers (animals). The example in Table 3.2,

Table 3.3. Relationship between true prevalence of disease and the predictive value of a positive test result

Sensitivity $= p(T+/D+) = 62\%$
Specificity $= p(T-/D-) = 99.5\%$

Example 1: $p(D+) = 3\%$

	$D+$	$D-$	Total
$T+$	186	48	234
$T-$	114	9652	9766
	300	9700	10,000

Predictive value $= p(D+/T+) = (186/234) \times 100 = 79.5\%$

Example 2: $p(D+) = 0.1\%$

	$D+$	$D-$	Total
$T+$	6	50	56
$T-$	4	9940	9944
	10	9990	10,000

Predictive value $= p(D+/T+) = 10.7\%$

Example 3: $p(D+) = 0.01\%$

	$D+$	$D-$	Total
$T+$	6	500	506
$T-$	4	99,490	99,494
	10	99,990	100,000

Predictive value $= p(D+/T+) = 1.18\%$

which is based on testing for visceral larva migrans, illustrates the relationship between predictive value, sensitivity, and specificity; the prevalence of disease being constant. The predictive value of this test is quite good (being at least 70%). This is only true because of the high prevalence proportion of visceral larva migrans of 37%.

The predictive value of a positive test result in a variety of circumstances can be estimated using the formula:

$$p(D+/T+) = \frac{p(D+) \times p(T+/D+)}{p(D+) \times p(T+/D+) + p(D-) \times p(T+/D-)}$$

Although valuable from a theoretical viewpoint, since it explicitly describes the factors influencing predictive value, the true prevalence of disease is rarely known, and hence this formula is not often used in practice. Its major value is to demonstrate what the predictive value would be if the test was used at a specified prevalence proportion.

Since the prevalence proportion of disease is usually below 0.2, the lack of specificity in most screening tests is responsible for the apparent prevalence of disease often being somewhat higher than the true prevalence of disease. This may be verified by comparing the apparent and true prevalence of disease for the data presented in Table 3.3. In general, the apparent prevalence is frequently not a good estimate of the true prevalence because of the false-negative and false-positive animals. However, if the sensitivity and specificity are known, the true prevalence may be estimated by:

$$p(D+) = \frac{p(T+) - p(T+/D-)}{1 - [p(T+/D-) + p(T-/D+)]}$$

Note that $p(T+/D-) = 1 -$ specificity, and $p(T-/D+) = 1 -$ sensitivity. For example, using the data in Table 3.3 example 2:

$$p(D+) = \frac{0.0056 - 0.005}{1 - (0.005 + 0.38)} = \frac{0.0006}{1 - 0.385} = 0.001 = 0.1\%$$

3.7.4 Methods for Improving Predictive Value

One method of improving the predictive value of a screening test is to screen only high risk populations; that is, populations likely to have a high rate of infection or disease. Observational studies (e.g., cross-sectional, cohort, and case-control) are used to identify subgroups with an elevated risk of infection or disease, and the screening program can then be concentrated on those individuals with a high risk, hence ensuring a relatively good predictive value.

A second method of improving the predictive value is to use more than one screening test. This may be done in several ways. The first example assumes that a relatively sensitive, inexpensive screening test is available for use on all animals in the population, and a more sensitive but expensive test is available for use on a limited number of individuals. Table 3.4 contains the expected results given that the initial test (with a sensitivity of 95% and specificity of 99%) is used on all individuals in the population, and the second test (with a sensitivity of 98% and specificity of 99%) is subsequently applied to the animals positive to the first test.

Table 3.4. Results expected after application of one test to all animals and a second test to all reactors from the primary test

Results of initial test:				Initial test:
	$D+$	$D-$	Total	
$T+$	95	99	194	Sensitivity 95%
$T-$	5	9801	9806	Specificity 99%
	100	9900	10,000	
Results of second test:				Second test:
	$D+$	$D-$	Total	
$T+$	93	1	94	Sensitivity 98%
$T-$	2	98	100	Specificity 99%
	95	99	194	

Note: Overall sensitivity = $(100 - 7)/100 = 93.0\%$
Overall specificity = $(9801 + 98)/9900 = 99.9\%$
Overall predictive value = $93/94 = 98.9\%$

The overall results of using these two tests is a combined sensitivity of 93% and a specificity of 99.9%. Notice that 5 diseased animals were missed on the first test and in order to reduce the number of false positives from the first test, an additional 2 infected animals were declared negative on the second test. However, the use of the second test reduced the number of false positives from 99 to 1. This demonstrates the general results to be expected utilizing tests in this manner. The actual results probably would not be this good, because if the two tests were biologically similar the results would be correlated; that is, they would tend to give similar results on samples from the same animal.

Another method of using multiple tests is to apply two or more tests simultaneously to all individuals. When tests are used in this manner, the resultant sensitivity and specificity are dependent on the way the results are interpreted. One method of interpretation used when a high sensitivity is required is known as parallel interpretation. Using parallel interpretation, an animal is considered positive if it reacts positively to one or the other or both tests. This increases the sensitivity but tends to decrease the specificity of the combined tests. This makes intuitive sense since it gives a diseased animal the greatest opportunity to react positively. The second method of interpretation used whenever a high specificity is required is known as series interpretation. In series interpretation, an animal must be positive to both of the tests to be considered positive. As mentioned, this will increase specificity but decrease sensitivity because the likelihood of a diseased animal reacting positive to both tests is less than the likelihood of it reacting positive to both, or positive to the first and negative to the second or vice versa.

The outcome from using series and parallel interpretation with two tests is shown in Table 3.5. The sensitivity of the first test is 50% and its specificity 98.7%. The sensitivity of the second test is 60% and its specificity 98.6%. When the tests are interpreted in parallel, 150 of the 200 diseased animals are considered positive for a resultant sensitivity of 75%. A total of 7620 of the nondiseased animals are considered negative and thus the specificity is 97.7%. When the results are interpreted in series, only 70 of the 200 diseased animals are considered positive for a resultant sensitivity of 35%. However, 7770 animals that are not diseased are considered to be negative for a specificity of 99.6%.

Obviously the above example could be expanded to include more than two tests and, again, the results would be similar to that indicated here — parallel interpretation increases sensitivity and series interpretation increases specificity. In general, the greater number of tests involved, the greater the increase in sensitivity or specificity depending upon the method of interpretation. To identify the optimal classification (i.e., minimizing the overall misclassification rates) requires the use of more elaborate techniques such as discriminant analysis; however, these are beyond the scope of this book.

Table 3.5.   Sensitivity and specificity of combined screening tests, with test results interpreted in series and in parallel

Test 1	Test 2	Diseased	Not diseased
+	−	30	70
−	+	50	80
+	+	70	30
−	−	50	7620
		200	7800
		Sensitivity	Specificity
Both tests in "parallel"		150/200 = 75%	7620/7800 = 97.7%
Both tests in "series"		70/200 = 35%	7770/7800 = 99.6%

3.7.5 Accuracy and Precision

Unlike sensitivity and specificity, which relate to the discriminatory powers of a test to differentiate healthy and diseased individuals, accuracy and precision relate more to quality control within the laboratory. Obviously if a test is inaccurate and lacks precision, the results will certainly influence the sensitivity and specificity of the test. However, for ease of discussion, accuracy and precision will be treated independently of sensitivity and specificity.

An accurate test gives a true measure of the substance, lesion, or structure of concern (i.e., the number of white blood cells, the level of blood sugar, the level of lead in blood, the size of follicles on ovaries). On the other hand, precision is the ability of the test to give a consistent measure upon repeated testing of the same sample. Each test will have its own inherent level of accuracy and precision.

Within limitations, accuracy is less important than precision in terms of screening tests. For example, if the extent to which a test tends to overestimate or underestimate the true level of the substance being measured is known, a correction for this may be made. When tests are not precise, more than one measurement should be made, and the average of the set of measurements used instead of just one test result.

Both precision and accuracy of a test are influenced by the variability of the test itself, the variability of the person who performs the test, and the differences between laboratories. This text is not concerned with how precision and accuracy of a test are evaluated. Nonetheless, a simple way of assessing the precision of a test performed by one person is to submit repeat samples in a blind manner and calculate the variability (variance) among results. (A blind technique is also essential when comparing test results for agreement and/or sensitivity and specificity. That is, the person performing test B should not have knowledge of the results of test A; otherwise, serious bias can occur.) Often, when using complicated tests requiring standardization on a daily basis, such a procedure will indicate that within-day precision is acceptable but between-day precision is poor. Hence paired sera (acute and convalescent) from the same animal should be tested on the same day.

The results of a study of intra- and inter-individual variation (precision) in the interpretation of canine chest radiographs are shown in Table 3.6 (Reif et al. 1970). The extent of agreement between the two radiologists was 74% and, on average, the radiologists agreed with their previous findings 82% of the time. Note the average sensitivity and specificity of chest radiographs for detecting pulmonary disease, assuming histologic diagnosis to be correct. Given the low specificity of only 87%, radiography would not be an appropriate method of screening canine populations for respira-

Table 3.6. Some findings on the sensitivity, specificity, and precision of radiographic techniques used to determine pulmonary disease in dogs

	Histological diagnosis	
	$D+$	$D-$
Radiographic $T+$	100	8
Interpretation $T-$	38	54
	138	62

$$\text{Sensitivity} = 100/138 = 72.4\%$$
$$\text{Specificity} = 54/62 = 87.1\%$$

In rereading 130 of the above radiographs, the two researchers disagreed with themselves 24 times and with each other 34 times, giving the following:

Intraindividual precision = 81.5% (18.5% error)
Interindividual precision = 73.9% (26.1% error)

Source: Reif et al. 1970.

tory disease if the true prevalence of disease was low. If used in this situation, the predictive value of positive radiographs would be extremely low.

3.8 Measuring Agreement

In many circumstances it is very difficult and costly to establish the true state of nature with regard to disease status. For example, the latter may require post mortem examinations, or as in the case of many viral diseases, culturing for the agent is both tedious and insensitive. Hence, in practice, veterinarians often have to utilize imperfect tests for which there are no quantitative estimates of sensitivity and specificity. In so doing, the tacit assumption is that the predictive values will be acceptable enough for practical purposes.

Under these circumstances, when a new test for disease is developed, its results are often compared to those from the current, standard, yet imperfect, test. A fictitious example of such a comparison is shown in Table 3.7. The standard test gives an apparent prevalence of 8%, the new test 10%, and both tests are positive in 4.2% of the animals. Note that these data do not directly indicate whether a positive test indicates disease (or infection) or a negative test indicates health (no infection). Thus, other than ascertaining if one test gives more positive responses than the other, all one can do is assess the extent of agreement between the test results.

An obvious measure of agreement is to calculate the observed percentage of agreemeent between the tests; in this example it is 90.4%. On the surface this seems quite good. However, in making this inference the implicit comparison level is no (i.e., 0%) agreement. This is incorrect, however, as there should be some agreement by chance alone. This is analagous

Table 3.7.   Agreement between two tests

		Standard test		Total	Apparent prevalence
		+	−		
New	+	42	58	100	0.1
Test	−	38	862	900	...
		80	920	1000	

Apparent prevalence,   0.08

Observed proportion agreement	$(42 + 862)/1000 = 0.904$
Chance proportion agreement (both +)	$0.1 \times 0.08 = 0.008$
Chance proportion agreement (both −)	$0.9 \times 0.92 = 0.828$
Chance proportion agreement	$0.008 + 0.828 = 0.836$
Observed minus chance agreement	$0.904 - 0.836 = 0.068$
Maximum possible agreement beyond chance level	$1 - 0.836 = 0.164$
Kappa	$0.068/0.164 = 0.41$

to tossing two coins and noting the percentage of tosses in which both coins land "heads" (representing positive) or both land "tails" (representing test negative). In coin tossing, the probability of obtaining a head is 0.5 for both coins; hence, one expects agreement 50% of the time (25% of the time for heads and 25% of the time for tails). In test comparisons the probability of being test positive is given by the apparent prevalence for each test. Hence, the probability of both tests being positive is given by the product of the two apparent prevalences. Similarly, the probability of both tests being negative is given by the product of 1 minus the apparent prevalence of each test. The sum of these two probabilities gives the level of agreement expected by chance alone, 83.6% in this example. The chance level of agreement is the explicit level of comparison for assessing agreement, the observed level being 6.8% higher than the chance level in this example. To evaluate the relative magnitude of this difference, it is divided by the maximum possible agreement beyond chance, which in this example is 16.4%. The quotient (often called kappa) is 0.41. No agreement beyond chance gives a kappa of 0, and a kappa of 1 indicates perfect agreement.

A qualitative assessment of kappa suggests that if it is high, the tests are measuring what they purport to measure. If kappa is low, much uncertainty exists and in the absence of sensitivity and specificity data it is difficult to say which test provides the more valid answers. In the comparison of tests, a kappa of at least 0.4–0.5 indicates a moderate level of agreement.

In recent years, kappa has also been applied to the assessment of agreement between clinical diagnoses and to measure the "repeatability" of a clinician's assessments on two separate occasions. Obviously, a blind technique should be used to prevent bias in these assessments. The study referred to in Table 3.6 contains sufficient data to assess between-clinician and within-clinician agreement in the interpretation of radiographs. The levels of precision cited reflect only observed levels of agreement, not the extent of agreement beyond chance. A fictitious example based on agreement between the diagnoses of front limb lameness in horses by two clinicians is shown in Table 3.8. In this example, the observed level of agreement was 84%, the expected level by chance was 54.8%, and kappa was 0.65. Although there is little data in veterinary medicine on this subject, a kappa of 0.5–0.6 would appear to be the level anticipated from experienced clinicians when attempting to diagnose conditions of moderate difficulty. Within-clinician agreement of diagnoses made on the same subjects on different occasions will likely be somewhat higher, resulting in kappa values of 0.6–0.8.

Elucidating reasons for disagreement may allow the improvement of the test's (or clinician's) ability to correctly detect the true state of nature. General reasons for disagreement in the results of serologic tests are the absence of certain antibody classes in animals during the very early or terminal stages of disease and the presence of microorganisms antigenetically similar to those of the agent the test is designed to detect. Disagreement in clinicians' diagnoses may reflect the lack of a standardized diagnostic workup procedure, a different knowledge base, being mislead by a biased history, or the inappropriate selection (or interpretation) of ancillary tests.

In any event, the application of sensitivity and specificity concepts as well as measures of agreement beyond chance to the evaluation of tests and clinician abilities should result in more refined tests and improved diagnostic ability.

Table 3.8. Agreement between two clinicians diagnosing reasons for front limb lameness in horses

		Clinician 2		Total	Apparent prevalence
		ND	OD		
Clinician 1	ND	26	4	30	0.3
	OD	12	58	70	. . .
		38	62	100	
Apparent prevalence,		0.38			

Observed proportion agreement	(26 + 58)/100 = 0.84
Chance proportion agreement ND	0.3 × 0.38 = 0.114
Chance proportion agreement OD	0.7 × 0.62 = 0.434
Chance proportion agreement	0.114 + 0.434 = 0.548
Observed minus chance agreement	0.84 − 0.548 = 0.292
Maximum possible agreement beyond chance level	1 − 0.548 = 0.452
Kappa	0.292/0.452 = 0.65

Note: ND = Navicular disease; OD = Other disease

References

Dodd, K. 1978. Estimation of the sensitivity, specificity and predictive value of the intradermal tuberculin test. Irish Vet. J. 32:87–89.

Elandt-Johnson, R. C. 1975. Definition of rates: Some remarks on their use and misuse. Am. J. Epidemiol. 102:267–71.

Glickman, L., P. Shantz, R. Dombroske, and R. Cypess. 1978. Evaluation of serodiagnostic tests for visceral larva migrans. Am. J. Trop. Med. Hyg. 27:492–98.

Green, A. 1982. The epidemiologic approach to studies of association between HLA and disease. I. The basic measures, concepts and estimation procedures. Tissue Antigens 19:245–58.

Kleinbaum, D. G., L. L. Kupper, and H. Morgenstern. 1982. Epidemiological Research: Principles and Quantitative Methods. Belmont, Calif.: Wadsworth.

Martin, S. W. 1977. The evaluation of tests. Can. J. Comp. Med. 44:19–25.

———. 1984. Estimating disease prevalence and the interpretation of screening test results. Prev. Vet. Med. 2:463–72.

Ransohoff, D. F., and A. R. Feinstein. 1978. Problems of spectrum and bias in evaluating the efficacy of diagnostic tests. New Eng. J. Med. 299:926–30.

Reif, J. S., W. H. Rhodes, and D. Cohen. 1970. Canine pulmonary disease and the urban environment. I. The validity of radiographic examination for estimating the prevalence of pulmonary disease. Arch. Environ. Health 20:676–83.

Robertson, T. G. 1963. Diagnosis of bovine tuberculosis. I. The evaluation of tuberculin tests. N.Z. Vet. J. 11:6–10.

Seiler, R. J. 1979. The non-diseased reactor: Considerations on the interpretation of screening test results. Vet. Rec. 105:226–28.

Williamson, N. 1980. Reproductive performance and recording systems. Proc. 13th Am. Assoc. Bov. Pract., November 19–22, Toronto, Canada.

PART II

Studying Disease in Animal Populations

C H A P T E R 4

Descriptive Epidemiology

Health represents the dynamic balance between the host and its environment. That this balance is frequently tipped against the host resulting in disease is obvious to all; a major role for the epidemiologist is the identification and description of the circumstances and factors leading to the imbalance. Like an ecologist, the epidemiologist is interested in the relationship between the factors (the host and the environment including the agent) and how the relationship changes. The occurrence of virtually every disease is influenced by factors representing each of the host, environment, and time categories. In addition to humane considerations, the effects of disease on productivity should be a feature when describing the epidemiology of a disease.

During the past century, the study of disease has primarily concentrated on the pathogenesis of disease, and many important epidemiologic features have been ignored. In many instances, the identification of the sources, transmission, survival, and effects of agents of disease was considered as describing the epidemiology of disease. However, epidemiologic investigations go beyond the agent and concentrate on the factors of host, environment, and time that alter the occurrence and/or severity of disease for groups of individuals. In these pursuits, epidemiology is essentially a holistic discipline, whereas most other medical disciplines are reductionistic. (This statement is not meant as a criticism of other disciplines, it merely points out two divergent views of health and disease. Society will be served best by cooperation and understanding between the proponents of each viewpoint.)

This chapter outlines and discusses those factors of the host, environment, and time that should be included when describing the epidemiology of disease; these factors are sometimes referred to as its natural history. Since epidemiology is a pragmatic discipline, it is hoped that subsequent to their identification a means of manipulating causal factors will exist so that the knowledge may be of practical value. At the very least, a thorough description of the natural history of disease should enhance the understanding of that disease. Although there are separate sections in this chapter for host, environment, and time factors, it is important to note that these categories are closely interrelated in terms of their effects on health.

Often, host factors are of secondary interest in epidemiologic studies. Despite this, it is important to describe the relationship of host factors to disease occurrence and, if necessary, to control the effects of host factors (e.g., by analytic methods such as standardization of rates—see 4.2). Otherwise, host factors may distort the observed association between environmental factors and disease. Only when it is known that host factors do not exert a significant effect on the occurrence of disease can they be ignored.

4.1 Host Factors

The major intrinsic host factors are age, sex, and breed. Depending upon the circumstances, other host factors such as species or physiologic state (e.g., pregnancy) should be considered. The occurrence of disease at different levels of these factors is best described by using incidence rates or prevalence proportions, rather than proportional morbidity rates or counts of cases. As mentioned previously, incidence rates and prevalence proportions provide estimates of the risk (probability) of disease occurrence at different levels of the host factor (e.g., in males versus females, intact versus castrated, old versus young, Holsteins versus Jerseys). On the other hand, case counts are influenced by the risk of disease and the number of animals in that host-factor category. Thus, the distribution of cases with respect to host factor(s) probably does not reflect the underlying risk of disease. Some veterinary medical texts describe the pattern of disease and make inferences about the risk of disease based solely on the number of occurrences, rather than adjusting for the population at risk. The reader should be alert to note and hesitant to accept inferences about risk of disease made in this manner. For example, although 60% of all cases of mastitis may occur in 4- to 7-year-old cows, one should not conclude that cows of this age are necessarily at increased risk of mastitis in comparison to other age groups. One must relate the age distribution of cases to that of the source population in order to make inferences about the risk of mastitis.

Sometimes the underlying population rates are unknown and cannot be estimated easily. In these instances the effects of host factors on the occurrence of disease can be described by comparing the relative frequency of the host factor in cases to its frequency in noncases. A formal statistic for this purpose is the odds ratio (see 5.3.1).

4.1.1   Age

Age is probably the most important host variable, because the risk of disease usually is more closely related to age than to other host factors. Thus, age should always be included when describing the distribution of disease. There are many factors, however, that can affect the pattern of disease occurrence with age. It is important to consider whether the distribution is due to age itself, the current effects of recent environmental exposures on animals of different current ages, or the different past environmental exposures of animals of different current ages. Techniques for separating these effects will be described later in this chapter (see 4.10). Whether age per se actually changes the risk of disease independent of the environmental factors is unknown. However, epidemiologists attempt to identify environmental factors that accompany but are separable from age that may alter the risk of disease. For example, the cumulative insults of machine milking may provide a more reasonable explanation for the progressive increase in risk of mammary gland infection as cows become older than age per se. Such a hypothesis is quite easily tested and if support for it is found, better milking machine design and/or more careful milking techniques should provide methods of preventing at least some of the increased risk related to age. Some unavoidable and unalterable changes in the mammary gland due to aging may persist however.

If age-specific rates are plotted (e.g., as a histogram), the shape of the resultant plot will depend on whether morbidity rates (incidence or prevalence), mortality rates, or the rates of other intermediate events such as culling are used. If age exerts a major influence on the risk of the disease in question, one would expect either a uniform increase or decrease—not necessarily linear—or a unimodal pattern of disease occurrence with age. For example, data on the occurrence of a number of syndromes in dairy cattle indicate that the incidence rate (risk) of most diseases increases with age. For many of the diseases the increase is consistent with a linear trend, whereas for others the pattern is curvilinear. Some diseases (e.g., various pneumonias in cattle) have a U-shaped age pattern (Dohoo et al. 1984b). That is, the disease occurs relatively frequently in young and old animals— probably either because of recrudescence or increased susceptibility—but with low frequency during the middle years. This pattern would probably be more pronounced if cohorts of cattle were followed from birth rather than from first calving.

Often, only prevalence data from periodic surveys are available, and this makes it difficult to determine the risk of acquiring infection or disease by age. Formulas are available to estimate age incidence from prevalence, but most are based on the assumption that the substance being measured (usually antibodies) is present for the life of the animal and that immigration and emigration in the population are minimal. Based on these assumptions, a constant probability (risk) of acquiring infection with age will produce a curvilinear age-specific prevalence pattern that increases with age. Similarly, it is difficult to make inferences about the risk of infection based on age-specific disease rates, or to make inferences about the risk of disease based on age-specific mortality rates. Nonetheless, knowing the age pattern of disease and mortality can help generate useful hypotheses about factors that might influence infection and disease respectively.

If the pattern of disease occurrence with age appears to be bimodal (i.e., two peaks are present), this may indicate that there are in fact two distinct syndromes present — although they may have clinical or pathological similarities — or that factors influencing disease occurrence in the different age groups differ. Apparently, bimodal patterns exist for feline leukemia (Essex 1982) and canine progressive retinal atrophy (Priester 1974). Infectious bovine rhinotracheitis (IBR) virus is associated with a number of syndromes, the frequency of which produces a bimodal or trimodal pattern with age. In calves less than 1 month of age, the virus produces an enteric syndrome. In older calves, 6–18 months of age, an upper respiratory tract syndrome is seen. In adult females, the virus is associated with both infertility and abortions. Since the same virus is common to these different conditions, the different syndromes probably reflect changes in the physiologic condition of animals as they age and differences in environmental conditions, rather than differences in the virus itself.

In humans, the young have a higher risk of most infectious diseases than do teenagers or adults, because the latter have an acquired immunity due to past exposure to the agents of these diseases, and because of physiologic and behavioral changes with age. Despite the higher rate of occurrence in the young, the severity of disease (chiefly under host control) often is less in the young than in the old. This is particularly true if the initial exposure of the young occurs while they have passive protection. The level and duration of passive protection in the young depend chiefly on the extent and timing of exposure of their mothers to the agent. When infections such as measles or poliomyelitis enter populations that have not been exposed for a number of generations, the differential rate of occurrence with age is absent and the increased severity of the disease in mature people becomes apparent.

The above age-related phenomenon probably occurs in animals also, but the pattern may be obscured for a number of reasons. First, a large percentage of domestic animals are slaughtered prior to reaching an age equivalent to adulthood in humans. Second, the hygienic standards on most farms facilitate the early exposure of animals to the more common pathogens, and vaccination programs may have altered the pattern of resistance in both adult and young populations. For example, if one observed cohorts of feral cats, the pattern of diseases such as panleukopenia would probably be quite different than the pattern in domesticated felines. These differences would reflect the divergent environmental exposures of these groups of cats, as well as possible inherent host differences such as genotype. Severe outbreaks of disease (such as infectious bovine rhinotracheitis or bovine virus diarrhea) in closed herds probably represent an analogy to the "island" outbreaks of human measles. Maintaining closed herds may free the owner from the everyday problems of endemic diseases; however, additional vigilance is required to prevent serious outbreaks following the introduction of infection to this highly susceptible population.

Most measures of productivity also are age related; examples range from racing ability in horses to milk production in dairy cows. Young animals appear to be more efficient than adults at converting feed energy into usable products, be it eggs or muscle protein. Despite this, there may be economic value in prolonging the life of certain animals. For example, the average survival time of dairy cows in Canada is about 4 years after their first calving. Since a cow's production potential does not decrease markedly between 7 and 10 years of age, the dairy industry might benefit if diseases leading to premature involuntary removal from the herd could be prevented. This is particularly true because of the large investment in rearing replacements for swine, beef, and dairy herds. Of course, this potential benefit must be balanced against the increased opportunity for genetic improvement afforded by replacement of culled stock. The economics of culling and purchasing or raising replacements should also be considered. As previously mentioned (see 3.6.1), because of the marked and consistent effect of age on the absolute level of production, some parameters (e.g., milk production in dairy cows) are standardized to facilitate direct comparisons of production in animals of different ages.

4.1.2 Sex

A number of diseases are associated with the sex of animals; for example, infectious diseases may occur more frequently, or with greater severity, in young male humans than in young females. On the other hand, female dogs have a much greater risk of diabetes mellitus than males (Marmor et al. 1982). This is also true of humans, and is an indication that dogs may be a good model for studying the pathogenesis of diabetes.

Many of the sex-associated diseases are directly or indirectly related to anatomic and/or physiologic differences between the sexes. Such diseases include parturient paresis (milk fever), mastitis, metritis, and cancer of the mammary glands in females, as well as sex-related behavioral problems such as abscessation as a result of fighting and urine spraying in male cats.

Neutering also may be associated with disease occurrence. These associations range from a sparing effect on the risk of mammary gland cancer in spayed bitches to an increased risk of laminitis in castrated ponies, the latter also being related to behavioral and husbandry changes. The risk of the feline urologic syndrome is increased in castrated males; however, not all of this increase is likely due to anatomic changes because spayed females also have a higher risk than intact females (Willeberg and Priester 1976). When investigating the effects of neutering, the age at neutering should be considered.

Sex of the animal also needs to be taken into account when productivity is being evaluated, since racing ability, weight gains, deposition of body fat, and feed efficiency may differ between sexes.

4.1.3 Breed

Breed differences in risk of disease and level of productivity are common, and breed effects should be considered and controlled (adjusted for) when studying the effects of other factors on disease occurrence or productivity. In general, breed differences may be separated into two components: differences due to genetic factors and differences due to phenotypic factors.

Population genetics, like epidemiology, is highly dependent on the collection and analysis of data from observational studies. Both disciplines are interested in determinants of disease, and as it is often unclear at the outset whether a disease has genetic determinants, there is much overlap between the two disciplines. Animal geneticists have developed a set of specialized analytic methods for identifying the heritability of continuous production traits. Recently these techniques have been modified to study the heritability of discrete traits such as the presence or absence of disease. The equivalence between these techniques and epidemiologic statistics such as the population attributable fraction (see 5.3.3) remain to be clarified. Although still in its infancy, one thing is clear: few diseases are determined solely by genotype or environmental factors. In fact, our current genetic make up is a result of the selection pressures exerted by the environment on our ancestors.

The close relationship between genetic and environmental determinants may be demonstrated by two avian diseases, yellow shanks and pendulous crops. Yellow shanks occurred when poultry with a specific genetic defect were fed yellow corn. If a farmer had only genetically defective birds and fed both yellow and white corn, the ration would appear to be the determinant, since only those fed yellow corn would develop yellow shanks. If a farmer had normal and genetically defective birds and fed only yellow corn, genotype would appear to be the determinant, since only genetically defective birds would develop the condition. In this syndrome both factors are required to produce the disease, and in the syntax of sufficient causes (see Chapter 5), the genetic defect and the specific environmental factor (yellow corn) would be considered necessary components of the sufficient cause (i.e., both must be present for the disease to occur). Pendulous crop in turkeys is slightly more complex in that three factors — genotype (bronze turkeys), environment (very hot weather), and excess water intake — combine to produce the syndrome. Assuming no restriction on water intake and only bronze turkeys being present, the disease appears to be environmentally determined. If two or more breeds are raised under hot conditions, the disease appears to be genetically determined. Again, genotype and environmental factors are components of a sufficient cause. Phenylketonuria represents an analogous disease in children in that both environmental and genetic factors are involved. In these examples, because both factors (genotype and environmental) are required for the disease to occur, the interaction between genotype and environmental factors is said to be complete.

The relationship between genotype and environment as determinants of many diseases is often not as obvious as in the previous examples. If the disease has determinants other than a particular genotype–environmental factor combination, the statistical interaction between genotype and environment is less than complete. Although feasible, it is more difficult to identify putative causes in these instances. In general, the sensible approach would be identifying the role that each factor plays as a determinant of the disease, and using this knowledge to prevent the disease in so far as the factors can be manipulated.

In some cases, diseases initially considered to be genetic in origin were later shown to be essentially determined by environmental factors. For example, detailed experiments were conducted to prove that a particular cyclopian malformation in sheep was caused by a genetic defect. The experiments failed, and later observational and experimental studies identified a poisonous plant, *Veratrum californicum*, as the major cause (Binns et al. 1962). In retrospect, careful analysis of the available observational data might have convinced the investigators of this without the need of expensive experimental studies. In this case, as well as in early Texas fever investigations, the observations of ranchers were eventually validated, although veterinary investigators initially ignored and sometimes ridiculed the initial observations.

Diseases due to genetic defects such as baldy calves, dwarfism, and spastic paresis in bulls (most following a Mendelian inheritance pattern) have been identified. The heritability of diseases following more complex patterns (e.g., Galtonian characteristics) has not been studied as well as the simpler Mendelian type characteristics. Certainly, resistance to infectious disease has a genetic component as demonstrated by experiments with laboratory animals (e.g., the selection and breeding of leukosis-resistant strains of poultry and Aleutian disease resistance in mink). However, identification of the heritability of most diseases of domestic animals must await the development of large, accurate data bases, similar to those currently available for recording production. Preliminary work suggests that diseases such as mastitis, atrophic rhinitis, and cystic ovarian disease have a genetic component, and that their heritability is sufficiently large so that sire and dam selection could reduce their incidence rate. Also, data from some swine herds indicate that the variability in the mortality rate in litters due to sire is quite large, varying from two to six times. This suggests that sire selection could reduce piglet mortality significantly (Straw et al. 1984).

In companion animals, the risk of many diseases including cancers, arthritis, and heart defects varies greatly among breeds. However, the proportion of this difference in risk that is genetically based is unknown. For example, phenotypic factors probably alter the risk of diseases such as hip dysplasia, with large breeds having an excess risk. Yet, there is a significant variation in the risk of hip dysplasia among dogs of the same general phenotype, and more than 25% of certain low-risk phenotype breeds develop dysplasia. Both of these facts suggest an important role of genotype. It has been shown that for some breeds, dogs owned by one person have significantly higher or lower rates of hip dysplasia than the breed average (Martin et al. 1980). This again supports the potential role of genotype and/or shared environment as determinants of this disease. To further complicate the issue, the effects of genotype and phenotype on the risk of hip dysplasia appear to be partially confounded with environmental factors, such as the amount of exercise the dog receives when young.

Phenotypic factors are believed to be important determinants in a number of diseases, ranging from bone cancer in dogs to displaced abomasum in dairy cows. A lack of pigmentation increases the risk of cancer-eye in Hereford cattle whereas gray coloration increases the risk of melanoma in horses. The underlying reasons for these associations are unknown in most cases. Data bases will be available in the near future that should allow an assessment of these types of multifactor problems. For example, one should be able to assess the impact of sire, phenotypic factors (e.g., size of cow, depth of chest, shape of abdomen), and other variables such as calving ease (which may be related to size of pelvic inlet and size of fetus) on the risk of abomasal displacement and other diseases.

Dogs have been and will continue to be studied intensively to aid understanding of the role of genotypic and phenotypic factors on disease occurrence and to identify models of human diseases. No other domesticated species has such a wide range of genotype and phenotype, and dogs share man's environment intimately and the occurrence of their diseases (such as bladder cancer) may be indicative of toxic substances in the environment of potential danger to man (Hayes et al. 1981).

As previously mentioned, host factors can distort the association between disease and factors of more immediate interest. For example, female canine diabetics were 16 times more likely to have a diagnosis of benign mammary tumor than female dogs with other endocrine diseases. When a summary statistic (odds ratio) adjusted for age was calculated (using the Mantel-Haenszel technique, see 5.4.1) the odds ratio was reduced to 5.6 (Marmor et al. 1982). This technique is used frequently in analytic studies to control for the effects of extraneous factors.

4.2   Standardization of Rates

Because host factors are often determinants of disease, host-attribute specific rates (e.g., age, sex, and/or breed specific rates) should be used to describe patterns of disease. Each level of the attribute is used to form a stratum; the stratum-specific rates should be studied carefully before any attempts are made to summarize them, since summary rates ignore and often oversimplify and/or distort the true pattern of disease in the study population. However, despite these drawbacks, it may be desirable to have a single, unbiased, summary statistic (free from the influence of host factors) to describe the frequency of disease. One method that can be used to produce such summary rates is standardization (or adjustment) of rates (Fleiss 1973, pp 155–64). Standardization can also be used to prevent distortion from factors other than host characteristics. (In this respect it is very similar to the Mantel-Haenszel technique discussed in 5.4.1; however, it is not as powerful and is used chiefly for descriptive purposes rather than for hypothesis testing.) The two methods of standardization are direct and indirect.

4.2.1   Direct Standardization

With direct standardization the observed stratum-specific rates (OBS R_i) must be known, and a standard population distribution (STD P_i), with respect to the factors being adjusted for, is used as the basis for adjustment. The STD P_i is the proportion of the standard population in each of the strata, the stratum indicator i ranging from 1 to the number of strata being considered. Each stratum represents each level of age, breed, sex, or combination thereof.

The choice of the standard population for direct standardization is not crucial; however, when possible it is desirable to select a standard that is demographically sensible. For example, if the disease rates in various areas of the country are to be compared and adjusted for age, the population-age distribution for the entire country would be an appropriate standard. If no obvious standard exists, construct a standard by taking the average distribution over all groups to be compared.

The general approach to direct adjustment of rates in each of the groups to be compared is:

direct adjusted rate = proportion of standard population in stratum *i*, multiplied by observed rate in stratum *i*, with the product summed over all strata

= sum of P_i (standard) $\times$ R_i (observed) over all strata

= Σ (STD P_i $\times$ OBS R_i)

This calculation is repeated for each group to be compared as shown in Table 4.1. The adjusted rate gives the rate expected if the observed stratum-specific rates applied in the standard population. Any differences between

Table 4.1. An example of direct standardization of rates

Suppose you are studying the association between source of cattle (ranch versus salesyard) and the occurrence of pneumonia in the 3-week period subsequent to arrival at the feedlot. Your initial study, based on random samples of 500 calves coming directly from ranches and 500 calves purchased at salesyards, gives the following results.

Source	Pneumonia	No pneumonia	Total	Incidence rate (%)
Salesyard	120	380	500	24
Ranch	25	475	500	5

Superficially, these results incriminate salesyards as a determinant of pneumonia. You are concerned, however, that these results might be distorted because of the age of cattle, since both calves and yearlings are purchased. The following method may be used to adjust the rates for the effect of age.

Source	Number of cattle	Observed distribution OBS(P_i)	Number developing pneumonia	Incidence rate OBS(R_i) (%)	Standard population distribution STD(P_i)
Salesyard					
Calves	400	.8	112	28	.45
Yearlings	100	.2	8	8	.55
Ranch					
Calves	50	.1	7	14	.45
Yearlings	450	.9	18	4	.55

It is obvious that age has a marked effect on the rate of pneumonia, but source also appears to have an effect. The standard population distribution was obtained by averaging the two observed distributions [i.e., $0.45 = (0.8 + 0.1)/2$].

The directly adjusted rates are found by multiplying the observed disease rate in each stratum by the standard population distribution in that stratum and adding the products over all the strata.

For the salesyard group: $(0.28 \times 0.45) + (0.08 \times 0.55) = 0.17$ or 17%
For the ranch group: $(0.14 \times 0.45) + (0.04 \times 0.55) = 0.085$ or 8.5%

The difference, 17% versus 8.5%, still suggests that source is a determinant of pneumonia. At the very least, the latter difference is not due to the effects of age; these effects having been removed by the process of standardization.

the adjusted rates must be due to factors other than those included in the adjustment procedure. Directly adjusted rates can only be compared to other directly adjusted rates when the same standard population distribution is used as the basis for standardization. Statistical tests are available to assess the likelihood that sampling variation can explain any differences among the group summary rates which remain after adjustment (Armitage 1971).

4.2.2 Indirect Standardization

Indirect standardization may be used if the strata-specific rates are unknown, provided the distribution (OBS P_i) of the factor(s) of interest (e.g., age) in the groups to be compared is known. It is also useful when the number of animals in the strata are small, and hence the stratum-specific rates are imprecise.

The adjustment is realized by using a set of stratum-specific rates from a standard population (STD R_i). The choice of the standard rates should be guided by the same general considerations as used in direct adjustment. However, it is very important that the standard population rates reflect what likely occurred in the groups being compared. The first step in indirect adjustment is to calculate the anticipated rate (overall expected rate), given that the standard population rates apply in each of the groups to be compared, as shown in Table 4.2. The general approach is:

> Overall expected rate = the proportion of the observed group in stratum i is multiplied by the rate in stratum i of the standard population, with the product summed over all strata
> = sum of P_i (observed) $\times$ R_i (standard) over all strata
> = Σ (OBS $P_i \times$ STD R_i)

Then, the observed crude rate is divided by the overall expected rate; the quotient is called a standardized morbidity/mortality ratio (SMR) depending on the endpoint (it may be another event such as culling). To complete the calculations, the indirect adjusted rate is found using the following formula:

> Overall average rate in standard population $\times$ SMR

Differences in indirect adjusted rates (or in the SMRs) are interpreted in a manner similar to direct adjusted rates; that is, any remaining differences are not due to the factors considered in the adjustment process. It should be noted, however, that indirect adjustment removes most but not

Table 4.2.   An example of indirect standardization of rates

Suppose that two random samples of dairy cattle, each obtained from a different area of the country, were obtained. A blood sample was taken from each animal and its age was also recorded. The blood samples were sent to a laboratory and tested for the presence of antibodies to bovine virus diarrhea virus. Three hundred of 575 animals from area A and 325 of 625 from area B had positive titers. Unfortunately, only the area was marked on the vials and hence it was not possible to calculate age-specific reactor rates. Nonetheless, you wish to remove any distortion in the overall rates due to age differences between the samples. The indirect method of adjustment may be used for this purpose.

| Age (years) | Number in sample | | | | Standard population rates (STD R_i) |
| | Area A | | Area B | | |
	No.	(OBS P_i)	No.	(OBS P_i)	
2–3.9	100	.17	25	.04	.3
4–5.9	200	.35	100	.16	.4
6–7.9	150	.26	250	.40	.5
8–9.9	75	.13	150	.24	.6
10+	50	.09	100	.16	.7
Total	575		625	Average reactor rate for	
Reactors	300		325	standard population is	
Crude rate	0.52		0.52	0.42	

Assume that a set of standard age-specific population reactor rates (STD R_i) is available and these will be used to obtain the expected rate of reactors. The rate expected if the standard rates applied in area A is:

$$0.17 \times 0.3 + 0.35 \times 0.4 + 0.26 \times 0.5 + 0.13 \times 0.6 + 0.09 \times 0.7 = 0.46$$

The rate expected if the standard rates applied in area B is:

$$0.04 \times 0.3 + 0.16 \times 0.4 + 0.40 \times 0.5 + 0.24 \times 0.6 + 0.16 \times 0.7 = 0.53.$$

These lead to standardized reactor ratios of $(0.52/0.46) \times 100 = 113\%$, and $(0.52/0.53) \times 100 = 97.7\%$ for areas A and B respectively.

The indirect adjusted rates are found by multiplying the standardized ratio for each area (expressed as a proportion) by the average rate for the standard population. This leads to indirect adjusted rates of $1.13 \times 42\% = 47.5\%$ for area A and $0.98 \times 42\% = 41.2\%$ for area B. This difference suggests that, after adjusting for differences in age, the prevalence of antibodies to bovine virus diarrhea virus is higher in area A than area B. At least the remaining difference is not due to differences in age structure of the animals in the two areas.

all of the effects of different distributions of the factors in each group. This is why the selection of the standard population rates to reflect the (unknown) rates in the groups being compared is important. The advantage of indirect standardization is that the stratum-specific rates in each group are not required, only the distribution of the host factors in the groups being compared. As mentioned, indirect standardization is preferred over direct methods if the number of individuals in the various strata is small.

Standardized morbidity or mortality ratios are often used in pictorial displays of disease occurrence in different geographic areas. This allows one to visually compare the level of disease in many areas without concern about the effect of differences in the underlying population structure.

As an example of the use of standardization, rate adjustment is used in the Danish pig health scheme. In this program, the observed rate of enzootic pneumonia in swine at abattoirs in different areas of the country is adjusted for herd size before making comparisons of the prevalence of pneumonia in these areas. (The adjustment is required because herd size has an important influence on the level of enzootic pneumonia, and the distribution of herd sizes differs from one area of Denmark to another. Therefore, in order to get a fair comparison of the rate of disease among abattoirs, without the comparison being distorted by herd size effects, it is necessary to adjust the rates for herd size [Willeberg et al. 1984].)

4.3 Immunity in Populations

Whether a disease spreads or persists depends not only on the nature of the causal agent, but also on the immunity of individuals and the structure and dynamics of the population (Fox et al. 1971; Yorke et al. 1979).

The ability of individual animals to resist infection, or to resist becoming diseased if infected, is referred to as immunity and may be either innate or acquired. Innate immunity is most often genetic in origin and is not dependent on previous contact with an agent by the individual or its parents. Examples include the resistance of horses to foot-and-mouth disease virus and current resistance of European rabbits in Australia to myxomatosis virus. Acquired immunity is resistance resulting from previous contact with an agent by the individual (active immunity), or resistance passed on from its mother (passive immunity) as a result of her contact with the agent. Contact with the agent may be natural or artificial (i.e., following vaccination). In simple terms, acquired immunity is humoral (antibody mediated) and/or cellular (cell mediated) in nature.

Immunity in individuals is relative rather than absolute, depending on the nature of the agent, the challenge dose, and the individual's environment. For purposes of discussion here, it will be classified as high, moderate, or low. From the viewpoint of the infecting organism, a host with high immunity presents a major stumbling block to survival since it is difficult to infect and hence the organism may die. A host with moderate immunity is more favorable to survival since it allows infection, some multiplication, and often shows little evidence of disease. Hosts with low or no immunity (i.e., highly susceptible individuals) are easily infected, and the organism may multiply freely, often resulting in disease in the infected host. This latter state may pose a great danger to other animals because of the increased challenge to their immunity. The best plan for survival for the organism might appear to be to invade highly susceptible individuals and multiply freely. However, if as a result of disease the host is killed and the host population is decimated, contacting a new susceptible host could become difficult, and the organism may die. Thus, a strategy appropriate for short-term survival of the organism in an individual is not necessarily appropriate for long-term survival in the population.

The ability of groups of animals to resist becoming infected or to minimize the extent of infection (i.e., the number and/or the severity of cases) is termed herd immunity. Like individual immunity, herd immunity may be innate or acquired and should be considered a relative rather than absolute state. In most groups of animals the distribution of individual immunity varies from very susceptible to very resistant. Frequency of contact between individuals within the herd plays a key role in determining the level of herd immunity. (In current models of herd immunity, such as the Reed-Frost model, frequency of contact is referred to as probability of adequate contact. The latter is the probability that an individual in the population will have contact with another individual; the nature of the contact varying with the disease but being sufficient to transmit the infection from an infected to a susceptible individual. (See 8.3.2 for details.) This factor together with the number of susceptible individuals in the herd plays the predominant role in determining the level of herd immunity. Just as individual immunity determines whether an organism can persist in the individual, herd immunity determines whether an organism can survive in the herd (Yorke et al. 1979).

The number of susceptible animals is chiefly influenced by population dynamics such as the number of births, deaths, additions, and removals from the population, as well as by past exposure of the population to the agent. To a large extent, the rate of contact is influenced by the husbandry, housing, and behavior of the animals. If the rate of contact between individuals in a population is low, or there are only a few susceptible animals in the population, most infectious agents will not spread; they may even die out. In contrast, if the rate of contact is high, or if there are many susceptible animals, the infectious agent can easily become widespread. Whether disease develops subsequent to infection is mainly influenced by immunity at the individual level, although population factors can serve to alter the amount of exposure and thereby change the likelihood of disease occurrence (see Fig. 11.3).

The initial experimental studies of herd-immunity phenomena (Topley and Wilson 1923) are both interesting and enlightening. One must recall that in the early years of the twentieth century it was generally believed the rise and fall of epidemics was due to a combination of increasing and then decreasing virulence of the organism, as well as the active immunization of individuals by chance exposure to small doses of the organism. During the 1920s and 1930s, experiments in laboratory-animal colonies were conducted to formally investigate some of the factors influencing the spread of agents in populations.

In general, the format of these experiments was to infect a number of laboratory animals (usually mice) and place them in a colony with other susceptible mice. The organisms used (generally *Salmonella typhimurium* or, more recently, *Ectromelia* virus) produce disease and/or death in a high proportion of infected animals, and thus the spread of infection through the colony was easily monitored (Yorke et al. 1979). The total number of mice in the colony, the number of susceptible mice in the colony, and the rate (frequency) of contact were varied. The rate of contact was altered by changing the type of housing or by forced mixing of the animals in one large pen for varying periods of time. The major results of these experiments may be summarized as follows: (1) For any given rate of contact the number of diseased animals or deaths was directly related to the number of susceptible animals; (2) If the number of susceptible animals was reduced below a critical level, the infection either failed to become established or died out; (3) Often, not all susceptible animals became infected during an outbreak nor did outbreaks always occur, although there were many susceptible animals in the population; (4) For any given number of susceptible animals, outbreaks of disease could be terminated or prevented by dispersing the mouse colony into a large number of groups, each containing only a small number of animals. (This effectively reduced the frequency of contact between members of the mouse population.)

These experiments demonstrated the key role played by the number of susceptible animals and the frequency of contact. The results also indicated that there was a genetic basis to disease resistance, and later experiments demonstrated that in heterogeneous groups of mice there was an interaction between nutrition and genetic factors and resistance to disease. More specifically, the resistance to infection was greater in certain genetic lines of mice on specified diets than was predicted, based on the general effect of that genetic line of mouse or diet. Recently it has been postulated that some of the increased susceptibility to disease following the mixing of mice in large colonies or the introduction of new, susceptible mice to the colony was the result of decreased immunity due to an adrenal-cortical stress reaction. For example, behavioral characteristics of the animals and disruptions in the social pecking order within the population are thought to be important features of individual and herd immunity.

The results of these early experiments have also been validated by numerous case studies and observational studies on human populations (e.g., the occurrence of measles and poliomyelitis). They have also proved invaluable in understanding the so-called island epidemics and the cyclical pattern of human diseases such as measles.

Undoubtedly, herd immunity is an important phenomenon in diseases of wild, companion, or domestic animals. For example, fox density (number of foxes per hectare) is a major determinant of rabies transmission in Switzerland (Steck and Wandeler 1980) and also in Canada. In Switzerland, rabies is rarely diagnosed in areas where the fox population is below 0.3 foxes per km^2. At the same time, fox vaccination campaigns that reach only about 60% of the fox population appear to be effective in halting the spread of rabies. If this is true, it may be that protecting about one-half of the foxes in an area decreases the number of susceptible foxes to below the critical density, thus preventing continued spread and perpetuation of the virus. As another example, the density of dogs appeared to influence the spread of parvovirus enteritis. In Stockholm, Sweden, where the dog density was high, parvovirus outbreaks were seen; whereas in other areas of the country with lower dog densities, the disease occurred only sporadically if at all (Wierup 1983).

Outbreaks of feline panleukopenia are probably influenced by the lack of herd immunity. In this case, large numbers of kittens are born in the spring and early summer. These kittens become susceptible through the loss of maternal antibodies at 3 to 4 months of age. This is also the time kittens become dispersed, in both feral- and pet-feline populations, and may explain the late summer–early fall outbreaks of feline distemper (Reif 1976).

Although not well documented, the lack of herd immunity may help explain the dual findings of increased disease occurrence (chiefly respiratory disease) in herds or pens containing large numbers of animals, and the negative impact of mixing animals from different sources. Exposure of these animals to new environments and/or adverse weather probably reduces the immunity of individuals also. Thus, under these conditions, organisms that are normally present without producing disease can become pathogens.

4.4 Environmental Factors

The environment includes all the biotic and abiotic components of a place, be it a pen within a barn or a large geographic area. Knowledge of the rate or risk of disease according to place is a first and essential step in understanding disease. In initial investigations the number of potential differences between areas where disease is frequent and where it is infrequent is so large that only general theories can be developed to explain its distribution. Subsequently, more detailed investigations of specific components of the environment may be pursued. General categories of environmental factors include features of the landscape or place, abiotic elements (i.e., air, soil, water, and climate), and biotic features including the flora and fauna. Immediate causes of disease, whether living organisms or toxicants, should also be sought and their importance as causes of the disease quantified. Whether one should concentrate initially on general features, such as air quality or the plant life of an area, or on the identification of specific agents depends on the setting and the nature of the problem. As a general suggestion one should not concentrate interest on specific agents to the exclusion of studying more general features of disease occurrence. Often, knowledge of the general features provides useful guidelines in generating a logical series of hypotheses about the involvement and nature of specific agents (Stallones 1972).

As an example of this approach, consider multiple sclerosis in humans, the ultimate cause of which still eludes researchers. The frequency of multiple sclerosis is directly correlated with latitude and increases dramatically with distance from the equator. Thus, one major thrust to current epidemiologic studies is to concentrate on cohorts of people who either enter or leave high- or low-risk areas. Since the change of risk of disease in these individuals appears to be related to their age at migration, the presence of a specific agent in high-risk areas is suggested (Nathanson and Miller 1978).

When disease occurs more frequently in certain areas than in others, the disease is said to be clustered. Disease may be limited geographically for a variety of reasons, many of which relate to forces that act upon the host, vector, or agent of disease. Geographic features such as rivers, lakes, and mountains can also serve to restrict the spread of disease. Sometimes disease is limited to traditional migration or market routes; this was true of Texas fever (bovine piroplasmosis). Although usually large, the geographic area of interest can vary in size from pens within a barn, to barns within a farm, to areas within a country. A recent serial provides data on the distribution of a variety of diseases and disease outbreaks in countries throughout the world (Commonwealth Agricultural Bureaux 1983).

Historically, knowledge that certain geographic markers (e.g., bogs or marshes) were predictive of increased risk of disease was used to prevent disease simply by avoidance of these areas. Some diseases like swamp fever (equine infectious anemia) are named after their association with these geographic features. During the 1800s, the observation that the distribution of Texas fever was analogous to that of the tick suspected of spreading the disease was instrumental in gaining support for further study of the role of the tick. The tick was subsequently shown to be the reservoir of the agent and capable of passing the infection by vertical transmission to succeeding generations of ticks. More recently, the study of the association between agents of disease and certain ecosystems or geographic markers has expanded and has been termed landscape epidemiology (Levine 1966).

There are a number of ways of determining spatial clustering, many of which are based on fairly rigorous mathematical procedures. For most practical purposes, simple graphic methods of detecting clustering are suitable. These include cartographic techniques such as spot maps, transparent overlays, isodemic maps, and grid maps.

4.4.1 Cartographic Methods

Spot maps are a basic tool for studying the geographic pattern of disease. Each occurrence of disease is plotted on a standard map, the scale of which depends on the investigation. Spot maps can be modified to show the change in distribution of disease over time. For example, different colors can be used to plot the occurrence of disease during different time periods, or each spot may be numbered to indicate the relative time of disease occurrence (see Fig 11.3).

Sometimes, instead of plotting each case individually, the average level of disease on a farm or in an area may be represented by different types of markings on black and white maps, or different colors on colored maps. Adjusted rates or, more frequently, standardized morbidity or mortality ratios may be plotted rather than unadjusted rates (host factors that may affect the level of disease are usually included in this adjustment). Although too elaborate for routine use, three-dimensional, computer-drawn maps (with the height proportional to the level of disease) provide tremendous insight into the geographic distribution of disease. The fox population of Switzerland has been displayed using this technique (Steck and Wandeler 1980).

Transparent overlays are also useful in mapping disease. One could describe the spread of a disease (such as rabies across a country) by plotting the extent of rabies in different time periods on separate transparencies; then the spread of disease can be displayed by sequentially overlaying the transparencies.

Grid mapping is not particularly useful for the practitioner, but it is useful when maps may be drawn using data in computer files. In this instance, each particular location is referenced by a specific x - y coordinate (a longitude and latitude marker). Using this technique, large volumes of data about the location of specific cases can be stored easily in computer files, and the same files can be utilized to create the map. The files may be updated regularly and maps easily redrawn as required.

One's ingenuity is the only real limitation to the usefulness of cartographic techniques. However, since the population at risk is frequently not uniformly or randomly distributed, one must be careful in interpreting clustering if only the distribution of cases is plotted. Steck and Wandeler (1980) provide many good examples of the use of cartographic techniques.

Isodemic mapping is a cartographic technique used to correct for non-random distribution of the population at risk. In ordinary maps, the area of different portions of the map reflects the actual physical area of the administrative unit. Thus, two counties of equal geographic size will be represented by equal-size areas on a map. In isodemic mapping each administrative area (e.g., a county) retains its original shape, but the size of each area when mapped corresponds to the relative magnitude of the population at risk, not the actual physical size of the area.

4.4.2 Analytic Methods

Often, a plot of infected premises may indicate clustering, suggesting farm-to-farm spread. However, in the absence of data on the distribution of all farms in the area such clusters are difficult to interpret. One way of assessing this apparent clustering is to compare the average distance between any two infected farms to the average distance between two randomly-selected noninfected farms, or to the distance between randomly-selected noninfected farms and the closest infected farm. The distance may be "by road" or "as the crow flies" depending on the situation. If automobiles or trucks are suspected of spreading the infection, road distance would be used. (This would not preclude the tracing of known vehicle movement and relating this to the distribution of affected farms.) If airborne spread were suspected, a straight-line distance would be more suitable. The latter can be obtained using calipers to measure the distance on an accurately plotted map of appropriate scale. If farm-to-farm spread is an important means of transmission, one would expect the average distance between pairs of infected farms to be less than the average distance between a noninfected farm and the closest infected premises. A similar method was used in a case-control study of brucellosis in two counties in Ontario, Canada. The case farms were infected farms identified from the district regulatory veterinarian's records. The controls were obtained by taking a random sample of herds with negative tests, provided the tests were conducted during the time period selected for the study. The average distance between the two closest infected farms was less than the distance between a noninfected and the nearest infected farm, supporting the hypothesis of farm-to-farm spread (Kellar et al. 1976; data not presented). This technique will not discriminate between "fence-line" and airborne spread, but it does provide an indication of whether the clustering is an artifact due to the distribution of farms or a real phenomenon.

4.4.3 Interpretation of Clustering

Once a relationship between a disease and geographical areas has been documented, it should be studied to see if characteristics of animals in the area can explain the association. If an explanation in terms of host factors can not be found, the following observations provide additional evidence that factors localized to a geographic area may be responsible for the association: animals leaving the high-risk area subsequently develop a lower risk of disease, and healthy animals entering the area experience an increased risk of disease; most animals of the herd or species of concern have a high rate of disease in the suspect area, and animals of the same breed or species do not have high rates of disease outside the suspect area; and animals of different breeds or species all have an increased rate of disease in the high-risk area. The latter observation is supportive but not essential, because only one breed of animal may be at risk of the disease. This could be due to inherent behavioral traits of the breed or to the system of husbandry imposed on it.

4.5　Abiotic Elements of Environment

Abiotic elements include the air, soil (rock), and water, plus the climate of the area. In developed countries, chemical air pollution also is a major concern from the standpoint of its effects on health and the environment. Outbreaks of fluorosis and lead poisoning have been recorded in animals pastured around fertilizer manufacturing and lead smelting plants. Historically, deaths of cattle at the Smithfield Fat Stock Show in England were early indications of the adverse effects of air pollutants; the chief pollutant being sulphur oxides resulting from the burning of coal (Schwabe 1984, p 563). These deaths preceded the first documented large-scale increases in mortality in humans by a number of years. The death of cats from mercury poisoning (Minamata disease) may similarly have predicted the adverse effects of pollution—in this case, water pollution—on humans (Goldwater 1971). Another example of the effect of unspecified air pollutants on health is the finding of more pulmonary disease in dogs living in polluted areas than in dogs living in relatively pollution-free areas (Reif and Cohen 1970; see Table 2.7). In fact, domestic and companion animals may serve as excellent sentinels of environments dangerous to man (Schwabe et al. 1971; Priester 1971; Hayes et al. 1976).

With regard to airborne transmission, droplet nuclei (1–2 microns in diameter) may contain living organisms or chemical pollutants. These nuclei do not "settle out" very rapidly, and they readily reach the lung when inspired. Noninfectious protein material may be transported to the lung in a similar manner and lead to hypersensitivity-type pneumonias. Despite the potential importance of airborne transmission of disease producing agents, two facts should be kept in mind. The nasal turbinates function to warm and filter in-coming air but apparently are not essential for the animal to have a normal lung. Pigs possessing moderately- to severely-distorted nares as a result of atrophic rhinitis appear to have only a slight increase in pneumonia over their penmates with normal turbinates (Takov 1983). Second, airborne transmission of some respiratory tract infections (e.g., human rhinoviruses) may be a less important route of transmission than direct contact and fomite transmission (Gwaltney and Hendley 1982). This may also be true of strangles in horses and pasteurellosis of cattle, as mentioned previously. When cattle lower their heads to drink, large volumes of infected nasal mucus and discharge may drain into the water. Although little evidence exists to support the hypothesis, it may be an important source of infection for other animals in the group.

Soil type can influence the survival of living agents as well as the availability of minerals (e.g., selenium) to plants and hence to animals. Zoonotic fungi such as *Histoplasma* and *Cryptococci* survive better in soils with high organic content. Anthrax bacilli appear to survive better in soils along river valleys. Soils containing limestone and dolomite are indicative of the likely presence of leptospiral organisms. A nationwide survey of soil in the United States for clostridial organisms has been conducted; 4 east-west transects were sampled at 50-mile intervals to ensure a representative country-wide sample. *Clostridium tetani* was present in approximately 30% of the samples regardless of soil type, whereas *Clostridium botulinum* appeared more frequently in some soil types than in others (Smith 1978). This points out the potential hazard of soil organisms including the potential for contaminating feed stuffs (such as honey) especially in areas where significant airborne soil erosion occurs. Recent large-scale outbreaks of botulism in human infants were concentrated in, but not restricted to, dry areas of the southwestern United States (Arnon et al. 1981). (The authors note, however, that the presence of large referral hospitals for children may have influenced this distribution.)

Water may carry toxic chemicals as well as infectious organisms. The temperature and flow pattern of water can also influence the concentration of intermediate hosts or vectors of infectious agents (Harris and Charleston 1977). Under certain environmental conditions, waterborne organisms may proliferate; in the case of blue-green algae, potent toxins leak into the water when the algae die and decompose. In other circumstances, humans and animals may defecate and urinate in irrigation ditches; infectious microorganisms and other parasites may thus contaminate food items, which then serve as sources of infection for other humans or animals.

Precipitation (rain or snow) "scrubs" the air, bringing infectious agents, radioactive particles, and pollutants to ground level. Contamination of pasture fields and crops can occur by this mechanism. The long-term damage from acid rain, one type of pollutant distributed by this mechanism, may be much more severe than any short-term problems.

Climate is an important determinant of many diseases. Adverse weather may affect the management and care of animals, stress the animal directly, or provide conditions suitable for survival of microorganisms and parasites or their vectors. Unfortunately, unraveling the effects of weather is not easy. Reasons for this include: its components are often very indirect determinants of disease; it may have multiple effects because there are a large number of weather components (e.g., minimum, maximum, and mean temperature; diurnal temperature fluctuations; day-to-day fluctuations; rainfall; humidity; windspeed); and it is difficult to separate the effects of various weather components. Further, the general macroclimate (for which data are available) may be quite different than the microclimate (i.e., weather within a barn or at ground level). Data on microclimate within various types of shelters are not readily available, and few studies on the effects of microclimate on disease and productivity have been reported. One study of microclimatic effects conducted in California dairies confirmed previous macroclimatic studies of the association between weather and the health status of calves (Thurmond and Acres 1975).

Despite the difficulties, even a cursory examination of data on respiratory disease in humans or animals indicates the potential impact of weather on disease occurrence. In California, where most calves are raised outdoors, adverse weather was shown to significantly increase calf mortality during mid-summer and mid-winter. Although management factors apparently accounted for most of the large variation in mortality rates among farms, the effect of weather was still apparent, even when the average level of mortality on a farm was low (Martin et al. 1975). Many feedlot owners and veterinarians believe weather exerts a significant effect on the health and productivity of their animals. Formal analyses tend to support this theory, although the percentage of disease explained by weather is small. Certainly, intensively reared animals (poultry, swine, or cattle) require careful control and manipulation of their microclimate to remain healthy and productive. Knowledge of the exact microclimatic requirements and the benefits of different types of housing and ventilation systems are lacking, however, partly because of the paucity of formal studies on this subject.

Another example of the effect of climatic factors is the demonstration of windborne spread of foot-and-mouth disease virus in England. Veterinarians in many European countries also believe that introduction of this and other infections into their countries may be due to windborne transmission. It is thought that wind is an important factor in spreading and prolonging outbreaks of Newcastle disease virus and infectious bronchitis virus of poultry; however, these theories remain to be adequately tested.

The importance of accurate and complete documentation of the geographic pattern of infected premises is demonstrated by the 1967 outbreak of foot-and-mouth disease in England. It might generally be thought that windborne spread would transmit the agent from infected premises to nearby farms. Although this pattern was present, it was also found, subsequent to the outbreak, that a meteorological phenomenon known as lee waves may have accounted for the 18- to 20-km downwind distances between clusters of infected farms (Tinline 1972). Had the outbreak not been well documented, in terms of time and location, the appropriate data to identify the lee wave spread would not have been available.

4.5.1 Bioclimatograms

A useful graphic method for investigating the relationship between two climatic factors and survival of parasites is the bioclimatogram (Schwabe 1969, p 621). For example, temperature may be plotted on the Y or vertical axis and precipitation on the X or horizontal axis. For each month of the year the average temperature and precipitation are plotted as one point. Each of these points is joined by a line beginning at January, connecting with February's point, and continuing to completion at December's point. If the temperature and moisture requirements for the survival and/or development of an agent or its vector are known, the bioclimatogram can provide a visual display of the months when the temperature and precipitation requirements are sufficient to allow survival and/or development of the particular agent. As an example, the rate of disease each month could be displayed directly on the bioclimatogram (or with the use of transparent overlays) to visually assess if the occurrence of the disease might be associated with temperature and precipitation. This knowledge could be applied, for example, to design housing for calves in a manner to lower the incidence of enzootic pneumonia. By plotting the average temperature and humidity requirements for the survival of an agent (such as mycoplasma) one could plan housing so that the temperature and humidity within the barn were consistent with conditions necessary to maintain calf health, but inconsistent with the environmental survival of mycoplasma agents.

4.6 Biotic Elements: Flora and Fauna

Because veterinarians focus their attention on only a few species of animals, it may be easy to forget that a large number of diseases in humans and animals are a result of a complex interplay between animal and plant species. Under natural conditions, the evolution of plant species directly influences the number and types of animals present in a defined ecosystem. This is less true today in our highly manipulated agricultural ecosystems, where the majority of foodstuffs may be grown some distance from the animal industry and transported to farms by truck and train.

4.6.1 Flora

Plants may be important as causes of disease because they form the basis of the ration or diet of most animals. The selection and processing of plants and their products to form a nutritious diet at minimal cost is now a highly specialized and competitive industry. Also, the availability and cost of major ration components (such as corn) may dictate the expansion or contraction of animal industries.

Not all plants are edible however. Plant toxicities (e.g., alkaloid toxicities from lupin species, Japanese yew, and *Crotalaria* or *Senecio* genera) occur commonly. Deficiency diseases (e.g., hypomagnesemia resulting from prolonged feeding of oats and/or barley; acute vitamin A deficiency in beef cattle resulting from grazing on inadequate pastures, and poor reproductive efficiency in cattle being fed inadequate amounts of energy, protein, and phosphorous) are well recognized. Dry hay may be a better roughage than corn silage for starting stressed calves because of the much higher levels of potassium in hay, and it is believed that the requirement for potassium is increased during periods of stress.

Plants may also be indirectly causally associated with a number of diseases. Facial eczema in sheep results from eating pasture heavily contaminated with fungi (*Pithomyces chartarum*). Sheep also become infected with metacercaria of liver flukes encysted on plants, as well as the larval forms of *Echinococcus granulosus*. Similarly, cattle may ingest the larval forms of *Dictyocaulus* from contaminated herbage. *Thermophilus* fungi contaminating hay may lead to interstitial pneumonia in humans and cattle (called farmer's lung); whereas other fungi produce toxins (often hepatotoxic) such as aflatoxin or ochratoxin as well as estrogenic substances such as zearalenone. Dicoumarol production by moldy sweet clover was at one time a major source of poisonings in North America. Today, low courmarin cultivars may allow renewed production of this very high-yielding legume. As mentioned previously, pollutants may settle onto fodder crops and be ingested in large doses.

Decaying plants may produce disease through the formation of toxic gases. Examples include silo-filler's disease (caused by the production and release of nitrous oxides in fermenting silage), and the effects of toxic gases such as methane, hydrogen sulphide, and ammonia released from decaying manure. The chronic effects of these gases on the health of livestock and the role they may play in predisposing the respiratory tract to infectious agents are of interest and concern for intensively reared livestock such as poultry, swine, and beef cattle.

Finally, feedstuffs of plant origin may serve as vehicles for a variety of microorganisms and parasites. Examples include *Listeria monocytogenes* in corn silage (perhaps because the organism grows well in silage, or because of the rodent concentration in silage), and the spread of toxoplasma cysts in grain, due to the habit of cats defecating in granaries while purportedly keeping the rodent population in check.

4.6.2 Fauna

With respect to animal species, and for most infectious diseases, any particular group of animals may be at risk of infection from other members of its own species or from members of other species of animals or invertebrates. The zoonoses (infectious diseases common to humans and animals) provide a good illustration of the complex way different species may combine to ensure the survival and transmission of infectious agents. For purposes of presentation, the zoonoses have been classified on the basis of their cycle of perpetuation as direct, cyclo-, meta-, and saprozoonoses (Schwabe 1984, pp 196–208).

4.6.2.1 DIRECT ZOONOSES. Direct zoonoses may perpetuate in a single host species. Examples include bovine brucellosis and tuberculosis; rabies in wild, domestic, and companion animals; and pseudorabies in swine. Although these diseases can survive in one species, there may be local exceptions.

Before pursuing this, a brief discussion of the distinction between reservoirs and carriers is in order. A reservoir is the species without which the agent is unlikely to perpetuate. A carrier, on the other hand, may silently (since it is subclinically infected) transmit the organism, but it is not necessary for the perpetuation of the agent. Thus, many species are carriers. For example, many species (including dogs, cats, and sheep) are susceptible to *B. abortus* infection but they are carriers only, not reservoirs, and do not sustain the infection for prolonged periods. Bovine tuberculosis essentially depends on the family *Bovidae* for survival, although local potential reservoirs (such as the badgers in England and opossums in New Zealand) are recognized. Cattle may be infected with the virus of pseudorabies, but again, they appear to be short-term carriers and usually develop clinical disease ("mad-itch") and are dead-end hosts. The major reservoir for rabies appears to vary with locale; for example, foxes are the reservoir in continental Europe, foxes and skunks in central Canada, and the raccoon in the southern United States. Bats (both insectivorous and bloodsucking) appear to be the primary reservoir of rabies in areas such as Mexico.

4.6.2.2 CYCLOZOONOSES. Cyclozoonoses require more than one vertebrate species for survival. Examples include the taeniad and echinococcal parasites. Hydatid disease, discovered fortuitously less than 20 years ago in California, depends on the dog-sheep cycle for survival. However, in California and probably other western states, the disease now has established itself in wildlife, particularly the coyote-deer cycle.

4.6.2.3 METAZOONOSES. Metazoonoses require a vertebrate and an invertebrate host for perpetuation. There is a long list of these diseases; chiefly parasitic, viral, rickettsial, and, less frequently, bacterial agents are involved. Examples of parasitic diseases include African trypanosomiasis with its devastating effects on animals and humans, and canine heartworm in North America. Heartworm has been recognized as endemic in the southeastern United States for many years, but only recently it has also been found to be hypoendemic in southern Ontario, Canada (Slocombe and McMillan 1979). In Ontario, mosquitoes are the presumed vectors and will sustain development of the parasites, although no locally trapped mosquitoes have been found to be infected.

Viral metazoonoses include eastern and western equine encephalitis and bluetongue. Avian species are the reservoir of the equine encephalitic viruses and bird-to-bird transmission is achieved by mosquitoes. It is fortunate for both humans and animals that these mosquitoes prefer to feed on birds. Had agricultural systems not encroached on the natural marshland ecosystem of the reservoir avian species, these viruses would likely have remained as only silent infections of birds. Bluetongue is currently a perplexing problem in North America because cattle are probably functional reservoirs. However, cattle are not unduly affected, and the virus is spread by biting insects, such as *Culicoides*. On the other hand, sheep develop severe clinical disease.

Plague is perhaps the most interesting of the bacterial metazoonoses. This infection is endemic in many ground squirrel colonies in the southwestern United States. It is spread primarily by fleas who prefer the ground squirrel to other species. Sporadically, however, dogs, cats, and humans may be infested and bitten by fleas, and hence become infected with bubonic plague. Outbreaks of plague may be observed subsequent to massive die offs in the squirrel colonies.

4.6.2.4 SAPROZOONOSES. Saprozoonoses require a nonanimal site, usually soil or water, to develop and/or survive. Many of the mycotic saprozoonoses do not require a vertebrate for their perpetuation, whereas most parasitic saprozoonotic agents require a vertebrate for at least part of their cycle of perpetuation. Examples of mycotic saprozoonoses include histoplasmosis, coccidiomycosis, blastomycosis, cryptococcosis, and aspergillosis. Parasitic saprozoonoses include coccidiosis, visceral larva migrans, ancylostomiasis, and ascariasis.

Although presented here to complete the classification of zoonoses, the survival and multiplication of the agents of saprozoonoses often is highly dependent on the structure and composition of the soil as mentioned in 4.5.

4.6.3 Within-Species Infections

Despite the importance of the zoonoses, the greatest problem facing the private veterinary practitioner is the threat and spread of infection among members of a species of animal. These diseases (some of which are zoonoses) greatly reduce the productive efficiency of domestic animals and threaten the health of companion animals. Examples include rinderpest, foot-and-mouth disease, brucellosis, and mastitis in cattle; strangles, corynebacterium pneumonia, and infertility in horses; distemper, parvovirus enteritis, kennel cough, and pneumonitis in companion animals; *Haemophilus* and *Mycoplasma* pneumonia in swine; and infectious laryngotracheitis and Newcastle disease in poultry.

Although all the above diseases have an agent as the proximate cause, feeding, housing, and management (including the use of quarantine) are probably important components of the causes of these diseases. Subsequent chapters contain methods and concepts that should prove useful in identifying causal factors that can be manipulated to prevent and/or control many of these diseases.

4.7 Agents of Disease

Most diseases have specific agents identified as one of their causes; in fact, many diseases are named on the basis of the agent (e.g., salmonellosis, brucellosis, lead poisoning, mercury poisoning). In other instances, organisms are named based on the signs of the syndrome with which they are associated (e.g., African swine fever virus, bluetongue virus, and equine infectious anemia virus). This linking of agents and disease has had much utility in terms of disease prevention and control; however, it also demonstrates some of the biases that have crept into nomenclature and conceptualization of the role of specific agents in disease processes. For example, meningococci normally reside in the pharynx and upper respiratory tract together with organisms called pneumococci; neither producing disease in this location. The names of these organisms reflect the anatomic location of the disease syndrome they cause when reaching the meninges or lungs respectively. The conditions under which the meningococci infect the nervous system are not totally understood; perhaps the genesis of this human syndrome is similar to the disease of the nervous system produced by *H. somnus* in cattle, an apparently normal resident of the respiratory tract and other mucosal surfaces. Pneumococci regularly enter and are removed from the lungs, but clinical disease may result in humans with lowered resistance.

The properties of living agents (including size, structure, and metabolism) and the properties of nonliving agents (such as size and chemical make up) are important to understanding specific diseases; however, these are the subject matter of other disciplines, particularly microbiology, parasitology, and toxicology. What the epidemiologist requires most frequently is an indication of whether a specific type of agent is present, where it is present (the host, vector, or vehicle), and the concentration of the organism (ie. organisms per gram of tissue, gram of feces, or ml of water). Obviously the sensitivity and specificity of the diagnostic procedures used are of interest, as well as the sampling procedure, including items such as how were samples collected or what animals were selected for obtaining swabs. Often, what is designated as "intermittent shedding" might more properly be termed "continuous shedding" because the nature of the sampling procedure is such that only infrequently would one expect to find the agent. Another example of this occurs with the dissection of vectors (e.g., mosquitoes) for the presence of parasites (e.g., heartworm larvae), or the culture of vectors for the presence of disease. The probability of finding the agent in one insect is extremely low; hence, pools of insects are examined. Mathematical procedures have been developed that provide assistance in deciding on the optimal number of insects per pool, as well as interpretation and extrapolation of results (Walter et al. 1980).

As yet, satisfactory sampling regimes to identify the presence of and concentration of agents in populations have rarely been applied. Hence, little is known of the distribution of most agents. Recently, a screening program was employed to identify the presence of selected bacteria (Salmonella, enteropathogenic Escherichia coli, and Campylobacter) on dairy farms (Waltner-Toews 1985). The program was based on fecal sampling of up to two calves less than 2 weeks of age at the time of visit. The sensitivity of this procedure for identifying infected premises is unknown (probably low); however, on the basis of this screening procedure, about 22%, 41%, and 13% of farms are known to be infected with Salmonella, E. coli, and Campylobacter respectively. The association between the presence of these infectious agents and disease occurrence is unknown at this time; however, the majority of culture-positive calves were normal at the time of sampling. This type of work together with multiphasic sero (cellular) epidemiologic screening needs to be greatly expanded to adequately establish the natural history of these agents and their associated diseases. Unfortunately, the latter activities are out of fashion for most microbiologists and immunologists; the leading technologies in these disciplines having shifted to more reductionistic activities directed at the basic biologic building blocks, including recombinant DNA technology.

The common sources of the agent should be identified when possible; again, it is useful to rank the sources in order of frequency (importance) rather than listing all possible sources and/or means of transmission. It is also important for the epidemiologist to investigate different methods of transmission. The possibility of water-bowl and feed-trough contamination as sources of infection for respiratory disease (such as strangles in horses and pasteurellosis in cattle) requires further study. Recently, it was demonstrated that rhinoviruses in humans are more likely to be spread by contact and/or vehicles than by aerosols (Gwaltney and Hendley 1982).

It is important to understand agents' requirements for survival or persistence. For nonliving agents this might include items such as whether it is bioconcentrated in the food chain, what form the chemical is most stable in, and whether it is affected by drying or by sunlight (Goldwater 1971). For infectious agents, it is important to know their optimal conditions for survival (including whether they survive outside living tissue), what vehicles provide protection for the organism, and its resistance to drying, sunlight, and antimicrobial agents, including disinfectants. As an example, the conditions for survival in aerosols of a number of viruses of cattle was investigated by Elazhary and Derbyshire (1979).

Finally, because of the dynamic nature of infectious agents and the lack of knowledge about their distribution, it is important to examine healthy animals as vigorously as diseased animals using the same test procedures. Because the overwhelming majority of organisms are ubiquitous, little importance can be attributed to the detection of a specific organism in diseased animals or tissues. With respect to investigations of the relationship between an agent and a disease, the question is usually not whether an organism can cause a specific disease (since this has often been demonstrated in laboratory studies), but rather, what evidence exists that the particular organism is an important cause of the disease under natural conditions. In addition, identifying the circumstances under which an agent can produce disease may be more useful in terms of preventing and controlling disease than relying primarily on directed action against the organism.

4.8 Temporal Factors

Just as the occurrence of disease is related to host and environmental factors, there are changes in the frequency of many diseases with time. These temporal patterns of disease occurrence should be elucidated clearly and detailed explanations for them sought using formal studies. In this section various graphic methods used to identify the pattern of the temporal changes in disease frequency are presented. Knowledge of temporal patterns may provide insight into factors affecting the balance between the host and agent. For example, in outbreaks of disease, the pattern of change (particularly its abruptness) may suggest an optimal method of investigation of the outbreak.

4.8.1 General Temporal Patterns

When plotting the number of cases or the rate of disease against time, the shortest practical time scale should be used. If the disease occurs infrequently and without discernable pattern, it is classified as sporadic. If the disease occurrence has a predictable pattern, it is classified as endemic. Seasonal or cyclical fluctuations in disease occurrence do not preclude the correct use of the term endemic, so long as the changes are predictable (i.e., occurring with regularity). The average frequency of endemic diseases may be low (hypoendemic), moderate (mesoendemic), or high (hyperendemic). If the level of disease occurrence is significantly greater than usual (more than two standard deviations above average) and the increase is not predictable, the disease pattern is classified as epidemic. If the epidemic occurs throughout a number of countries, it may be termed pandemic.

The three patterns of disease occurrence (sporadic, endemic, and epidemic) provide useful information about the host-agent balance. Sporadic patterns suggest that the agent either infrequently infects the host, or the agent is usually present and clinical disease results from the effects of other factors. Clinical mastitis in dairy cows and infectious thromboembolic meningoencephalitis in feedlot cattle are diseases which occur sporadically. The infectious agents of these diseases usually are present, but clinical disease occurs infrequently and is not readily predictable. Some evidence indicates that meningoencephalitis tends to be associated with outbreaks of respiratory disease, and the stress and physiologic changes resulting from the respiratory disease may allow the *Haemophilus* organisms to enter the circulatory system, subsequently producing lesions in the central nervous system. It could be argued that a large percentage of infectious diseases seen by veterinarians are sporadic in nature and probably result from unknown factors tipping the agent-host balance in favor of the agent, rather than from intrinsic properties of the agent per se.

Endemic diseases are a result of a predictable, probably long-term balance between the agent and host. The lower the level of disease (degree of endemicity), the better the balance between the host and agent. The balance is quite dynamic, however, and both the level and the stability of the balance can be influenced by environmental as well as host factors. Subclinical mastitis is mesoendemic in North American dairy cows and dairy calf mortality is mesoendemic in California dairy farms. The increase in disease (chiefly respiratory disease) that occurs after feedlot cattle are assembled should also be termed endemic because of its predictability. The level of endemicity is less certain, but it appears that management is a major determinant of it. Although it is almost always fatal for individual foxes, rabies is endemic in the Canadian fox population and increases in occurrence, quite predictably, in the fall of each year when the fox kits leave their home and search for new territory.

Epidemic patterns suggest a gross imbalance with the agent having the upper hand. This imbalance is common when a new strain of organism is produced (e.g., by mutation), or during the initial exposure of the host to an organism. Currently, no adequate explanation of the pandemic of canine parvovirus enteritis exists.

All the above patterns of disease with time relate to explicit geographic limits. Diseases (such as foot-and-mouth disease) that may be endemic in some areas of the world, may produce epidemics in other areas, even though the number of cases in the epidemic area might be far less than in the area designated as endemic.

It is a general epidemiologic tenet that over time the relationship between a host and agent changes from the parasitic (favoring the agent) to a commensal state (favoring neither host nor agent). Thus, given time and a stable environment, the pattern of disease changes from epidemic to endemic and finally to sporadic. In the natural state the more resistant hosts have an increased probability of survival. From·an ecologic viewpoint, the production of disease or death rarely favors the perpetuation of the agent; thus natural selection favors less pathogenic organisms. Rabies and plague are notable exceptions to this rule. Thus, although in the short-term there usually is a positive correlation between the level of infection, disease, and death, this will not likely be true over a long period. Rather, the number of cases or deaths relative to the number of infected animals declines with the passage of time. Under laboratory conditions it is possible to select for increased virulence by repeated passages of the agent, usually in the same species. This does not contradict the previous principle, and is primarily due to the unnatural selection—if the previous process is called natural selection—of the sickest individuals for culture and repeated passage of the isolated agent. Under these restricted artificial conditions, the more virulent strains of organisms have a marked selection and survival advantage.

The history of the biological control efforts aimed at the European rabbit, *Oryctolagus cuniculi*, in Australia provides an excellent opportunity to examine the evolution of a host-parasite relationship. The rabbit was introduced into the southern part of Australia by Thomas Austin in 1859. In the ensuing years, because of the lack of natural predators, it advanced at a rate of approximately 70 miles per year over large parts of the country. By 1887 the rabbit population had multiplied so proficiently that the government offered a reward for a method that would exterminate it (Fenner 1954).

Although it had been previously observed that myxomatosis was very lethal for *Oryctolagus*, the first to suggest the use of myxoma virus as a method of biological control was a Brazilian investigator named Aragao. Experiments were subsequently carried out to determine whether the virus would be harmful to other Australian animals. It was not, and myxoma virus was deliberately introduced into the rabbit population in 1950. Within 10 months, infected rabbits were found over an area of approximately 500,000 square miles. By the third year following virus release it was estimated that the original rabbit population of approximately 500 million had been reduced by 80–90%. However, within several years of its initial release, the virus being isolated in the field was less virulent (the case fatality rate decreased from 99% to approximately 90%), and the time between infection and death had increased (Burnet and White 1972). Change in the resistance of the rabbit was slower to develop but was also evidenced by 1957. By this time, the rabbit population in some locations had been exposed to five successive epidemics each having at least a 90% case fatality rate. Using virus that killed approximately 90% of rabbits selected from previously unexposed areas, the case fatality rate in the latter repeatedly exposed population was less than 50%. This degree of protection was not due to any acquired immunity due to previous exposure, as the vast majority of these rabbits and their parents had never encountered the virus although their ancestors had. The changed resistance was innate and inheritable — an example of natural selection in a very intensive form acting to favor gene mutations (Burnet and White 1972). By 1965 it was estimated that the rabbit population and the virus had evolved to a state with the rabbit population at around 20% of their numbers before the advent of myxomatosis (Fenner and Ratcliffe 1965).

4.8.2 Graphic Techniques

The temporal patterns of morbidity and/or mortality may be investigated and displayed by appropriate graphic techniques. Initially, one can plot the number of events of interest or, more preferably, the rate (incidence, prevalence, or mortality) against time. Patterns may be obvious at that point. By general agreement, secular trends describe changes over many years or decades; cyclical changes are those with a periodicity of 2–5 years; and seasonal changes have a periodicity of 1 year or less.

Often the random variation in disease occurrence can obscure temporal patterns. A technique known as a moving average is useful to remove the unwanted fluctuations and allow visual identification of any underlying patterns. Moving averages of 3 to 5 months are useful for investigating seasonal patterns; 15- to 25-month moving averages for cyclical patterns; and 37-month moving averages for long-term (secular) trends. To plot a 3-month moving average, the rates for January, February, and March are averaged and plotted against February, the temporal midpoint for the average. Then, the rates for February, March, and April are averaged and plotted on March. This continues until all the data have been included. Obviously, many years of data are required to adequately identify cyclical or secular patterns.

When interpreting secular changes, one should look for marked trends or abrupt changes, since useful explanations (hypotheses) often may be found. When attempting to explain the changes, it is important to assess whether other factors (e.g., differences in diagnostic accuracy, completeness of reporting, changes in duration of disease, differences in host characteristics) can explain the disease pattern. Indications that the trend is real may be found by identifying different trends in different breeds, or different trends in different diseases of equal diagnostic difficulty. In addition, if a disease is not fatal, its prevalence among necropsied animals and/or abattoir specimens over a period of time can be used to assess long-term changes. Gradual changes in disease occurrence are difficult to interpret and rarely suggest useful explanations for the change because a large number of differences (particularly in environment) may have occurred during that time.

When cyclical changes are noted, a likely explanation is that herd immunity underlies the pattern. This might involve alterations in the immune percentage (due to lack of exposure or the birth of susceptible animals) or changes in the probability of contact, possibly because of variations in population size.

Seasonal variations in disease occurrence may have a number of different causes, ranging from direct effects of weather on the agent or host, to indirect effects of weather due to changes in flora and fauna, or to management and housing changes of animals in relation to weather. Diseases in which wildlife with seasonal habits serve as reservoirs or carriers and those transmitted by insect vectors tend to have seasonal patterns. It is also possible for dramatic yearly increases in the susceptible population to lead to seasonal patterns of disease. This may explain the seasonal occurrence of feline panleukopenia. However, usually more than one birth cohort is required to increase the number susceptible to the point where a disease outbreak is likely to occur. This would explain the 2–5 year periodicity for cyclical changes.

4.9 Disease Occurrence in Absolute Time

In this approach for describing the temporal pattern of disease occurrence, the time of disease occurrence is displayed relative to one or more events of interest; (MacMahon and Pugh 1970, pp 169–73) the calendar date of occurrence is ignored, since it is not important in this context. Figure 4.1 is an example of this approach, in which the rate of treatments in groups of calves is graphed with respect to the time after arrival in a feedlot. The day of arrival becomes day 0, the next day, day 1, and so forth. The shape of the epidemic curve and the time after arrival when the treatment rate is highest can be noted. The day on which the cumulative proportion of treatments reaches 50% is called the median day and may be used to demarcate the midpoint of the outbreak.

As another example, parturition in a number of species appears to directly or indirectly lead to a number of diseases; that is, the diseases cluster temporally around parturition. Obvious examples include milk fever and retained fetal membranes; less obvious clustering exists for clinical mastitis and abomasal displacements. Recently, the average time to post-

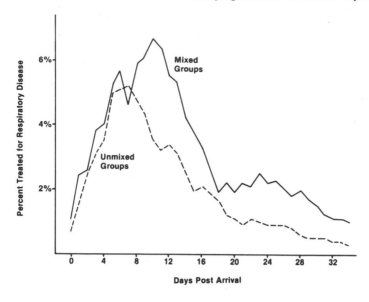

4.1. Prevalence proportion of animals treated in Bruce County feedlots by days post arrival.

partum occurrence of a number of diseases was determined (Dohoo et al. 1984a, 1984b) and provided indirect evidence of clustering for some of them (Table 4.3). Use of the more formal approach as follows to validate these observations and identify if the occurrence of other diseases (such as foot diseases) are temporally associated with parturition also is suggested. If they are temporally associated, new avenues of study to elucidate the pathogenesis of the syndromes may be opened.

The simplest approach to a formal evaluation of time clustering occurs when there is only one suspect causal factor (e.g., parturition) that seems worth investigating. Initially, the variability among the dates of onset of the disease (the standard deviation of the period between the day of onset and the median day of the outbreak) is calculated. This is then compared to the variability (standard deviation) of the period between exposure to the suspect factor and disease occurrence. If the variability of the latter is less than the variability of the date of onset, this would support the hypothesis that the factor may have been the cause of the disease.

A recent report stated that 70% of all cases of parvovirus enteritis in vaccinated dogs occurred within 2 weeks of vaccination (Sabine et al. 1982). This time clustering of cases is certainly suggestive of a temporal clustering between the vaccination regime and clinical disease. A formal investigation of this hypothesis could be made by calculating the variance

Table 4.3.   Counts and incidence rates of first diagnosis of selected dairy cattle diseases by 7-day intervals, up to 56 days postpartum (2711 lactations)[a]

Days postpartum	Abomasal displacement	Ketosis	Severe mastitis
0–7	15[b] (0.6)[c]	77 (2.8)	30 (1.1)
8–14	8 (0.3)	44 (1.7)	3 (0.1)
15–21	2 (0.1)	39 (1.5)	1 (0.0)
22–28	1 (0.1)	13 (0.5)	3 (0.1)
29–35	2 (0.1)	10 (0.4)	1 (0.0)
36–42	0 (0.0)	5 (0.2)	1 (0.0)
43–49	0 (0.0)	3 (0.1)	1 (0.0)
50–56	0 (0.0)	3 (0.1)	2 (0.1)

Source: Dohoo et al. 1984a.
[a]37% of all foot problems were diagnosed within 60 days of parturition.
[b]Number of incident cases of the disease diagnosed in the time period.
[c]Incidence rate (%).

of dates of onset of parvovirus enteritis relative to the date of vaccination, and comparing this to the variance of the time between the date of vaccination and the date of onset of enteritis in other dogs in the same areas. If the latter was greater than the former, it would support the hypothesis. Two possible explanations for this clustering are that animals were incubating the infection at the time of vaccination, or that they contracted the infection while at the veterinary clinic for vaccination. (The reader might consider how to retrospectively assess each of these factors as explanations of this temporal clustering.) It should also be noted that vaccination may trigger clinical disease occurrence in some vaccinated individuals, while at the same time be effective in preventing disease. Hence, the above approach does not shed light on the overall potential value of a vaccine.

This approach may be extended to identify the most likely cause of an outbreak when all animals are exposed to the putative causal factor(s). (This latter situation precludes the comparison of exposed and unexposed groups to identify the most likely reason for the outbreak.) The variability of the period between exposure to the true cause of the disease and subsequent disease occurrence should be less than the variability of the period between disease occurrence and exposure to noncausal factors. As an initial step, the time between exposure to each putative factor(s) and the occurrence of disease in that individual is calculated. (If groups of animals constitute the sampling units, the median time of the outbreak is noted and the time between the median day and exposure to the putative factor(s) is calculated.) Then, the average time period and the standard deviation of the period between disease occurrence and exposure to each suspect factor is determined. If the average periods are approximately the same duration, the factor having the smallest standard deviation (or variance) is the most likely cause or source of the problem. If the averages differ greatly in magnitude, the coefficient of variation (standard deviation divided by the average) should be used for making this inference.

10   Age and Time Interrelationships

As mentioned earlier, the patterns of disease with age can assist in generating hypotheses to explain disease occurrence. However, care is required when interpreting these patterns.

The existence or occurrence of an event (i.e., disease, death, or culling) may be affected by age per se, and/or by factors acting temporally close to the occurrence of the event (the current environment), and/or by factors that existed at some time prior to the occurrence of the event (the past environment). For example, the current milk production of dairy cows is related to the probability of being culled and may be influenced by current age, current environmental factors (such as the presence or absence of mastitis in the herd) and past environmental factors (such as whether or not the cows had pneumonia as calves). The problem is to identify which of these factors plays an important role in the level of production and hence of culling.

The usual method of examining age patterns (such as those of culling) implicitly relates the occurrence of the event to a current time period; that is, the rates portray the age pattern of occurrence currently existing. This method of calculating rates has been called periodic, cross-sectional, or current; the latter being preferred here. Current rates for a specified calendar time period have the following general form which is similar to that used for most rates:

$$\frac{\text{no. animals of age } X \text{ with event in current time period}}{\text{average no. animals of age } X \text{ at risk in current time period}}$$

The formula may be modified depending on what is being studied (i.e., prevalence or incidence, mortality, culling). When interpreting current rates, assume the event of interest is influenced by the current environment; however, the effects of age cannot be separated from the effects of the current environment, and the effects of past environment must be ignored.

If the age pattern of disease occurrence could be influenced by past environmental experience (including the animal's history with regard to previous disease occurrence) another approach known as cohort analysis is useful. Cohort analysis describes the rate of the event of interest in a defined cohort over a series of time intervals. Cohort analysis uses rates calculated as for risk rates and have the following general format for each time period:

$$\frac{\text{no. animals of age } X \text{ with event of interest}}{\text{no. animals of age } X \text{ initially at risk in cohort}}$$

Again, this formula should be modified depending on what is being measured. All the animals in the numerator are a subset of the initial cohort of animals. Cohorts are usually defined on the basis of time of birth (month or year), time of entry to the herd, or on the basis of experiencing an event of interest such as parturition.

To separate age effects from effects of current environmental factors and from effects of past environmental factors, the results from at least three surveys conducted in different calendar time periods should be available. Age effects are present when the disease pattern varies by age, regardless of cohort; cohort effects are present when the disease pattern varies by cohort, regardless of age. Current effects are present when the disease pattern varies by calendar time regardless of age and cohort (Kleinbaum et al. 1982, pp 130–33; Susser 1973, pp 81–86).

An example of this approach (using fictional data describing current culling rates in dairy cows, based on a series of yearly surveys) is given in Table 4.4. Consider the data relating to 1973; note the general increase in the rate of culling with age, and the peak in the 2- to 3-year-old cows. An interpretation of the increased risk of culling with age might be that cows "wear out" as they get older. The peak in the 2- to 3-year-old cows might be explained as an age effect (cows are more likely to be culled in their first lactation) or that environmental factors existing in 1973 exerted a greater harmful effect on 2- to 3-year-old cows than cows of other ages. It is not possible without additional data to discriminate between these possibilities.

Suppose that in 1978, another periodic study of culling was performed in the same population. Again, note the general increase in rate of culling with age, and the peak risk in 7- to 8-year-old cows. How does one interpret this peak? Is it an age effect or is it due to current environmental factors

Table 4.4. Hypothetical dairy cattle culling rates, by age and calendar year

Age	Year of Survey									
	1970	1971	1972	1973	1974	1975	1976	1977	1978	1979
0<1	.05	.10	.05	.05	.05	.05	.05	.05	.05	.05
1<2	.10	.10	.20	.10	.10	.10	.10	.10	.10	.10
2<3	.15	.15	.15	.30	.15	.15	.15	.15	.15	.15
3<4	.20	.20	.20	.20	.40	.20	.20	.20	.20	.20
4<5	.25	.25	.25	.25	.25	.50	.25	.25	.25	.25
5<6	.30	.30	.30	.30	.30	.30	.60	.30	.30	.30
6<7	.35	.35	.35	.35	.35	.35	.35	.70	.35	.35
7<8	.40	.40	.40	.40	.40	.40	.40	.40	.80	.40
8<9	.45	.45	.45	.45	.45	.45	.45	.45	.45	.90
9<10	.50	.50	.50	.50	.50	.50	.50	.50	.50	.50

being particularly detrimental to the survivorship of 7- to 8-year-old cows? The answer is not obvious.

Since the past environment of cows might affect the current probability of culling, it is desirable to examine rates based on the cohort approach. As in this example, the cohorts usually are defined and the cohort rates calculated, retrospectively, from the available data.

The culling rates of each birth cohort are shown in Table 4.5. Note the general increase in risk of culling with age, similar to what was observed in the current surveys. Note also that the cohort born in 1971 has twice the risk of culling of other cohorts. Now, armed with the results of both approaches, it is easier to logically interpret the effects of age and current and past environment on culling. Since the risk of culling increases with age in the cohort approach, it seems logical to accept this as an underlying biologic association. Also, since the increased risk of culling in the 1971 birth cohort explains the peaks noted in the 1973 and 1978 surveys, it seems reasonable that factors active in this birth cohort of calves (perhaps an outbreak of enteric or respiratory disease with permanent tissue damage) explain the peaks of culling. (The disease pattern is consistent in this cohort regardless of age.) Since no other patterns are noted in the cohort rates, one may conclude that the current environment had little effect on culling.

Usually, the patterns of disease are not as clear as those given in this fictional example; however, veterinarians should realize the potential value of the cohort approach. Table 4.6 contains the results of four current surveys, conducted at yearly intervals, to determine the reactor rate to bovine leukemia virus (BLV) in a dairy herd (Huber et al. 1981). Notice that the prevalence proportion decreases with time from 23% in 1977 to 11.8% in 1980. (This feature is sufficient to indicate that both current and cohort analyses should be used. If there is no secular trend in the frequency of the event of interest with time, the age pattern will be the same in both the current and cohort approaches, as it was in the previous example of cull-

Table 4.5. Hypothetical dairy cattle culling rates, by age and birth cohort

Age	Year of birth									
	1970		1971		1972		1978		1979	
0<1	.05	1970	.10	1971	.05	1972	.05	1978	.05	1979
1<2	.10	1971	.20	1972	.10	1973	.10	1979	...	
2<3	.15	1972	.30	1973	.15	1974	...		...	
3<4	.20	1973	.40	1974	.20	1975	...		...	
4<5	.25	1974	.50	1975	.25	1976	...		...	
5<6	.30	1975	.60	1976	.30	1977	...		...	
6<7	.35	1976	.70	1977	.35	1978	...		...	
7<8	.40	1977	.80	1978	.40	1979	...		...	
8<9	.45	1978	.90	1979	...		...		...	
9<10	.50	1979	...		...		...		...	

Table 4.6. Prevalence of antibodies to BLV in a purebred Holstein herd, by age and calendar year

Age (months)	1977 No.	1977 Percent	1978 No.	1978 Percent	1979 No.	1979 Percent	1980 No.	1980 Percent
<24	9/53[a]	17.0	2/47	4.3	2/85	2.4	0/29	0.0
24–35	24/94	25.5	16/65	16.9	3/92	3.3	6/128	4.7
36–47	9/31	29.0	19/79	24.1	9/57	15.8	5/76	6.6
48–59	13/55	23.6	5/20	25.0	18/72	25.0	6/34	17.6
>60	6/32	18.8	13/56	23.2	14/59	23.7	23/73	31.5
	61/265	23.0	50/267	18.7	46/365	12.6	40/340	11.8

Source: Huber et al. 1981, with permission from Am. J. Vet. Res.
[a]Numerator = number positive; denominator = number tested.

ing.) The reactor rates also appear to increase with age, except for the lack of an obvious pattern in 1977. Assuming these changes reflected the effect of current environment and age, the changes are consistent with horizontal spread of an endemic infection. That is, the older animals get, the more likely they are to have contacted the endemic infectious agent and have antibodies to BLV. An explanation for the decrease in prevalence with time is not obvious.

Table 4.7 portrays the same data using a cohort format. Note that there is only a slight increase in prevalence, according to age, within each cohort. (The cohorts are birth cohorts, but due to the method of testing there are missing data; some cohorts were 4-years-old before they were tested.) Note also that the prevalence proportion decreases in the more recent cohorts. Taken together, the results of the current and the cohort analyses imply a large cohort effect, a small increase in prevalence with age, and no effect of current environment. (Recall the conditions described earlier for age, cohort, and current effects.) There appears to be minimal spread of infection among cohorts in this herd. Why each succeeding cohort should have a lower prevalence of reactors than its predecessor (in the

Table 4.7. Prevalence of antibodies to BLV, by age and birth cohort of Holstein cows

Birth cohort	Initial test	Age at testing (months) <24 No.	<24 Percent	24–35 No.	24–35 Percent	36–47 No.	36–47 Percent	48–59 No.	48–59 Percent	>60 No.	>60 Percent
1977	1979	2/85[a]	2.4	6/128	4.7	...	...	...	...	...	...
1976	1978	2/47	4.3	3/92	3.3	5/76	6.6	...	...	...	...
1975	1977	9/53	17.0	11/65	16.9	9/57	15.8	6/34	17.6	...	...
1974	1977	...	...	24/94	25.5	19/79	24.1	18/72	25.0	23/73	31.5
1973	1977	...	...	...	...	9/31	29.0	5/20	25.0	14/59	23.7
1972	1977	...	...	...	...	...	...	13/55	23.6	13/56	23.2

Source: Huber et al. 1981, with permission from Am. J. Vet. Res.
[a]Numerator = number positive; denominator = number tested.

absence of a control program) is an interesting question to ponder; although there is no obvious explanation for it, the cohort effect is nonetheless real.

These data are not intended as the final word on BLV in dairy herds. Many people believe (primarily based on current rates) that the prevalence rate increases with age as a result of horizontal transmission of the virus. A recent prospective cohort analytic study investigated the time(s) at which horizontal spread of BLV appeared greatest (Thurmond et al. 1983); the data from this study indicated an increasing prevalence of BLV antibodies with age (i.e., a true age effect).

References

Armitage, P. 1971. Statistical Methods in Medical Research. New York, N.Y.: John Wiley & Sons.

Arnon, S. S., K. Damus, and J. Chin. 1981. Infant botulism: Epidemiology and relation to sudden infant death syndrome. Epidemiol. Rev. 3:45–66.

Binns, W., L. F. James, T. L. Shupe, and E. T. Thacker. 1962. Cyclopian type malformation in lambs. Arch. Environ. Health 5:106–13.

Burnet, M., and D. O. White. 1972. Natural History of Infectious Disease. Cambridge, England: Cambridge Univ. Press.

Commonwealth Agricultural Bureaux. 1983. Animal Disease Occurrence, C.A.B. Farnham House, Farnham Royal, Slough, U.K.

Dohoo, I. R., S. W. Martin, A. H. Meek, and W. C. D. Sandals. 1984a. Disease, production and culling in Holstein-Friesian cows. I. The data. Prev. Vet. Med. 1:321–34.

Dohoo, I. R., S. W. Martin, I. McMillan, and B. W. Kennedy. 1984b. Disease, production and culling in Holstein-Friesian cows. II. Age, season and sire effects. Prev. Vet. Med. 1:655–70.

Elazhary, M. A. S. Y., and J. B. Derbyshire. 1979. Effect of temperature, relative humidity and medium on the aerosol stability of infectious bovine rhinotracheitis virus. Can. J. Comp. Med. 43:158–67.

Essex, M. E. 1982. Feline leukemia: A naturally occurring cancer of infectious origin. Epidemiol. Rev. 4:189–203.

Fenner, F. 1954. The rabbit plague. Sci. Am. 190:30–35.

Fenner, F., and F. N. Ratcliffe. 1965. Myxomatosis. New York: Cambridge Univ. Press.

Fleiss, J. L. 1973. Statistical Methods for Rates and Proportions. Toronto, Canada: John Wiley & Sons.

Fox, J. P., L. Elveback, W. Scott, L. Gatewood, and E. Ackerman. 1971. Herd immunity: Basic concepts and relevance to public health immunization practices. Am. J. Epidemiol. 94:179–89.

Goldwater, L. J. 1971. Mercury in the environment. Sci. Am. 224:3–9.

Gwaltney, J. M. Jr., and J. O. Hendley. 1982. Transmission of experimental rhinovirus infection by contaminated surfaces. Am. J. Epidemiol. 116:828–33.

Harris, R. E., and W. A. G. Charleston. 1977. An examination of the marsh microhabitats of Lymnaea tomentosa and L. columella (Mollusca: Gastropoda) by path analysis. N.Z. J. Zool. 4:395–99.

Hayes, H. M. Jr., R. Hoover, and R. E. Tarone. 1976. Bladder cancer in pet dogs: A sentinel for environmental cancer? Am. J. Epidemiol. 114:229–33.

Huber, N. L., R. F. DiaGiacomo, J. F. Evermann, and E. Studer. 1981. Bovine leukemia virus infection in a large Holstein herd: Cohort analysis of the prevalence of antibody-positive cows. Am. J. Vet. Res. 42:1474–76.

Kellar, J., R. Marra, and W. Martin. 1976. Brucellosis in Ontario: A case control study. Can. J. Comp. Med. 40:119–28.

Kleinbaum, D. G., L. L. Kupper, and H. Morgenstern. 1982. Epidemiologic Research: Principles and Quantitative Methods. Belmont, Calif.: Wadsworth.

Levine, N. D., ed. 1966. Natural Nidality of Transmissible Diseases. Urbana: Univ. Illinois Press.

MacMahon, B., and T. F. Pugh. 1970. Epidemiology: Principles and Methods. Boston, Mass.: Little, Brown.

Marmor, M., P. Willeberg, L. T. Glickman, W. A. Priester, R. H. Cypess, and A. I. Hurvitz. 1982. Epizootiologic patterns of diabetes mellitus in dogs. Am. J. Vet. Res. 43:465–70.

Martin, S. W., C. W. Schwabe, and C. E. Franti. 1975. Dairy calf mortality rate: Influence of meteorologic factors on calf mortality rate in Tulare County, California. Am. J. Vet. Res. 36:1105–09.

Martin, S. W., K. Kirby, and P. W. Pennock. 1980. Canine hip dysplasia: Breed effects. Can. Vet. J. 21:293–96.

Nathanson, N., and A. Miller. 1978. Epidemiology of multiple sclerosis: Critique of the evidence for a viral etiology. Am. J. Epidemiol. 107:451–61.

Priester, W. A. 1971. Cats are pollution sentinels. Science. Sept. 24, 1971.

_____. 1974. Canine progressive retinal atrophy: Occurrence by age, breed, and sex. Am. J. Vet. Res. 35:571–74.

Reif, J. S. 1976. Seasonality, natality and herd immunity in feline panleukopenia. Am. J. Epidemiol. 103:81–87.

Reif, J. S., and D. Cohen. 1970. Canine pulmonary disease and the urban environment. II. Retrospective radiographic analysis of pulmonary disease in rural and urban dogs. Arch. Environ. Health. 20:684–89.

Sabine, M., L. Herbert, and D. N. Love. 1982. Canine parvovirus infection in Australia during 1980. Vet. Rec. 110:551–53.

Schwabe, C. W. 1969. Veterinary Medicine and Human Health. 2nd ed. Baltimore, Md.: Williams & Wilkins.

_____. 1984. Veterinary Medicine and Human Health. 3rd ed. Baltimore, Md.: Williams & Wilkins.

Schwabe, C. W., J. Sawyer, and W. Martin. 1971. A pilot system for environmental monitoring through domestic animals. Am. Inst. Aero. and Astro. No. 71–1044.

Slocombe, J. O. D., and I. McMillan. 1979. Heart-worm in dogs in Canada in 1978. Can. Vet. J. 20:284–87.

Smith, L. D. 1978. Occurrence of *Clostridium botulinum* and *Clostridium tetani* in the soil of the United States. Health Lab. Sci. 15:74–80.

Stallones, R. A. 1972. Environment, ecology and epidemiology. Pan. Am. Health Org. Sci. Pub. No. 231.

Steck, F., and A. Wandeler. 1980. The epidemiology of fox rabies in Europe. Epidemiol. Rev. 2:71–96.

Straw, B. E., A. D. Leman, M. R. Wilson, and J. E. Dick. 1984. Sire and breed effects on mortality in the offspring of swine. Prev. Vet. Med. 2:707–14.

Susser, M. 1973. Causal Thinking in the Health Sciences: Concepts and Strategies in Epidemiology. Toronto, Canada: Oxford Univ. Press.

Takov, R. 1983. Swine respiratory disease: Their interrelationships and relationship to productivity. M.S. thesis, Univ. of Guelph, Ontario, Canada.

Thurmond, M. C., and S. D. Acres. 1975. The effect of climate on neonatal calf mortality. Paper submitted as partial fulfillment for MPVM degree, University of California, Davis.

Thurmond, M. C., K. M. Portier, D. M. Puhr, and M. J. Burridge. 1983. A prospective investigation of bovine leukemia virus infection in young dairy cattle, using survival methods. Am. J. Epidemiol. 117:621–31.

Tinline, R. R. 1972. Lee wave hypothesis for the initial spread during the 1967–68 foot-and-mouth epizootic. *In* Medical Geography, ed. N. D. McGlashan. London Methuen.

Topley, W. W. C., and G. S. Wilson. 1923. The spread of bacterial infection: The problem of herd immunity. J. Hyg. 21:243–49.

Walter, S. D., S.W. Hildreth, and B. J. Beaty. 1980. Estimation of infection rates in populations of organisms using pools of variable size. Am. J. Epidemiol. 112:124–28.

Waltner-Toews, D. 1985. Dairy calf management, morbidity, mortality and calf-related drug use in Ontario Holstein herds. Ph.D. thesis, Univ. of Guelph, Ontario, Canada.

Wierup, M. 1983. A canine parvoviral epidemic in relation to the population at risk. Proc. 3rd Int. Sym. Vet. Epidemiol. Econ., Sept. 1982. Arlington, Va.

Willeberg, P., and W. A. Priester. 1976. Feline urological syndrome: Associations with some time, space and individual patient factors. Am. J. Vet. Res. 37:975–78.

Willeberg, P., M. A. Gerbola, B. Kirkegaard Petersen, and J. B. Andersen. 1984. The Danish pig health scheme: Nation-wide computer-based abattoir surveillance and follow-up at the herd level. Prev. Vet. Med. 3:79–91.

Yorke, J. A., N. Nathanson, G. Pianigiani, and J. Martin. 1979. Seasonality and the requirements for perpetuation and eradication of viruses in populations. Am. J. Epidemiol. 109:103–23.

Disease Causation

Causation in one form or another is of central interest in most epidemiologic studies. However, because most epidemiologic studies are observational in nature and are conducted in the field outside of direct or indirect control of the investigator, proving causation is difficult if not impossible. Thus, inferring cause and effect based on the results of observational studies and field trials is, to an extent, a matter of judgment (Susser 1977). Therefore, a set of widely accepted guidelines is required to ensure a common basis for making inferences about causation.

5.1 Introductory Guidelines

The requirement for guidelines to assess causation is not a new or unique problem (Evans 1978; Susser 1973). In the early years of the microbiologic era, guidelines were required to help evaluate whether an organism should be considered the cause of a syndrome or disease. The Henle-Koch postulates became widely accepted and have served this purpose for the past century. In summary form they are: (1) the organism must be present in every case of the disease; (2) the organism must not be present in other diseases, or in normal tissues; (3) the organism must be isolated from the tissue(s) in pure culture; and (4) the organism must be capable of inducing the disease under controlled experimental conditions.

As far as is known, Koch did not believe in following all these postulates slavishly; although he did believe that a causal agent should be present in every case of the disease and should not be present in tissues of normal animals. These guidelines led to the successful linking of organisms and disease syndromes, and this allowed a dramatic improvement in our ability to prevent and control a large number of so-called infectious diseases. If the use of the Henle-Koch postulates has had a drawback, it probably lies in the narrowing of the thought process about causation. Each disease was perceived as having a single cause, and each agent was perceived as producing a single disease. On this basis, many diseases have been classified and named according to the agent associated with them. For example, *Escherichia coli* is the cause of colibacillosis, and salmonella organisms are the cause of salmonellosis. Although functional and in agreement with Koch's postulates, the linking of agents and diseases in this manner represents circular reasoning and may not be as meaningful as one might first think. Furthermore, it is now accepted that many factors in addition to microorganisms are responsible for infectious diseases.

Partly because of the limitations of the Henle-Koch postulates to deal with multiple etiologic factors, multiple effects of single causes, the carrier state, nonagent factors such as age that cannot be manipulated experimentally, and quantitative causal factors, epidemiologists and other medical scientists have looked for different guidelines about causation. Examples of these are the rules of inductive reasoning formulated by philosopher John Stuart Mill (MacMahon and Pugh 1970; Susser 1973). His canons (extensively paraphrased) may be summarized as the methods of agreement, difference, concomitant variation, analogy, and residue:

Method of Agreement. If a disease occurs under a variety of circumstances but there is a common factor, this factor may be the cause of the disease. (This method is frequently used to identify possible causal factors in outbreak investigations; one attempts to elucidate factors common to all or most occurrences of the disease.)

Method of Difference. If the circumstances where a disease occurs are similar to those where the disease does not occur, with the exception of one factor, this one factor or its absence may be the cause of the disease. (This is the basis of traditional experimental design; namely, keeping all factors constant except the one of interest. It also provides the rationale for contrasting the characteristics and environments of diseased and nondiseased animals in the search for putative causes.)

Method of Concomitant Variation. If a factor and disease have a dose-response relationship, the factor may be a cause of the disease. (A factor whose strength or frequency varies directly with disease occurrence is a more convincing argument for causation than simple agreement or difference.)

Method of Analogy. If the distribution of a disease is sufficiently similar to that of another well understood disease, the disease of concern may share common causes with the other disease. (This method is treacherous to use, except as a general principle.)

Method of Residue. If a factor explains only X% of disease occurrence, other factors must be identified to explain the remainder, or residue (i.e., $100 - X\%$). (This is often used in study design. For example, when studying the association between factor B and disease and if it is known that factor A causes some of the disease, it may prove useful to perform the study in animals or units not exposed to factor A.)

Although rarely used by epidemiologists in their original form, these rules form the basis for many of the guidelines to be discussed. Formulating, evaluating, and testing hypotheses is central to epidemiologic research.

The basic problem in attempting to establish causation between a specific factor and a disease in observational field studies lies in the inability of the investigator to ensure that other factors did not cause the event of interest. In laboratory experiments, it is possible to demonstrate with a great deal of certainty that a factor causes a disease, because of the ability to control all the conditions of the study. Hence, in a well-designed laboratory experiment, if the difference in the rate of disease between exposed and unexposed animals is statistically significant, most would accept a cause and effect relationship has been established (Method of Difference). In a field trial, despite the control provided over allocation to experimental groups, other unknown factors may influence the outcomes. Hence, it is not possible to state with the same degree of certainty that other factors did not cause the event of interest. Thus, additional evidence, usually provided by other workers repeating the study in their area and finding similar results, is required. In observational studies a large number of known and unknown factors including sampling biases could lead to a difference in rates of outcome in exposed and unexposed animals. One should not be dismayed at this possibility, but to compensate for it the design of observational studies may have to be more complex than field trials. Also, some additional guidelines are required to develop causal inferences based on the results of observational studies.

A thorough discussion of current concepts on causation is beyond the scope of this text. However, a unified set of guidelines has been published (Evans 1978) and can be summarized as follows:

1. The incidence and/or prevalence of the disease should be higher in individuals exposed to the putative cause than in nonexposed individuals.

2. The exposure should be more common in cases than in those without the disease.

3. Exposure must precede the disease.

4. There should be a spectrum of measurable host responses to the agent (e.g., antibody formation, cell mediated immunity). (This guideline refers particularly to proximate causes of disease such as infectious and noninfectious agents.)

5. Elimination of the putative cause should result in a lower incidence of the disease.

6. Preventing, or modifying, the host's response should decrease or eliminate the expression of disease.

7. The disease should be reproducible experimentally.

The last step is often extremely difficult to fulfill, particularly if a number of cofactors in addition to the proximate agent are required to produce the disease. Evans (1978) concludes with a plea to direct attention not only to those factors that produce disease but also to those that produce health. It is of paramount importance that veterinarians accept and act on this plea, particularly for those involved in domestic animal industries.

The initial steps used by epidemiologists for assessing causation were outlined in Chapter 1. Basically, the sequence is to demonstrate that a valid association exists, to assess the likelihood (using judgment criteria) that a causal association exists, and, if possible, to elaborate the nature of the causal association.

5.2 Statistical Associations

For a factor to be causally associated with a disease, the rate of disease in exposed animals must be different than the rate of disease in those not exposed to the factor. This is equivalent to requiring that the frequency of the factor in diseased individuals must be different from its frequency in nondiseased individuals. Similarly, for a disease to cause a change in production, the level of production must differ between animals having the disease and those not having the disease. These conditions are necessary but not sufficient for establishing causation (see 5.6.2). Since epidemiologists frequently choose a qualitative variable such as disease occurrence, death, or culling as the outcome (dependent variable), the format for displaying these data and their relationship to a putative causal factor having two levels (e.g., exposure or nonexposure to an agent; or possessing or not possessing a factor, such as male versus female) is shown in Table 5.1. The proportions or rates usually contrasted are also shown.

To evaluate the probability that sampling error might account for the observed differences, a formal statistical test is required. If the observed differences are deemed significantly different, it implies that chance variation due to sampling error is unlikely to have produced the observed differences. Under these conditions one would say that the factor and the disease were associated.

In declaring a difference to be statistically significant, one does not imply that the difference was due to the exposure (independent variable); it only implies that sampling error was unlikely to have produced the difference. Other factors besides chance or the independent variable could have caused the differences.

Table 5.1. A 2 × 2 table displaying the relationship between two dichotomous variables, one the factor, the other the disease

The numbers of individuals (sampling units) in each of the four possible factor-disease categories may be displayed using the following format:

		Diseased $D+$	Not diseased $D-$	Total
Exposed (factor positive)	$F+$	a	b	$a + b$
Not exposed (factor negative)	$F-$	c	d	$c + d$
		$a + c$	$b + d$	$n = a + b + c + d$

Lowercase characters indicate values are derived from a sample, whereas capital characters indicate population (census) values. Hence, for rates and proportions given below p indicates an estimate (a statistic) from a sample, whereas P indicates the corresponding population value (the parameter).

Proportion or rate of interest	Sample notation	Calculated using
Exposed	$p(F+)$	$(a + b)/n$
Diseased	$p(D+)$	$(a + c)/n$
Diseased and exposed	$p(F+ \text{ and } D+)$	a/n
Diseased in the exposed group	$p(D+/F+)$	$a/(a + b)$
Diseased in the nonexposed group	$p(D+/F-)$	$c/(c + d)$
Exposed in the diseased group	$p(F+/D+)$	$a/(a + c)$
Exposed in the nondiseased group	$p(F+/D-)$	$b/(b + d)$

Note: As mentioned in Chapter 2, not all sample statistics are valid estimates of population parameters in cohort and case-control studies. See Table 2.5 for details.

If only a few individuals or sampling units are included in a study, it is quite likely that differences will be declared statistically nonsignificant (i.e., there is >5% probability the observed differences might have arisen because of sampling variation). In this situation, if the observed differences could be of biologic importance one should not ignore the findings. Instead, one should act judiciously and assume the difference is real until future studies either validate or refute the observation. On the other hand, in extremely large samples trivial differences of no biologic importance would be declared statistically significant because sampling error would be minimal.

In selecting a statistical test, consider the type of data (qualitative and quantitative) as well as the design of the study (Snedecor and Cochran 1980). Qualitative data (such as rates or proportions) are derived by counting events (the qualitative factors) and dividing by the appropriate population at risk as discussed in Chapter 3. For risk rates, the chi-square test provides the probability that differences as large or larger than observed in the sample would arise due to chance alone, if there were no association (i.e., no real difference) in the population. By convention, if this probability is less than 5%, one may say the rates are significantly different; hence the factor and the disease are statistically associated. The result of the chi-square test is influenced by the magnitude of the difference as well as the sample size. Example calculations for the chi-square statistic for testing differences between two independent or two correlated proportions are shown in Tables 5.2 and 5.3 respectively.

For those wishing a faster method of calculating the Yates-corrected, chi-square statistic (for testing differences between independent proportions), the following formula may be used for 2×2 tables:

Table 5.2. The chi-square test applied to differences between two independent proportions

The following data relate the type of ventilation of swine herds to the level of pneumonia detected at the abattoir. The herd prevalence of pneumonia was considered high if $> 5\%$ of marketed pigs had pneumonia (herds are the units of concern).

	Herd pneumonia prevalence		
Ventilation	High	Low	Total
Fan	91	73	164
No fan	25	60	85
	116	133	249

The first step is to calculate the expected number of herds in each ventilation type–pneumonia level category. For any cell in the table the expected number may be found by multiplying the corresponding row and column totals and dividing by the total number of units. For the a cell (row 1, column 1) we have:

$164 \times 116/249 = 76.40$

The expected numbers in the b, c and d cells may be calculated using the same approach or by subtraction, since the marginal totals remain the same. The four expected values are:

$$76.40 \qquad 87.60$$
$$39.60 \qquad 45.40$$

A value is calculated for each cell by subtracting the expected (Exp) value from the corresponding observed (Obs) value, making the difference positive (if necessary) and subtracting one-half (Yates-corrected), squaring this quantity, and then dividing the result by the expected value. The chi-square statistic is then found by adding these four numbers together. The formula is: $\chi^2 = \Sigma[(|Obs - Exp| - 0.5)^2/Exp]$ where sigma (Σ) indicates "the sum of" over all cells.

In this example we have:

$$\frac{(|91 - 76.4| - 0.5)^2}{76.4} + \frac{(|73 - 87.6| - 0.5)^2}{87.6} + \frac{(|25 - 39.6| - 0.5)^2}{39.6}$$
$$+ \frac{(|60 - 45.5| - 0.5)^2}{45.5} = 14.3$$

The critical values of chi-square at the 10%, 5%, and 1% levels of significance (for comparing two proportions) are 2.71, 3.84, and 6.64 respectively. Since the calculated value of chi-square exceeds 3.84, there is less than a 5% probability that differences as large or larger than observed would arise due to sampling error. Thus, one could assume that ventilation type and level of pneumonia were associated in the population from which these data were obtained; that is, significantly more herds with fans had a high prevalence of pneumonia than herds with no fans.

$$X^2 = \frac{[|(a \times d) - (b \times c)| - 0.5\ n]^2 \times n}{(a + b) \times (c + d) \times (a + c) \times (b + d)}$$

Except for rounding errors, this gives the same answer as the previous method. When used on 2×2 tables, all chi-square statistics have 1 degree of freedom; hence, the critical value for significance at the 5% level is 3.84.

Quantitative data are based on measurements and are summarized by means, standard deviations, and standard errors. Student's t-test provides information about differences between two means that is similar to that provided by the chi-square test for differences between two rates. Example calculations for testing the difference between two independent or two correlated means are shown in Tables 5.4 and 5.5 respectively. The probability

Table 5.3. The chi-square test (McNemar's) applied to differences between two correlated proportions

If two observations are made on the same individual, or if two individuals or units were paired (either by matching prior to selection in observational studies, or by blocking prior to randomization in experiments) the test is modified to take any correlation between the two observations into account.

The following data were obtained by testing blood samples for antibodies to Brucella abortus using the tube agglutination (TAT) and the complement fixation (CFT) tests. All intermediate level titers were designated as positive for current purposes.

		CFT		
		+	−	Total
TAT	+	38	29(s)	67
	−	21(r)	1749	1770
		59	1778	1837

Note that the cell entries are pairs not individuals (i.e., 38 samples were positive on both tests).

The question in this example is whether the proportion positive in the TAT (67/1837) is significantly different from the proportion positive in the CFT (59/1837). The chi-square statistic is calculated using the two numbers r and s, representing the number of discordant pairs.

$$\chi^2 = (|r - s| - 1)^2/(r + s)$$
$$\chi^2 = (|21 - 29| - 1)^2/(21 + 29) = 7^2/50 = 0.98$$

Since this is much less than 3.84, there is little evidence to suggest that the rates differ, so one should act as if they are the same.

The odds ratio (Table 5.6) is used to describe the strength of association, and for matched data (portrayed as above) it is calculated as s/r; in this instance 29/21 = 1.38. The interpretation is that the cattle in this sample were 1.38 times more likely to be positive to the TAT than the CFT. However, since the chi-square statistic was not significant, one should assume an equal likelihood (an odds ratio of 1) of being positive to the TAT and the CFT.

(As a generalization of this format, in a case-control study, TAT would represent the cases and CFT the controls. + and − would represent the exposure status. In a cohort study, TAT would represent the exposed group and CFT the unexposed group. + and − would represent the diseased and nondiseased animals respectively.)

Table 5.4.   Student's t-test applied to differences between two independent means

Suppose one wished to compare the 305-day milk production (Y) of cows with clinical mastitis ($M+$) to the production of cows without clinical mastitis ($M-$). The milk production is expressed as breed-class-average (BCM) and all cows are from the same herd.

Group 1 $M+$	Group 2 $M-$
128	143
133	145
123	138
141	148
129	137
...	154
...	140
$\bar{y} = 130.8$	143.6
$s^2 = 45.2$	36.3
$n = 5$	7

Pooled $s_p^2 = [(n_1 - 1)s_1^2 + (n_2 - 1)s_2^2]/(n_1 + n_2 - 2)$
$\quad\quad\quad = (4 \times 45.2 + 6 \times 36.3)/10$
$\quad\quad\quad = 39.86$

The formula is:

$t = (\bar{y}_1 - \bar{y}_2)/[s_p^2 \times (1/n_1 + 1/n_2)]^{1/2}$
$\quad = -12.8/[39.86 \times (1/5 + 1/7)]^{1/2}$
$\quad = -12.8/3.70 = -3.46$

The critical value of t changes with the sample size; with type 1 error of 0.05 and 10, ($n_1 + n_2 - 2$) degrees of freedom it is 2.23. Thus, since the calculated value of t is greater (in absolute magnitude) than 2.23, there is less than a 5% probability that differences as large as or larger than observed are due to sampling variation. Therefore, one may act as if the difference is real; that is, clinical mastitis and level of milk production are associated in the population.

that chance variations may account for the observed differences in the sample when no real differences exist in the sampled population is referred to as the type I error. One minus the type I error provides the confidence level. For simplicity, a type I error of 0.05 (i.e., 5%) is assumed throughout this text.

5.3   Epidemiologic Measures of Association

As discussed, statistical significance is a function of the magnitude of difference, the variability of the difference, and the sample size. Once the decision is made that sampling variation (chiefly a function of sample size) is not a probable explanation for the difference observed, the epidemiologist will apply other measures of association. Unfortunately, there is a plethora of terms for these epidemiologic measures, and currently there is

Table 5.5. Student's t-test applied to differences between two correlated means

Suppose that in the previous example the control cows (those without mastitis) were maternal siblings of the affected cows. On the average, this matching should increase the power of our test because two cows from the same dam should have more similar levels of milk production than two randomly chosen cows from the same herd. To take advantage of this, use the within-pair difference as the basic test statistic.

Assume that the following data were obtained.

Group 1 $M+$	Group 2 $M-$	Difference d
128	142	-14
133	143	-10
123	134	-11
141	155	-14
129	141	-12
$\bar{y} = 130.8$	143.0	$-12.2\ (\bar{d})$
$s^2 = \ \ 45.2$	57.5	$3.2\ (s^2_{\bar{d}})$

The formula is:

$$t = \bar{d}/(s^2_{\bar{d}}/n)^{1/2}$$
$$= -12.2/(3.2/5)^{1/2}$$
$$= -15.3$$

The critical value of t with type 1 error $= 0.05$ and $n - 1 = 4$ degrees of freedom is 2.78. Since the calculated value exceeds (in absolute magnitude) the critical value, there is less than a 5% chance that sampling error produced the difference of 12.2 units. Therefore, one should assume that the difference is real; specifically, cows with mastitis produce less milk than maternal siblings without mastitis in this population.

little agreement on the usage of these terms (Waltner-Toews 1983). The terminology used in this text is, in the main, consistent with historical use, but modifications to reflect recent concepts have been included (Kleinbaum et al. 1982). These measures are independent of sample size and include the strength of association, the effect of the factor in exposed individuals, and the importance of the factor in the population. Formulas for these measures are contained in Table 5.6; an example of their calculation and interpretation is contained in Table 5.7.

5.3.1 Strength of Association

The strength of association between a factor and a disease is known as relative risk (RR); it is calculated as the ratio between the rate of disease in the exposed and the rate of disease in the unexposed group. Other terms for this measure include risk ratio, incidence rate ratio, or prevalence ratio, depending on the statistics being compared. If there is no association between the factor and the disease, the relative risk will be 1, excluding variation due to sampling error. The greater the departure of the relative risk

Table 5.6.   Epidemiologic measures of association for independent proportions in 2 × 2 tables

Measure	Calculate using	Comments
Strength		
Relative risk (RR)	$= [a/(a + b)]/[c/(c + d)]$	Not applicable in case-control studies
Population relative risk (RR_{pop})	$= [(a + c)/n]/[c/(c + d)]$	Only use in cross-sectional studies
Odds ratio (OR)	$= ad/bc$	Applicable in all study types
Population odds ratio (OR_{pop})	$= \dfrac{d \times (a + c)}{c \times (b + d)}$	Only use in cross-sectional or case-control studies, if controls are representative of nondiseased population
Effect		
Attributable rate (AR)	$= [a/(a + b)] - [c/(c + d)]$	Not applicable in case-control studies
Attributable fraction (AF)	$= AR/[a/(a + b)]$ $= (RR - 1)/RR$	For use in cross-sectional or cohort studies (often expressed as a percentage)
Estimated AF	$= (OR - 1)/OR$	For use in case-control studies
Total effect (importance)		
Population attributable rate (PAR)	$= [(a + c)/n] - [c/(c + d)]$ $= [(a + b)/n] \times AR$	For use in cross-sectional studies, or when frequency of disease in the population is available
Population attributable fraction (PAF)	$= PAR/[(a + c)/n]$ $= (RR_{pop} - 1)/RR_{pop}$	
Estimated PAF	$= 1 - \dfrac{c \times (b + d)}{d \times (a + c)}$ $= (OR_{pop} - 1)/OR_{pop}$	Only use in case-control studies if controls are representative of the nondiseased population

from 1 (i.e., either larger or smaller), the stronger the association between the factor and the disease. Since the relative risk is the ratio of two rates of disease, it has no units (Table 5.6). In terms of disease causation, if the relative risk is less than 1, the factor may be viewed as a sparing factor; whereas if the relative risk is greater than 1, the factor may be viewed as a putative causal factor.

The relative impact of the factor in the population is calculated by dividing the estimate of the overall rate of disease in the population by the rate of disease in the unexposed group. This measure is known as the population relative risk (RR_{pop}) and adjusts the ordinary relative risk for the prevalence of the factor in the population.

Relative risk cannot be calculated in case-control studies because the rates of disease in the exposed and unexposed groups are unknown. However, another measure known as the odds ratio (OR) is used in its place. The calculation of the odds ratio shown in Table 5.6 is quite simple and, because

Table 5.7.   **Examples of the chi-square test and measures of association.** [Data derived from a cross-sectional study of the relationship between dry cat food (DCF) and feline urologic syndrome (FUS)]

	FUS+	FUS−	Total	Rates of FUS
DCF+	13	2163	2176	5.97 per 1000
DCF−	5	3349	3354	1.49 per 1000
	18	5512	5530	3.25 per 1000
Proportion DCF+	0.72	0.39	0.39	

Chi-square statistic = 6.85

Since this is greater than 3.84, one may safely assume that the observed differences are unlikely due to chance; that is, act as if DCF and FUS are associated in the cat population.

Epidemiologic measures of association	Interpretation of measure
RR = (5.97)/(1.49) = 4.01	The rate of FUS in DCF exposed cats is 4.01 times greater than the rate of FUS in non-DCF exposed cats.
OR = (13 × 3349)/(5 × 2163) = 4.03	Interpret as above.
RR_{pop} = (3.25)/(1.49) = 2.18	The rate of FUS in the cat population is increased 2.18 times because of DCF exposure.
OR_{pop} = (18 × 3349)/(5 × 5512) = 2.19	Interpret as above.
AR = 5.97 − 1.49 = 4.48 per 1000	The rate of FUS in DCF exposed cats that may be attributed to DCF is 4.48 per 1000.
AF = (4.48)/(5.97) = 0.75	75% of FUS in DCF exposed cats is attributable to DCF.
PAR = 3.25 − 1.49 = 1.76 per 1000	The rate of FUS in the cat population that may be attributed to DCF is 1.76 per 1000. That is, we would expect the rate of FUS to decrease by 1.76 per 1000 if DCF were not fed.
PAF = (1.76)/(3.25) = 0.54	54% of all FUS in the cat population is attributable to DCF.

Source: Willeberg 1977, with permission.

of the manner of calculating it, has been referred to as the cross-products ratio. In veterinary literature the odds ratio often has been termed the approximate relative risk, because if the disease in the population is relatively infrequent (< 5%), the odds ratio is very close in magnitude to what the relative risk would be if it could be calculated. In this situation, a is relatively small and b approximates $a + b$; thus $a/(a + b)$ approximates a/b. Similarly $c/(c + d)$ approximates c/d. (The method of calculation of the odds ratio when matching is used in the study design is shown in Table 5.3.) The odds ratio is interpreted exactly the same as relative risk and has an advantage over the relative risk in that it may be used to measure the strength of association irrespective of the sampling method used. The odds ratio is also a basic statistic in more powerful methods known as log-linear and logistic modeling.

Just as there is a population analog for relative risk, there is also one for the odds ratio. Besides indicating the relative impact of the factor in the population, it may be used to derive the rate of disease in the factor-positive and factor-negative groups, if an outside estimate of the rate of disease in the population is available. For example, the rate of disease in the factor-negative group is found by dividing the estimate of the population rate $P(D+)$ by the population odds ratio. The rate of disease in the factor-positive group is found by multiplying the rate of disease in the factor-negative group by the odds ratio. This procedure is not exact, but sufficient for practical purposes if the disease is relatively infrequent ($<5\%$), since the odds ratio approaches the relative risk under these conditions.

When disease is the factor and production is the dependent variable, the relative effect of the disease on production may be found by dividing the level of production in the diseased group by the level in the nondiseased group.

5.3.2 Effect of Factor in Exposed Group

Since there is usually some disease in the factor-negative group, not all of the disease in the exposed group is due to the factor; only the difference between the two rates is explainable by or attributable to the factor. In calculating the attributable rate, one assumes that the other factors which lead to disease in the factor-negative group operate with the same frequency and intensity in the factor-positive group. This absolute difference is called the attributable rate (AR) and is determined by subtracting the rate of disease in the unexposed group from the rate in the exposed group. The attributable rate has the same units as the original rate and is defined as the rate of disease in the exposed group due to exposure. The larger the attributable rate, the greater the effect of the factor in the exposed group (Table 5.6).

Sometimes it is desirable to know what proportion of disease in the exposed or factor-positive group is due to the factor. This fraction is called the attributable fraction (AF) or etiologic fraction (in the exposed group), and may be calculated from first principles or from either the relative risk or odds ratio statistics as demonstrated in Table 5.6.

One interesting and practical application of using the attributable fraction is in estimating the efficacy of vaccines. By definition, vaccine efficacy (VE) is the proportion of disease prevented by the vaccine in vaccinated individuals (Varughese 1981). (This is equivalent to saying the proportion of disease in unvaccinated individuals that is attributable to being unvaccinated is the attributable fraction when nonvaccination is the factor.) Thus in order to calculate vaccine efficacy, subtract the rate of disease in vaccinated animals from the rate in unvaccinated animals and express the difference as a fraction or percentage of the rate of disease in unvaccinated animals. If these rates are available, vaccine efficacy is easily calculated. However, there are a number of instances where these rates are unavailable although estimates of vaccine efficacy would be quite useful. One example is the determination of the efficacy of oral vaccination of foxes against rabies. If the oral rabies vaccine was marked with tetracycline, it is possible to assess whether an animal ate the vaccine by noting fluorescence in the bones or teeth of these animals. Thus, regular fox kills and/or foxes found dead can be examined for the presence of rabies and their vaccine status. The results can be portrayed in a 2 × 2 table, as per a case-control study, and the percent of rabid foxes that were unvaccinated can be compared to the percent of nonrabid foxes that were unvaccinated, using the odds ratio. An estimate of the vaccine's efficacy is then obtained from the odds ratio using the formula for estimated attributable fraction (Table 5.6). For example, suppose the following data were obtained:

| | Health status of foxes | |
	Rabid	Nonrabid
Unvaccinated	18	30
Vaccinated	12	46
	30	76

The odds ratio is 2.3. Hence VE = AF is 57%. That is 57% of the rabies in unvaccinated animals was due to not being vaccinated. A major assumption in using this method is that vaccinated animals are no more or less likely to be submitted to the laboratory (in this instance, found dead or killed by hunters) than unvaccinated animals. Provided this assumption is reasonable, this approach should benefit veterinarians in private practice as well as those in diagnostic laboratories. In both instances, by noting the history of vaccination of cases and comparing this to the history of vaccination in noncases, some idea of the potential efficacy of vaccines under field conditions could be obtained.

When production is the dependent variable, the effect of the disease on production is measured by the absolute difference between the level of production in the diseased and nondiseased group.

5.3.3 Effect of Factor in Population

When disease is the dependent variable, the importance of a causal factor in the population is determined by multiplying its effect (the attributable rate) by the prevalence of the factor. This is called the population attributable rate (PAR), and it provides a direct estimate of the rate of disease in the population due to the factor (Table 5.6). In cross-sectional studies, the PAR may be obtained directly by subtracting the rate of disease in the unexposed group from the estimate of the average rate of disease in the population.

The proportion of disease in the population that is attributable to the factor is called the population attributable fraction (PAF) or etiologic fraction. This is easily calculated from data resulting from cross-sectional studies, and also may be estimated from case-control studies provided the control group is representative of the nondiseased group in the population. (This is unlikely to be true if matching or exclusion were used in selecting the groups under study.) Neither the population attributable rate nor fraction is obtainable directly in cohort studies unless the prevalence (or incidence) of exposure or disease in the population is known.

The total impact of a disease on production is found in an analogous manner; the effect of the disease is multiplied by the total number of cases of the disease.

5.4   Causal Inference in Observational Studies

Although the previous measures of association are easily calculated, their interpretation is based upon certain assumptions. When interpreting attributable rates and attributable fractions, one assumes that a cause and effect relationship exists. However, since a statistical association by itself does not represent a causal association, these statistics need to be interpreted with caution.

A first step in determining causation is to note the sampling method used to collect the data, because some sampling methods are better for demonstrating causation than others. For example, cohort studies are subject to fewer biases than case-control studies, and the temporal relationship between the independent variable (factor) and the dependent variable (disease) is more easily identified than in case-control or cross-sectional studies.

Second, note how refined the independent and dependent variables are. One may refine dependent variables by using cause-specific outcomes rather than crude morbidity, mortality, or culling statistics. This refinement should strengthen the association between the factor and outcome of interest if the association is causal. For example in calves, ration changes might be strongly associated with death from fibrinous pneumonia but not with death from infectious thromboembolic meningoencephalitis (ITEME). Thus, an original association between crude mortality rates and ration changes would become numerically stronger for mortality from fibrinous pneumonia and weaker or nonexistent for mortality from ITEME. At the same time, the independent variable can be refined to make it more specific. Such refinement could take many dimensions. The timing of exposure (e.g., ration changes) could be restricted to specified intervals, the energy content of the ration might be calculated and compared, or the total intake of ration might be noted. All of these refinements are designed to localize and identify the timing, nature, and possible reasons for the association under investigation.

The third step is to seek other variables that might produce or explain the observed association or lack of association. A search may reveal more direct causes of disease whereas in other instances, variables that can distort the association may be discovered. The latter are called confounding variables.

5.4.1 Confounding Variables and Their Control

As a working definition, a confounding variable is one associated with the independent variable and the dependent variable under study. Usually, confounding variables are themselves determinants of the disease under study, and such variables if ignored can distort the observed association. Preventing this bias is a major objective of the design and/or analysis of observational studies.

Confounding is a common phenomenon, and many host variables (such as age and sex) may be confounding variables. For example, age is related to castration and to the occurrence of some diseases such as feline urologic syndrome. Thus, the effects of age must be taken into account when investigating possible relationships between castration and feline urological syndrome. Age is also related to the occurrence of mastitis and the level of milk production in dairy cows. Thus, age must be considered when examining the effect of mastitis on milk production.

An example of confounding is shown in Table 5.8. Although the data are fictitious, the example is concerned with an important problem: how to identify the association between one organism and disease in the presence of other microorganisms, using observational study methods. The objective of the study is to investigate the possible association between the presence of staphylococci and mastitis in dairy cows. Streptococcal organisms represent the confounding variable, in that they are associated with the occurrence of mastitis and with the presence or absence of staphylococcal organisms. A cohort study of the association between the presence of staphylococci and mastitis that ignores the presence of streptococcal organisms will yield biased results; a relative risk of 4 is obtained, when the true value is 3. (The same bias would occur in cross-sectional or case-control studies.) The amount of bias in this example is not too serious in biological terms, because the distortion is not large. However, confounding may produce an association that is apparently very strong or mask a real association. Thus, it is important to prevent this distortion whenever possible.

In observational studies, three methods are available for controlling confounding: exclusion, matching, and analysis. The methods are not mutually exclusive, and two or more of them may be used in the same study.

Table 5.8. Population structure with respect to the distribution of staphylococci (STA), streptococci (STR) and mastitis (M) in dairy cows

Organisms		Number of cows		
STA	STR	with mastitis	Number of cows	Rate of mastitis (%)
+	+	4800	40,000	12
+	−	1200	20,000	6
−	+	400	10,000	4
−	−	600	30,000	2
		7000	100,000	7

In this fictitious population, the rate of mastitis actually is tripled by STA infection (i.e., 12/4 or 6/2); however, this result is obtained only after knowing and accounting for the distribution and effects of STR. If STR is ignored, it would appear that the presence of STA quadruples the rate of disease (10%/2.5%). (10% is the average rate of mastitis in STA-infected cows and 2.5% is the average rate of mastitis in STA-free cows.) For example, suppose a cohort study is performed using $n = 2000$; i.e., 1000 cows STA + and 1000 STA −. For the time being, the status of each cow with respect to STR will be ignored and it is also assumed that there is no sampling error. Under these conditions the anticipated results are:

	$M+$	$M-$	Total	Rate of $M+$ (%)	RR
STA +	100	900	1000	10	4
STA −	25	975	1000	2.5	...

STA apparently quadruples the rate of $M+$. The unknown but unequal numbers of STR + and STR − cows within each STA category have confounded or biased the results. If the STR status of each cow in the sample had been noted, the data could be displayed as follows:

		$M+$	$M-$	Total	Rate of M (%)	RR
STR +	STA +	80	587	667	12	3
	STA −	10	240	250	4	...
		90	827	917		
STR −	STA +	20	313	333	6	3
	STA −	15	735	750	2	...
		35	1048	1083		

By stratifying the data according to the levels of the confounding variable STR (prior to analysis), the distortion due to the distribution and effects of STR has been prevented.

Exclusion (i.e., restricted sampling) may be used to prevent confounding by selecting animals or sampling units with only one level of the confounding variable. Since all units possess (or do not possess) the confounding variable(s), any effects due to these variables are excluded, and no distortion can occur. In general, units that do not possess the confounding variable are preferable over those that do. Exclusion may be used in all study designs, but since the resulting sample is no longer representative of the total population, inferences about the importance of the association — as measured by population attributable fraction — cannot be made unless additional data are available.

Matching may be used to equalize the frequency of the confounding variable in the two groups being compared, effectively neutralizing the distorting effects of the confounding variable(s). Only a few variables known to be strong determinants of the disease should be selected for matching, or it may be difficult to find units with the appropriate combination of variables. Matching is not applicable to cross-sectional studies.

In cohort studies, the usual procedure for matching is to select the exposed group (possessing the putative cause) and then to select the unexposed group in an appropriate manner to balance the distribution of the confounding variable(s) in the exposed and unexposed groups. One method is to select as the first nonexposed unit a unit with the same level(s) of the confounding variable(s) as the first exposed unit. The second unexposed unit is matched to the second exposed unit and so on, until the unexposed group selection is completed. In case-control studies an analogous procedure is used, the cases being selected first and then the controls; the selection of the latter being restricted to noncases possessing the appropriate level(s) of the confounding variable(s). In prospective studies the unexposed (or nondiseased) group can be selected in concert with the exposed group; there is no need to wait until the exposed (or diseased) group is completely selected before selecting the referent group. Matching in case-control studies may not prevent all distortion from confounding variables, although the remaining bias is usually small. In case-control studies, care is required when identifying variables for matching, since if the variables identified as potential confounding variables are not true determinants or predictors of the disease, the power of the statistics (chi-square) may be reduced. Matching is also used in experiments to increase precision and is referred to as "blocking." When matching is used, the analysis of results should be modified to take account of the matching; for example, by using the chi-square and t-tests for correlated data (see Tables 5.3 and 5.5).

The third method, analytic control of confounding, is frequently used in observational studies. When data are collected about the study units concerning the putative factor and/or disease, data are also collected on the presence or absence of the potential confounding variable(s). The data are then stratified and displayed in a series of 2×2 tables; one table for each level of the confounding variable, as was done in the mastitis example in Table 5.8. Each table is analyzed separately and, if deemed appropriate, a summary measure of association may be used.

The most frequently used method to summarize associations in multiple tables is known as the Mantel-Haenszel technique, and its use is demonstrated in Table 5.9 (Mantel and Haenszel 1959; Kleinbaum et al. 1982). By setting out the appropriate column headings and displaying the data in the manner shown, the calculations required for this procedure are easily performed. (The odds ratio is used as the measure of association because it may be applied to data resulting from any of the three observational analytic study types.) The summary odds ratio is often called an adjusted odds ratio, and the confounding variable(s) controlled in the analysis should be explicitly stated when reporting results. For example, using the data in Table 5.8 one can calculate an odds ratio describing the association between staphylococcal organisms and mastitis, controlling for the effects of streptococcal organisms. (You can verify from Table 5.9 that the summary odds ratio will have a value close to 3.) An advantage of this technique is that the strength of association between streptococcal organisms and mastitis (controlling for staphylococci) may be determined using the same data. A disadvantage is that it requires very large data sets if the number of confounding variables is large; otherwise, many of the table entries will be zero. Also,

Table 5.9.   The Mantel-Haenszel method for calculating a summary odds ratio

Since there will be two or more 2×2 tables, the data display in the ith table will be:

	Diseased	Nondiseased	Total
Exposed	a	b	$a + b$
Unexposed	c	d	$c + d$
	$a + c$	$b + d$	$n = (a + b + c + d)$

The subscript i which accompanies each of the above cell frequencies or totals has been omitted for clarity.

In each 2×2 table the expected value of a is $E(a) = (a + b) \times (a + c)/n$ and the variance of a is $V(a) = (a + b) \times (c + d) \times (a + c) \times (b + d)/n^2(n - 1)$.

For each table calculate $E(a)$, $V(a)$, ad/n and bc/n as well as their respective sums; the summation being across all of the tables.

The summary odds ratio is:

$$OR = (\Sigma ad/n)/(\Sigma bc/n)$$

and the overall chi-square statistic with one degree of freedom is:

$$\chi^2 = (|\Sigma a - \Sigma E(a)| - 0.5)^2/\Sigma V(a)$$

The latter tests whether the sample OR departs significantly from the null value of one. Applying these calculations to the data in Table 5.8 one obtains

Table(i)	a	$E(a)$	$V(a)$	ad/n	bc/n	OR
1	80	65.50	16.11	20.94	6.40	3.27
2	20	10.76	7.22	13.57	4.34	3.13
	100	76.26	23.33	34.51	10.74	

Summary: $OR = 34.51/10.74 = 3.21$
$$\chi^2 = (|100 - 76.26| - 0.5)^2/23.33 = 23.2$$

Because of the size of the calculated χ^2 versus 3.84, we can safely conclude that STA and M are associated, specifically that STA-infected cows are 3.21 times more likely to have M than STA-negative cows. (The reason this is not 3 exactly is because, although the tables both have RR = 3, the OR are not equal, being 3.27 and 3.13 respectively, and their weighted average becomes 3.21.)

because each table provides an odds ratio statistic, it is sometimes difficult to know if differences in odds ratios between tables are due to sampling error or real differences in degree of association. Tests have been developed to evaluate the significance of differences in odds ratios among tables (Kleinbaum et al. 1982). In general, one should be reasonably sure that the strength of association is similar in all tables before using the Mantel-Haenszel technique for summarization purposes.

5.5 Criteria of Judgment in Causal Inference

If an association persists after careful consideration of the study design, a search for additional variables, and control of confounding variables, the following guidelines may be used to assess the likelihood that an association (arising from an analytic study) is causal. (Here "likelihood" is used in a qualitative rather than a quantitative sense.) These criteria of judgment are in addition to the guidelines set out earlier (5.1). In fact, these criteria resulted from attempts to logically assess the association between smoking and lung cancer. Further details on judgment criteria are available (Susser 1973, 1977).

5.5.1 Time Sequence

It is obvious that for a factor to cause a disease it must precede the disease. This criterion is automatically met in experiments and well-designed prospective cohort studies. However, in many cross-sectional and case-control studies it is difficult to establish the temporal relationship. For example, many studies have indicated that cystic ovarian disease is associated with high milk production in dairy cows. Yet in terms of causation, the question is whether cystic ovarian follicles precede or follow high milk production, or whether they are both a result of a common cause. Another example is the association between ration changes and increased morbidity rates in feedlot cattle. For causation, the question is whether the ration changes precede or follow increased morbidity rates. In this instance and perhaps others involving feedback mechanisms, both may be true.

5.5.2 Strength of Association

In observational analytic studies, strength is measured by relative risk or odds ratio statistics. The greater the departure of these statistics from unity, the more likely the association is to be causal. Although no explicit statistic is used when production is the dependent variable, the relative difference in level of production between animals with and without a particular disease may be used to assess the likelihood of the disease producing the observed differences. Strength is used as an indication of a causal association because for a confounding variable to produce or nullify an association between the putative factor and the disease, that confounding variable must have just as strong an association with the disease. In this event, the effects of the confounding variable would likely be known prior to the study, and some effort to control its effects would be incorporated into the study design. Although the attributable fraction and/or the population attributable fraction are not used as direct measures of strength, they should be borne in mind when interpreting the size of the relative risk or odds ratio. Thus, a given odds ratio could be given more credence if the population attributable fraction was large rather than small.

5.5.3 Dose-Response Relationship

This criterion is an extension of Mill's canon concerning the method of concomitant variation. An association is more likely to be causal if the frequency of disease varies directly with the amount of exposure. (This argument was used in the previous chapter when making inferences about patterns of disease with age.) Also, changes in productivity should directly follow the severity of the disease if the disease is a cause of decreased production. Thus, if eating large volumes of concentrates is a causal factor for left displaced abomasum in dairy cows, one would expect a higher rate of left displaced abomasum in cows fed relatively large amounts of concentrates compared to those fed relatively small amounts of concentrates. This criterion is not an absolute one, because there are some diseases where one would not necessarily expect a monotonic dose-response relationship (e.g., where a threshold of exposure was required to cause the disease).

5.5.4 Coherence

An association is more likely to be causal if it is biologically sensible. However, an association that is not biologically plausible (given the current state of knowledge) may still be correct, and should not be automatically discarded. Further, since almost any association is explainable after the fact, it is useful to predict the nature of the expected association and explain its biological meaning prior to analyzing the data. This is particularly important during initial research, when one is collecting information on a large number of unrefined factors to see if any are associated with the disease.

5.5.5 Consistency

Consistency of results is a major criterion of judgment relative to causal associations, and in many regards is the modern equivalent to Mill's "method of agreement." An association gains credibility if it is supported by similar findings in different studies under different conditions. Thus, consistent results in a number of studies are the observational study equivalent of replication in experimental work. (Also, because field trials are not immune to the effects of uncontrolled factors, replication of field trials is sometimes required to provide additional confidence that the results are valid.)

As an example of using the consistency criterion consider that in the first year of a health study of beef feedlot cattle, an association between feeding corn silage within 2 weeks of arrival and increased mortality rates was noted. Such a finding had not been reported before and was not anticipated. Thus, the likelihood it was a causal association was small. During the second year of the study, this association was again observed, giving increased confidence that the association might be, in fact, causal. During the third year, no association was noted between morbidity or mortality rates and feeding of corn silage. On the surface this tended to reduce the validity of the previously observed association. However, it was noted that during the third year of the health study the majority of feedlot owners using corn silage had delayed its introduction into the ration until the calves had been in the feedlot for at least 2 weeks. Thus, because of this consistency it was considered very likely that the association between early feeding of corn silage and increased levels of morbidity and/or mortality in feedlot calves was causal in nature (Martin et al. 1981, 1982).

5.5.6 Specificity of Association

At one time, perhaps because of the influence of the Henle-Koch postulates, it was assumed that an association was more likely to be causal if the putative cause appeared to produce only one or a few effects. Today, this criterion is not widely used because it is known that a single cause (particularly if unrefined) may produce a number of effects. Specificity of association may be of more value in studies where the factor and disease variables are highly refined. In initial studies when variables are often composite in nature, the application of this criterion is likely to be unrewarding.

The previous criteria of judgment should be helpful when inferring causation based on results of analytic observational studies. These criteria are less frequently applied to results of experiments, although with the exception of time sequence they remain useful guidelines for drawing causal inferences from experimental data also.

5.6 Elaborating Causal Mechanisms

If an association is assumed to be causal, it should prove fruitful to investigate the nature of the association. There are a variety of ways of doing this; some are highly correlated with the manner of classifying the disease. Nonetheless, knowledge of details of the nature of an association can often be helpful in preventing the disease of concern.

Initially, it is useful to sketch out conceptually or on paper the way various factors are presumed to lead to disease. Such models invariably are quite general, but can be progressively refined and appropriate details added as new information is gained. As an aid to this modeling process, the concepts of indirect and direct causation as well as necessary and sufficient causes will be described.

5.6.1 Indirect versus Direct Causes

For a factor to be a direct cause of a disease there must be no known intervening variable between that factor and the disease, and both the independent and dependent variables must be measured at the same level of organization. All other causes are indirect causes (Susser 1973). Although researchers often seek to identify the most direct or proximate cause of a disease, it may be easier to control disease by manipulating indirect rather than direct causes. For example, although living agents or toxic substances are direct causes of many diseases, it may be easier to manipulate indirect factors such as management or housing to prevent the disease. Furthermore, whether intervening variables are present often represents only the current state of knowledge. In the 1800s the lack of citrus fruits was correctly considered a direct cause of scurvy in humans. Later with the discovery of vitamin C, the lack of citrus fruits became an indirect cause of the disease. Finding the more direct cause of the condition allowed other avenues of preventing the disease (e.g., synthetic ascorbic acid), but did not greatly reduce the importance of citrus fruits per se in preventing scurvy.

The second condition for direct causation—that the independent and dependent variables be measured at the same level of organization—may need some elaboration. If one is interested in the cause(s) of a disease of pigs as individuals, and the study has used pens of pigs or some other grouping as the sampling unit, the factor under investigation can, at best, be an indirect cause of that disease. For example, a study might find that pigs housed in buildings with forced air ventilation systems have more respiratory disease than those housed in buildings without forced air ventilation systems. This finding might be regarded as a direct cause of the difference in the rate of respiratory disease among groups of pigs, but only as an indirect cause of respiratory disease in individual pigs. In addition, while it may make sense to say that a particular group of pigs had more respiratory disease because they were raised in a building with a forced air ventilation system, it makes less sense to say that a particular pig had respiratory disease because it was raised in a building with a forced air ventilation system. The study has failed to describe the effect of ventilation on the occurrence of the disease at the individual pig level. Despite this lack of knowledge, however, respiratory disease might easily be controlled by manipulating the ventilation system.

Many diseases have both direct and indirect effects on productivity.

Consider retained fetal membranes, postpartum metritis, and their effects on the parturition-to-conception interval. Retained membranes appear to have a direct adverse effect on the ability to conceive; this effect being present in cows without metritis. Retained membranes also have a large indirect effect on conception; this effect being mediated via postpartum metritis. Thus, if it was possible to prevent retained fetal membranes, conception would be improved and the occurrence of postpartum metritis greatly reduced. If it was possible to prevent only postpartum metritis, the negative indirect effects of retained membranes could be prevented.

5.6.2 Necessary and Sufficient Causes

Another dimension for classifying determinants is as necessary or sufficient causes (Rothman 1976). A necessary cause is one without which the disease can not occur. Few single factors are necessary causes, except in the anatomically or etiologically defined diseases. For example, pasteurella organisms are a necessary cause of pasteurellosis but not of pneumonia; *E. coli* is a necessary cause of colibacillosis but not of diarrhea. (Pneumonia and diarrhea are manifestationally not etiologically classified syndromes.) In contrast to a necessary cause, a sufficient cause is one that always produces the disease. Again, single factors infrequently are sufficient causes. Today it is accepted that almost all sufficient causes are composed of a grouping of factors, each called a component cause; hence most diseases have a multifactorial etiology. By definition, necessary causes are a component of every sufficient cause. In general usage, *Pasteurella* spp. are "the cause" of pasteurellosis, yet a sufficient cause of pasteurellosis requires at least the lack of immunity plus the presence of pasteurella organisms.

In practical terms, the identification of all the components of a sufficient cause is not essential to prevent the disease, just as it is not essential to know the direct cause of a disease in order to prevent it. If one key component of the sufficient cause is removed, the remaining components are rendered insufficient and are unable to produce the disease. Most putative causal factors are components of one or more sufficient causes.

A description of hypothetical necessary and sufficient causes in the context of pneumonic pasteurellosis of cattle is presented in Figure 5.1. In sufficient cause I, it is argued that an animal that lacks humoral immunity to pasteurella, that is stressed (e.g., by weaning and transportation), and that is infected with pasteurella will develop pneumonic pasteurellosis. Sufficient cause II implies that an animal infected with viruses or mycoplasma and pasteurella and lacking pasteurella-specific antibodies will develop pneumonic pasteurellosis. Sufficient causes III and IV have similar components, with lack of cellular immunity replacing lack of humoral antibody as a component. Note that the four sufficient causes all contain the necessary cause, pasteurella organisms. Thus, this method of conceptualizing a suffi-

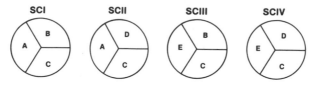

5.1. Hypothetical sufficient causes (SC) for pneumonic pasteurellosis. A = lack of specific globulins; B = adrenal stress of environmental origin, i.e., weather, water, energy, social; C = presence of *Pasteurella* spp; D = presence of viral/mycoplasma agents; E = lack of cellular immunity.

cient cause, although greatly oversimplified, provides a formal, rational way of conceptualizing and understanding the multietiologic causation of pneumonic pasteurellosis. A similar approach can be used with other diseases.

The concept of sufficient causes (SC), each composed of two or more components, has practical utility in relation to explaining quantitative measures of a factor's impact on disease occurrence, such as the population attributable fraction. Using the example in Figure 5.1, assume that SCI produces 40% of all pasteurellosis, SCII 30%, SCIII 20%, and SCIV 10%, and that these sufficient causes account for all occurrences of pneumonic pasteurellosis. The percentage explained by or attributable to each of the factors is:

A: 40% + 30% = 70%
B: 40% + 20% = 60%
C: 40% + 30% + 20% + 10% = 100%
D: 30% + 10% = 40%
E: 20% + 10% = 30%

Each of these represents the population attributable fraction ($\times 100$) for each factor; factor C, being a necessary cause, explains all of the occurrence of pasteurellosis; whereas adrenal stress (factor B) explains only 60% of pasteurellosis. The total percent explained by the five factors exceeds 100% because each factor is a member of more than one sufficient cause. Using this concept of PAF, one could estimate that preventing infection with viruses or mycoplasma (e.g., by vaccination) would reduce the total occurrence of pasteurellosis by 40%.

5.6.3 Path Models of Causation

Path models represent another way of conceptualizing, analyzing, and demonstrating the causal effects of multiple factors. In a path model, the variables are ordered temporally from left to right, and causal effects flow along the arrows and paths. Statistical methods are used to estimate the relative magnitude (path coefficients) of each arrow. In addition to the knowledge acquired by constructing them, path models give increased power to the analysis and interpretation of the data.

The previous component causes of pasteurellosis are displayed in a path model in Figure 5.2. In this model, stress is assumed to occur before (and influence) humoral and cellular immunity, which occur before viral and bacterial infection of the lung. The model implies that factors A and E (humoral and cellular immunity) are independent events (i.e., the presence or absence of one does not influence the presence or absence of the other). Because C is a necessary cause, all the arrows (causal pathways) pass through it.

Numerical estimates of the magnitude of the causal effect (passing along each arrow) are determined using a statistical technique known as least-squares regression analysis; odds ratios may be used in simple models. If the magnitude of an effect is trivial, it may be assumed to be zero and the model can then be simplified. The value of these coefficients is influenced by the structure of the model itself, as well as the causal dependency between factors, thus emphasizing the importance of using a realistic biologic model. Path models actually describe the logical outcome of a particular model; they do not assist materially in choosing the correct model.

An example of a simple path model, relating waterflow, percentage of the stream bottom that was bare mud, and the softness of the mud (flocculence) to the number and species of snail in that stream is shown in Figure 5.3 (Harris and Charleston 1977). The snails serve as intermediate hosts for *Fasciola hepatica*, and a quote from the authors describes the reasons for the structure of the chosen model:

Water was assumed to affect snail numbers directly, as well as via mud and flocculence, since both these factors are partly determined by the amount of water present. The amount of mud was also expected to influence snails directly, but

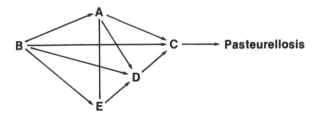

5.2. Structural model of pneumonic pasteurellosis based on the causal factors in Fig. 5.1.

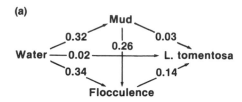

(a)

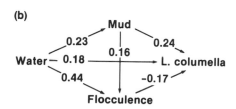

(b)

5.3. Path diagrams of the hypothesized effect of water, mud, and flocculence on population density of (a) *L. tomentosa* and (b) *L. columella* in March microhabitats. (Source: Harris and Charleston 1977)

larger areas of mud were less likely to contain vegetation and so were more likely to be flocculent; hence the indirect path from mud to snails via flocculence.

Broadly speaking, the results of the path models substantiated these assumptions. However, the authors' specific comments are informative and point out the value of this approach; they report

The main difference between snail species is the association with flocculence; flocculent mud appears to favor *L. tomentosa*, whereas *L. columella* seem to prefer firm mud. The overall effect of mud on snail numbers appears to operate differently too. The proportion of bare mud influences *L. columella* numbers directly, but the main effect on *L. tomentosa* is indirect, via the increased flocculence of muddy habitats. Increasing water cover affects *L. tomentosa* numbers indirectly, by increasing the area of flocculent mud. Water has some direct effect on *L. columella* as well as an indirect effect via mud; the indirect path via flocculence has a negative effect.

5.6.4 Displaying Effects of Multiple Factors

Methods for displaying rather than investigating the effects of two or three variables on the risk of disease need to be utilized and improved as an aid to communicating the effects of multiple factors between researchers, and between practitioners and their clients. One method is based on the Venn diagram approach and is particularly useful when the risk values increase steadily with increases in the number of putative causal factors. Examples are shown in Figures 5.4 and 5.5. Basically, the method involves

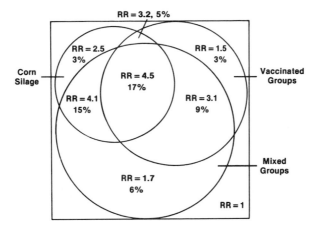

5.4. Association between number and type of factor and risk of excessive mortality in feedlot calves. Area of each circle represents proportion of calf groups experiencing that factor. RR = relative risk of mortality. Percentage of deaths attributable to each factor grouping is shown; approximately 57% of deaths were attributable to the 3 factors. (Source: Martin et al. 1981, with permission)

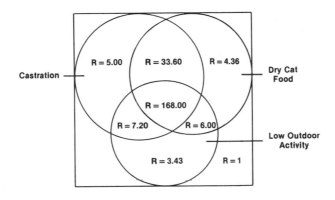

5.5. Venn diagram of 3 high risk factors for feline urological syndrome in male cats. Area of each circle represents proportion of cats experiencing that factor. R = estimated relative risk. (Source: Willeberg 1977, with permission)

calculating the relative risk or odds ratio of disease for each possible combination of variables relative to the lowest risk group. The diameter of the circle representing each factor is drawn proportional to the prevalence of that factor, and one attempts to keep the overlap (the area of intersection) proportional to the prevalence of that combination of variables.

References

Evans, A. S. 1978. Causation and disease: A chronological journey. Am. J. Epidemiol. 108:249–58.

Harris, R. E., and W. A. G. Charleston. 1977. An examination of the marsh microhabitats of *Lymnaea tomentosa* and *L. columella* (Mollusca: Gastropoda) by path analysis. N.Z. J. Zool. 4:395–99.

Kleinbaum, D. G., L. L. Kupper, and H. Morgenstern. 1982. Epidemiologic Research: Principles and Quantitative Methods. Belmont, Calif.: Wadsworth.

MacMahon, B., and T. F. Pugh. 1970. Epidemiology: Principles and Methods. Boston, Mass.: Little, Brown.

Mantel, N., and W. Haenszel. 1959. Statistical aspects of the analysis of data from retrospective studies of disease. J. Natl. Cancer Inst. 22:719–48.

Martin, S. W., A. H. Meek, D. G. Davis, J. A. Johnson, and R. A. Curtis. 1981. Factors associated with morbidity and mortality in feedlot calves: The Bruce County beef project, year two. Can. J. Comp. Med. 45:103–12.

_____. 1982. Factors associated with mortality and treatment costs in feedlot calves: The Bruce County beef project, years 1978, 1979, 1980. Can. J. Comp. Med. 46:341–49.

Rothman, K. J. 1976. Causes. Am. J. Epidemiol. 104:587–92.

Snedecor, G. W., and W. G. Cochran. 1980. Statistical Methods. 7th ed. Ames: Iowa State Univ. Press.

Susser, M. 1973. Causal Thinking in the Health Sciences: Concepts and Strategies in Epidemiology. Toronto, Canada: Oxford Univ. Press.

_____. 1977. Judgment and causal inference: Criteria in epidemiologic studies. Am. J. Epidemiol. 105:1–5.

Varughese, P. 1981. Vaccine efficacy. Can. Dis. Weekly Rep. 7:47–48.

Waltner-Toews, D. 1983. Evaluating risk from a 2×2 table: Five useful measures. Can. Vet. J. 24:86–88.

Willeberg, P. 1977. Animal disease information processing: Epidemiologic analyses of the feline urological syndrome. Acta Vet. Scand. Suppl. 64:1–48.

C H A P T E R __6__

Surveys and Analytic Observational Studies

All epidemiologic studies involve data collection, manipulation, and analysis. In general, the more organized these functions are, the easier the task will be. Also, appropriate data collection can improve the accuracy and precision of the data. Thus, the basic considerations necessary for the design of observational studies are described in this chapter. A discussion of the uses and limitations of animal disease surveillance is provided in Chapter 11, and applications of analytic studies are presented in Chapter 12.

6.1 Principles of Surveys and Data Collection

The nature of the study and the setting in which the data will be collected will influence the design and structure of the data recording form or questionnaire (Woodward et al. 1982). At the very least, all studies require a well-planned data collection form. Simple forms will suffice if the investigator is collecting and recording data from only a few sources (such as medical history sheets) or for recording the results of field experiments. More care and planning are required when the data to be collected are complex or the investigator is not in direct control of data (e.g., in a survey involving personal interviews or in a mailed questionnaire). For reasons described subsequently, the investigator may not wish to specify the actual objective of the study on the survey form; nonetheless objectives should be stated explicitly as part of the investigator's plan of research.

6.1.1 Title of the Study

Appearing at the top of the survey form, the title should be clear and sufficiently detailed to inform collaborators of the general purpose of the survey. Consider the following two titles as examples: "Sow Survey" versus "Diseases of Sows During Pregnancy." In most cases, the latter title would be preferred. It is not necessary however to provide specific details in the title. In fact, sometimes it is desirable to keep the collaborators blind as to the exact purpose of the survey in order to prevent biased answers. For example, questions in the survey might relate to a number of diseases as well as management or housing factors, although one syndrome (say metritis, mastitis, or agalactia) is the primary objective of the study. If the survey form is mailed to collaborators, a brief cover letter should be included.

6.1.2 Questions

Frequently the most important step in solving a problem is knowing what question(s) to ask. Questions should be clearly worded, straightforward, and necessary (Woodward and Chambers 1980). Initially, it is useful to list all of the factors about which information is required; then structure the questions so that the answer(s) to each question provides the appropriate data. If ventilation is of interest, the investigator must consider what specific information about ventilation is required. The presence or absence of fans would provide some information, the number and sizes of fans other information, and the method of controlling the fans still other information. At least one question would be required to obtain data on each of these dimensions that describe the ventilation.

Another useful approach to identify needed questions is to construct in advance the tables necessary to meet the study objectives, then cross-check these with the data that will be obtained from the recording form. This will help ensure that the appropriate questions are asked, and that all questions asked are required.

Often in preliminary studies where questions concern a broad range of factors (so-called "data snooping surveys") it is useful to record in advance the interpretation to be placed on all of the associations that may be observed. That is, should the number of fans be positively or negatively correlated with the rate of disease? Why? Should the rate of disease differ depending on whether automatic or manual switches are used to control the fans? If so, how should it differ? The rationale behind this exercise is the more questions asked the greater the likelihood of finding at least one factor significantly associated with the disease. Most associations between unrefined factors and disease are explainable after the fact; yet there must be some explanations that are, a priori, more sensible than others. For example, one might initially hypothesize an inverse relationship (a negative correlation or an odds ratio of less than one) between the presence of fans and the level of respiratory disease. Presumably such a hypothesis relates to the maintenance of acceptable temperature and humidity levels, as well as the removal of dust and microorganisms from the air. However, suppose a positive association is observed. How does one interpret it? In general, it is preferable not to ignore observed associations, but associations running counter to the initial explanation should be viewed with some skepticism until they are validated.

6.1.3 Sequence of Questions

Questions should be grouped according to subject matter or another logical basis such as the temporal relationship of events. This will help orient the collaborator's mind to the task at hand. General surveys might be structured on the basis of major factor categories such as housing, ration, management, etc. On the other hand, if the survey is concerned with events related to the neonatal period or to the period after arrival in the herd, flock, or feedlot, sequencing the questions on a temporal basis might be more useful.

6.1.4 Format of the Record Form

The layout of the recording form should assist the analysis and/or computer entry of data. Excess transcription of data should be avoided; each time a number is written down the probability of introducing an error increases. A useful format guideline is to keep the answers in an obvious column, usually at the extreme right side of the page. Also, to ease data entry it is useful to record the column number from the computer file next to the datum when using fixed field data entry. In other cases, the question number can specify the column where the datum is to be located in the file. If a recording form contains a lot of data that will not be analyzed (at least initially), the data to be entered may be highlighted with special colored pens. Although recent advances in interactive computer programs reduce data entry problems, these suggestions will be useful nonetheless.

6.1.5 Framing the Questions

Asking questions correctly is as much an art as it is a science (Woodward and Chambers 1980). Nonetheless, certain principles should be followed. Avoid asking leading questions; the question should begin with "Do you," not "You do." Make sure there is an obvious answer to each question, usually by providing a list of acceptable answers. In general, open-ended questions should be avoided. For example, the question "Ventilation system?" is too vague. It could be interpreted as requiring a yes-no answer for the presence or absence of a ventilating system, a judgment of the system's adequacy, a description of the fans, inlets, etc., or a host of other interpretations.

The terminology used in the question should be appropriate for the collaborators. For example, one probably should not ask a dairy farmer, Did the cow abort? but rather, Was the calf born dead? and How many months was the cow pregnant? Besides providing more detailed information, these two questions avoid confusion about the meaning of the term abortion. Usually, animal owners may be questioned about clinical entities (such as scours or coughing) but not about entities classified on the basis of pathologic criteria (such as enteritis or pneumonia).

Some questions will have a set of mutually exclusive and exhaustive categories of answers (i.e., there is only one acceptable answer to a question and all possible answers are included). For example, in specifying "breed," each animal must fit into one and only one category. Thus all possible breeds should be specified, or the more common breeds might be listed with a final category of "other breed." If more than one answer is acceptable (e.g., an Angus-Hereford cross), nonexclusive categories are required. Other examples of nonexclusive categories relate to questions about ration content or the signs of disease. These are nonexclusive because the ration usually has more than one component, and there is usually more than one sign of disease. Although nonexclusive categories simplify the design of the recording form, they present problems in the analytic phase because of the potentially large number of combinations of answers.

A partial solution to these problems is that it may be sufficient to collect data only on the major ration component(s) or the major presenting sign(s). In other instances, a set of nonexclusive answers can be made exclusive (e.g., by asking Is the animal coughing? or Is the animal eating normally?). Another way of circumventing this is to list all possible combinations of categories (although this is usually not advisable because the list becomes too long). In the latter instance one can assign a numeric code to each possible single answer in such a manner that the sum of all possible answers produces a unique number, representing each particular combination of individual factors. For example, if there are five possible breeds, they could be coded 1, 2, 4, 8, and 16. Crossbred animals may be identified by using the sum of the numbers denoting the appropriate breeds. If an animal is a cross between the first and third breed listed, it would be coded as 5. The latter is more useful when cross-tabulation procedures will be used for analysis than when other methods such as linear regression are planned. Thus, each situation should be assessed individually.

When possible, it is desirable to record the answer as a continuous variable (e.g., the actual age, weight, titer). Grouping can be used if necessary later on. Most computer programs allow the specification of category limits, allowing a more powerful and flexible approach to the analysis than initially using categories such as $2 < 4$, $4 < 6$, and $6 < 8$. Unless it is desired to use a free-field format, when continuous variables are recorded they should be right justified. In a two column answer for age, a 9-year-old should be recorded as –9, or 09, not 9–, since the latter may be read as 90 years old. (A decimal placing could be specified, but this gives an upper limit of 9.9 years on the age if the field has only two columns.)

With numeric codes or answers, missing data must be differentiated from no answer or "unknown." If there can be no answer, the column may be left blank, but if an answer should be given and is not available, a missing value code that will not be confused with valid answers should be used (e.g., 99 or −9 might be used to code for missing age values).

When a long list of possible answers is available, studies have shown a tendency for collaborators to select answers placed early in the list. Two solutions are offered. First, keep the list of answers short. Second, one may use two or three forms of the same questionnaire, and the order of the possible answers can be randomized within each form.

6.1.6 Editing the Data

All recording forms should be edited manually before and/or during computer data entry or manual analyses. Initially, make sure that all required questions are answered and that no inappropriate answers are recorded. This procedure is often necessary when a hierarchy of questions is used. For example, "if the answer is 'yes,' answer the specified subquestions; if the answer is 'no,' proceed to the next major question." (The question number may be specified.) Thus, manual editing should ensure that all appropriate subquestions are answered, and it should also detect any inappropriate answers (e.g., the number of fans may have been recorded although the farmer had stated that none of them was operative).

In large surveys, computer assisted editing can enhance data validity. For example, programs can be devised to check that a cow name and number are valid, that the animal's reported age is consistent with the recorded birth date, that the event specified is biologically feasible, etc. That is, if the cow is recorded pregnant, a diagnosis of metritis is not feasible unless the event "abortion" or "calving" was specified. Computer editing can be expensive however, and judgment is required in the extent of its use. It should not be performed automatically in all cases. The setting in which data entry will occur and the likelihood of entering incorrect data should be considered prior to instituting computer assisted editing. In many cases no computerized editing is necessary; in others, it should be an essential component of data entry.

6.1.7 Pretesting the Survey

Few people can design a perfect survey form in one attempt. Rather, iterative restructuring and rethinking of the questions and layout are required. A guideline about the time required to produce a useful survey is to make an initial careful estimate and then multiply by four or five.

Although framing the questions is an art, the evaluation of the survey during the pretest should be as scientifically rigorous as possible. Initially, one should check to see if the survey is too long, too detailed, or unclear. Then, some attempt should be made to establish the precision (reproducibility) of the survey. This may be done by asking the same question twice during the same interview, or at a different interview. In a mail survey, attempts to elicit the same answer with two different but similar questions may provide evidence on reproducibility and validity of responses.

Note also that each question has its own sensitivity, specificity, and predictive value. Suppose the factor one wishes to obtain information on is the use of a specific vaccine. The sensitivity of the question, Do you use the vaccine? is the proportion of those who actually use the vaccine that answer affirmatively. The specificity is the proportion of those who don't use the vaccine that answer negatively. The predictive value, on the other hand, is the proportion of those who answer affirmatively who actually use the vaccine.

In order to assess the sensitivity and specificity of a question, an independent means of establishing the true state of nature is required. This may require investigative assessments (e.g., a search of the drug pail, inspection of the housing, or examining the feed bunks). One requires both care and tact in these assessments so as not to offend the collaborator. It is useful to remember that all memory (including our own) is often faulty, more frequently by omission than by deliberate action. Although it is best to evaluate a survey keeping the collaborators blind to the evaluation, in many instances it may be necessary to inform the respondents of the pretest.

6.1.8 Analysis

The details of the analysis will depend on the type of data collected as well as on the objectives of the survey. Nonetheless, one should not rush into detailed analyses before inspecting the data thoroughly and performing several simple summaries. This principle should be followed no matter how analytically adept the investigator.

When performing an analysis on a large data file, use only a portion of the data set initially. This will minimize costs if errors exist in the data set or in structuring the analytic program. Also at this stage, it is important to verify that the appropriate number of cases is present for each analysis or subanalysis.

6.1.9 Final Thoughts

Choose a time for data collection convenient for the collaborators. Sometimes this is not possible (e.g., if data relating to events in the period after arrival of calves in a feedlot are required, this is always a busy time). Be aware that the timing of the survey can affect the results. For example, if dairy farmers from California were asked to rank disease in order of importance, calf losses would likely be ranked as important if the interview was in the winter or summer, but less important if the interview was in the early summer or fall. This is due to the seasonal nature of calf losses, not its overall importance.

To ensure consistency, decide who should answer the questions (i.e., should it be the owner, the person who feeds the animals, or the farm manager). Make sure all personnel involved know what is expected of them. Even if only two people administer the study, regular meetings to rehearse the data collection strategies, clear up problem areas, or to reinforce procedures will prove useful.

Finally, every effort should be made to obtain a high level of cooperation. Mail surveys often produce only a 40–50% response rate, whereas more than 80% cooperation is often obtained in personal interview surveys. Unfortunately, the results of a survey with a return rate of less than 70 or 80% are suspect. The reason is that the collaborators are self-selected volunteers and could very well have different opinions, management styles, and levels of disease than those who refuse to collaborate. Thus the general strategy is to select a practical number of individuals for the study and attempt to obtain a high rate of collaboration, rather than selecting two or three times as many potential collaborators and using the results of the 30–40% who choose to volunteer. Strong associations are unlikely to be reversed if the cooperation rate is high; this may be shown by assuming the opposite association exists among all nonrespondents. All associations are suspect if the cooperation rate is low; hence, it should be noted that it is the proportion of prospective collaborators who cooperate, not the absolute number of cooperators, that is important in terms of obtaining valid data.

An excellent critique of the methods used in national surveys of disease occurrence in animals is available (Leech 1971). The use of questionnaire data in smaller scale field studies has also been described (Selby et al. 1973, 1976; Ruppaner 1972; Ruppaner and Goodger 1979). It is particularly interesting to note that observers from different sectors of the industry may rank diseases quite differently in terms of their importance (Ruppaner 1972). An example of the use of mail questionnaire data and its validation are provided by Hutchings and Martin (1983).

6.2 Analytic Observational Studies

A general classification of the types of studies used to test hypotheses are shown in Figure 6.1. A more detailed description of analytic observational study methods is contained in Figure 6.2. General considerations regarding the selection of study type and the sampling schemes appropriate to each study type were explained in Chapter 2. The remainder of this chapter provides an outline of key items to be considered in the design and performance of each type of analytic observational study.

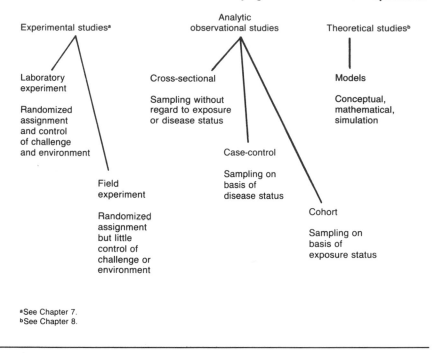

Experimental studies[a]

Laboratory experiment

Randomized assignment and control of challenge and environment

Field experiment

Randomized assignment but little control of challenge or environment

Analytic observational studies

Cross-sectional

Sampling without regard to exposure or disease status

Case-control

Sampling on basis of disease status

Cohort

Sampling on basis of exposure status

Theoretical studies[b]

Models

Conceptual, mathematical, simulation

[a]See Chapter 7.
[b]See Chapter 8.

6.1. Types of studies to test hypotheses.

A chief advantage of analytic studies is that they are directed toward the species of concern in its natural environment. This greatly reduces the problems associated with extrapolating results from a particular study to the target population. It also allows the investigator to test a much broader range of hypotheses than would be possible under controlled experimental conditions. However, it is often necessary to place restrictions on the source and selection of animals, for practical limitations and in order to make the groups to be contrasted comparable, although these restrictions may reduce any investigator's ability to extrapolate results beyond the sample. As a specific example, it is important to concisely and clearly describe the criteria used to define the status of the sampled units with respect to the independent and dependent variables. Although the specific criteria might lead to the exclusion of a few sampling units, without them there would be an increased probability of misclassification of the sampling units, and the validity of the results might be questioned.

For the observational studies discussed here, it is assumed that exposure and disease status are expressed as dichotomous or binary variables. Hence the chi-square test may be used to analyze the relationship between the putative causal factor and disease. In veterinary medicine, since it is also extremely important to quantify the effect of disease on the level of

Type of study		Time	
	Previous	Current	Future
Cross-sectional		n ⟵ $\begin{array}{l} F+?--D+? \\ F-?--D+? \end{array}$	
Prospective longitudinal*		n ⟶ $\begin{array}{l} F+?--D+? \\ F-?--D+? \end{array}$	
Retrospective longitudinal*	$\begin{array}{l} F+?--D+? \\ F-?--D+? \end{array}$ ⟶ n		
Case-control	$\begin{array}{l} F+? \\ F+? \end{array}$ ⟵ $\begin{array}{l} D+ \\ D- \end{array}$		
Prospective cohort		$\begin{array}{l} F+ \\ F- \end{array}$ ⟶ $\begin{array}{l} D+? \\ D+? \end{array}$	
Retrospective cohort	$\begin{array}{l} F+ \to D+? \\ F- \to D+? \end{array}$		

*Implies follow-up over a period of time.

F: presence of factor
D: presence or acquisition of disease
n: arbitrary sample size
?: unknown event at time of initiation of study

6.2. Types of analytic observational studies, according to sampling strategy and temporal events related to the factor and/or disease. F = presence of factor; D = presence or acquisition of disease; n = arbitrary sample size; and ? = unknown event at time of initiation of study.

production, many studies have disease status as the independent variable and level of production as the outcome or dependent variable. In this instance the outcome variable is continuous and the chi-square test is inappropriate (unless one divides production into categories). If the impact of production level on disease occurrence was being investigated, level of production would be the exposure variable and disease occurrence the outcome of interest. Here the independent variable is continuous, and again the chi-square test is inappropriate. Nonetheless, the general methodology of observational studies is easily transposed to the latter studies and the t-test (described in Chapter 5) is suitable for the preliminary analysis of data from studies of this type.

Throughout this chapter the term sampling unit is used rather than individual, because in many epidemiologic studies a group of animals (e.g., a herd or flock) is the sampling unit rather than the individual. Although this makes the grammar somewhat formal, the distinction between individuals versus aggregates as sampling units is very important to note. Many reports fail to make this distinction, rendering their results of little or no value.

Finally, a current biologic problem will be used to give substance to the discussion of study types. Suppose the objective is to study the association between the presence of ureaplasma in the vagina and infertility in dairy cows. (It is assumed that ureaplasma can cause infertility; the objective here is to determine the extent to which ureaplasma and infertility are associated under field conditions.) Further assume that individual cows will be the sampling units, and that only 2 cows per farm are included in a study; this will prevent bias from farm-size related effects. Prior to performing the study, the method(s) and timing of culturing cows for ureaplasma would need to be decided and standardized, and infertility would need to be defined in a workable, concise manner. The actual definitions and procedures could differ depending on the type of analytic study selected, but these differences will be ignored for illustrative purposes.

6.3 Cross-Sectional Study Design

In the example, a cross-sectional study would require that a random sample of dairy cows be made (the sampling frame would need to be defined and a sampling method, probably multistage, selected), accompanied by an assessment of the current ureaplasma and infertility status of each cow. Subsequent to this, comparisons could be made between the prevalence of existing infertility in cows currently infected with ureaplasma and the prevalence of infertility in noninfected cows.

Technically, cross-sectional studies provide a snapshot of events at a particular time. The point of time may range from an instant ("at the time of sampling") to longer periods (such as "during the past year"), although all are treated as static, point-in-time events. For purposes of causal interpretations, cross-sectional studies are best suited to studying permanent factors (such as breed, sex, or blood-type), since such factors can not be altered by the passage of time or by the presence or absence of disease. When the independent variable is a nonpermanent factor (as in the ureaplasma example), one can never be sure whether the factor status is influencing disease occurrence or vice versa. That is, perhaps infertility allows ureaplasma to colonize and multiply in the vagina.

If random selection of sampling units is used and applied with adequate rigor, the key features relating to validity of cross-sectional study results are the accuracy of the data regarding the factor and disease status. Thus, criteria for classifying the sampling units as exposed and/or diseased should be clearly stated. In particular, one usually attempts to exclude potential false-positives when specifying these criteria. That is, if misclassification of sampling units may occur, it is better to have a few exposed (diseased) units classified as nonexposed (nondiseased) than to have nonexposed (nondiseased) units classified as exposed (diseased). This makes the study results more conservative, but gives credence to any observed differences in rates of disease according to exposure status.

If the information about the factor and disease status may be biased by knowledge of the reason for the study, collaborators need not be informed of the major objective of the study. For example, in a study to identify ration factors associated with the occurrence of left displaced abomasum in dairy cows, questions were asked relating to nonration factors as well as the occurrence of diseases other than displaced abomasum (Pearson 1978). It was hoped that this prevented the farmers from keying on the ration-displaced abomasum relationship and perhaps biasing the answers depending on their beliefs about the subject. Also, useful data to answer secondary objectives were obtained.

Sometimes the original sample is obtained by cross-sectional methods; then the sampling units are observed over a period of time, and changes in exposure and/or disease status are noted. These studies are known as longitudinal studies, combining the benefits of cohort study methods (the ability to determine the factor status prior to disease occurrence and thus obtain incidence data) with the benefits of cross-sectional sampling (the knowledge of the frequency of the factor and/or disease in the source population). Thus, the distinction between study types becomes blurred, particularly since longitudinal studies may be performed in a prospective or retrospective manner as described in Figure 6.2. Many studies reported in the veterinary literature are longitudinal in type, although most have used purposive or convenience samples rather than a true probability sample, reducing the ability to generalize beyond the sample data.

Questionnaire-based surveys, studies relating ancillary data to the results of immunologic, microbiologic, or toxicologic testing, and slaughterhouse surveys are common examples of cross-sectional studies. Examples of longitudinal studies include a California survey investigating pulmonary emphysema in cattle (see Table 2.6), a mail survey on factors associated with morbidity and mortality in feedlot calves (see Table 6.1), a retrospective study of diseases and productivity in dairy cattle (see Table 6.2), a prospective study of diseases and productivity in dairy cattle (see Table 6.3), and a study of respiratory disease in racing standardbred horses (see Table 6.4). (See 12.4.3 for other examples.)

6.4 Case-Control Study Design

In case-control studies, separate samples of units with (cases) and without (controls) the specified disease are selected. Then the relative fre-

Table 6.1. Summary of the effects and importance of CALFNO, ANTIMICROBIAL, and RUFCHANGE on mortality rates in feedlot calves

Factor(s)						
CALFNO	ANTI-MICROBIAL	RUFCHANGE	$P(F_i)^a$	Mortality rate[b]	Relative[c] risk (RR)	PAR%[d]
+	+	+	.133	1.185	3.5	12.0
+	+	−	.031	2.039	6.0	5.6
+	−	+	.251	1.230	3.6	23.7
−	+	+	.046	1.990	5.9	8.1
+	−	−	.097	1.198	3.5	8.9
−	+	−	.046	0.751	2.2	2.0
−	−	+	.195	0.791	2.3	9.4
−	−	−	.200	0.330	1.0	0.0

[a]Proportion of farms treated in this manner.

[b]Mortality rates derived from the mean of $\log_{10}$ transformed rates.

[c]Mean mortality rates in each grouping divided by the rate of mortality in "small farm, no antimicrobial added to water on arrival and major roughage source not changed within four weeks" group. The relative risk of the latter group is arbitrarily set to "1."

[d]Population attributable risk % describes the percentage of all deaths that is attributable to each of the CALFNO-ANTIMICROBIAL-RUFCHANGE groups. This is calculated by the formula:

$$\frac{100p(F_i) \times [p(D+/F_i) - p(D+/F_0)]}{p(D+)}$$

Source: Hutchings and Martin 1983, with permission.

Notes: Where $p(D+)$ is the overall mortality rate and $p(D+/F_i)$ is the mortality rate in a specific grouping of factors; CALFNO was dichotomized into >155 per farm and ≤155 per farm; ANTIMICROBIAL indicated whether prophylactic antimicrobials were added to the water supply; and RUFCHANGE indicated whether or not the type of roughage was changed within one month of arrival.

Note the general increase in RR as the number of risk factors present increased. Also note that the importance (PAR%) is affected by the RR and the prevalence of the factors; hence two factor groupings can have nearly similar RRs, but quite different PAR%. Note that PAR% is called population attributable fraction (PAF) in this text.

quency of the factor in each of these groups is compared using the odds ratio. Often all units with the disease and an equal number of controls are selected. In the present example, all infertile cows in a defined area might be used as cases, and an equal number of fertile cows selected as controls. (Matching for herd, age, and level of production might be used to increase the comparability of these groups.) Each cow's current ureaplasma infection status would be determined, and the proportion of infertile cows infected with ureaplasma would be compared to the proportion of fertile cows infected with ureaplasma. If the rate of infection were higher in infertile cows, this would support but not prove the hypothesis of ureaplasma producing infertility.

Since a number of biases can affect the results of case-control studies, key items are the criteria and methods used in the selection of cases and

Table 6.2. Decomposition of estimated bivariate associations into direct, indirect, and common cause components (810 Holstein lactations; 20 ROP-herd health herds; 1970–1975)

Variables		Association				
		Causal			Correlation	
Independent	Dependent	Direct	Indirect	Spurious	Estimated	Observed
Retained placenta	Metritis	.47	.00	.00	.47	.47
Retained placenta	Cystic follicle	.00	.06	.02	.08	.09
Retained placenta	Luteal cyst	.11	.01	.00	.12	.12
Retained placenta	Calving inter-val	.00	.06	.04	.10	.13
Retained placenta	BCM	.00	.01	.01	.02	.02
Retained placenta	Days in milk	.00	.04	.05	.09	.14
Metritis	Cystic follicle	.12	.00	.01	.13	.13
Metritis	Luteal cyst	.00	.01	.06	.07	.03
Metritis	Calving inter-val	.12	.02	.01	.15	.15
Metritis	BCM	.00	.02	.01	.03	.03
Metritis	Days in milk	.00	.10	.02	.12	.15
Cystic follicle	Luteal cyst	.12	.00	.01	.13	.14
Cystic follicle	Calving inter-val	.14	.01	.03	.18	.18
Cystic follicle	BCM	.09	.02	.00	.11	.14
Cystic follicle	Days in milk	.00	.13	.04	.17	.16
Luteal cyst	Calving inter-val	.08	.00	.03	.11	.11
Luteal cyst	BCM	.00	.01	.01	.02	.08
Luteal cyst	Days in milk	.00	.06	.02	.08	.09

Source: Erb et al. 1981, with permission.
Note: Using path analysis (see 5.6.3), the observed correlations between two variables (left hand columns) were decomposed into direct and indirect causal effects and spurious (the result of confounding variables) effects.

controls, the comparability of cases and controls, and an accurate unbiased history of exposure to the factor of interest.

6.4.1 Selection of Cases and Controls

In addition to being clear and concise, the criteria required to be a case should be highly specific in order to exclude false-positive units. If by design, certain types of sampling units are to be excluded from the case group (e.g., cases with known causes other than the factor of interest), these units should be excluded from the study; they should not be included in the control group even if not diseased.

In most studies, lists of cases are obtained from one or more clinics or

Table 6.3.   **Average probabilities of a cow being culled in the first 150 days of lactation (without and with selected diseases) and the relative risk (RR) and
population attributable fraction (PAF) associated with those diseases**

Disease	Average probability of being culled	Estimated RR	Estimated PAF (%)
None	.012	1.0	0.0
Severe mastitis	.956	79.7	53.2
Milk fever—stage 3	.350	29.2	64.7
Foot-leg disease	.373	31.1	38.7
Teat injury	.425	35.4	19.4
Mild mastitis	.045	3.8	19.2
Respiratory disease	.107	8.9	8.0

Source: Dohoo and Martin 1984, with permission.
Note: The presence of each of the above diseases increased the risk (RR) of a cow being
culled. The importance (PAF) of a disease in terms of its effect on the risk of culling is
influenced by its RR and prevalence. More than 100% of culling is explained because the
diseases were components of the same sufficient cause (see 5.6.2).

Table 6.4.   **Relationship between upper respiratory tract disease and anti-influenza
(E1) titers in Standardbred horses**

Antibody titer	Probability of disease	
	1974	1975
640	.003	.092
320	.009	.124
160	.027	.124
80	.108	.232
40	.265	.295
20	.519	.366
10	.694	.704

Source: Sherman et al. 1979, with permission.
Note: Anti-influenza titers appear to be protective since there is an indirect relationship
between titer and the probability of disease. However, even horses with high titers acquire
upper respiratory tract disease, probably because other factors in addition to antibody presence are required for protection, and/or other agents may have been the proximate cause of
disease in these horses.

diagnostic laboratories. Except for specified exclusions, all cases first
diagnosed in a specified time period can be included in the study. Usually
there is a very large number of potential controls. If little or no effort is
required to obtain the history of exposure to the factor(s) of interest, then
all noncases or all noncases with specified other diseases may be used as
controls. Whether explicit sampling of noncases is used depends on the
time and expense required to obtain the factor status for each unit selected.
When sampling from a large number of potential controls, random or
random systematic selection is preferred, provided no matching of cases
and controls is to be used.

When both of the study groups are obtained by purposive selection from laboratory or clinic records, the cases and/or controls may not be representative of all cases and noncases in the source population. In particular, the prevalence of the factor(s) of interest in the available controls may not reflect its prevalence in the source population as it ought to, particularly if valid estimates of the importance of the association are desired. If there is doubt about the representativeness of the cases and/or controls, additional data should be obtained to help evaluate the situation. Unfortunately, in practice only qualitative data are readily available to test how representative the groups are, and these deficits should be borne in mind when interpreting and extrapolating the results.

A particular form of unrepresentative sample that gives rise to biased estimates of association arises when the rate of admission to the laboratory or clinic is associated with both the factor(s) of interest and the disease status. When these records are used in a subsequent study, the differential admission rate acts as a confounding variable and can bias the true association between the factor(s) and disease. This phenomenon is often called Berkson's fallacy after the person initially describing it. A classic example of Berkson's fallacy occurred in a study of the association between cancer and tuberculosis based on human autopsies (Pearl 1929). The initial study results indicated less tuberculosis in autopsied cancer victims than in autopsied people dying from diseases other than cancer; thus suggesting a sparing effect of tuberculosis on cancer. It was later found that the autopsy series contained a disproportionately large number of tuberculosis cases because the latter were more likely to be autopsied, and when this was taken into account the association between tuberculosis and cancer disappeared.

Documented instances of Berkson's fallacy in veterinary medicine are rare; however, the effects of differential admission rates may have been observed, using hospital records, in a case-control study of the relationship between clinical mastitis and age of dairy cows. No association between age and mastitis was found in the case-control study; yet in a subsequent longitudinal study in the population of cows giving rise to the data for the case-control study, the rate of mastitis was found to increase significantly with the cow's age. The difference in results was due to the fact that many diseases of dairy cows increase in frequency with age, and thus the population of cows with diseases (the hospital population) was older than the average age in the source population. Hence, only diseases whose frequency increased with age more rapidly than the average of other diseases were observed to have a significant association with age in the case-control study. Thus in this example, submission rate for diagnosis was related to both age and diagnosis and biased the association between these two variables (Erb and Martin 1978; 1980).

The likelihood of admission rate bias can be assessed by comparing the characteristics of the control group(s) to independent samples from the source population; if the control group and population appear to have similar distributions with respect to a number of factors, admission rate bias is unlikely. Also, the probability of admission bias occurring may be reduced by selecting controls from all available noncases. It may be slight comfort that the majority of case-control study results apparently have not been unduly affected by this phenomenon. In some studies (e.g., the association between lung cancer and smoking based on hospitalized patients), when the effects of admission rate are removed, the association between smoking and lung cancer becomes stronger because smokers are more likely to be hospitalized than nonsmokers, and lung cancer patients are more likely to be hospitalized than non–lung cancer patients. Thus the observed association based on hospital data is weaker than the association in the source population. Further, admission rate biases are unlikely to explain strong associations (relative risk > 3) and are unlikely to explain a gradient of risk with different levels of exposure. This is an additional reason for inclusion of these two items when considering the likelihood that an observed association is causal.

When using noncase patients from a clinic as controls, it is advisable to select the controls from all noncase patients rather than a specific subset of other diagnoses. It is possible to select different sets of controls from a number of diagnostic categories—one set from all noncase patients and another from patients with diseases X, Y, or Z. When this is done, it is advisable to record biologically reasonable interpretations for all possible associations prior to conducting the study. Often, logical explanations for some possible differences in associations between different control groups are not apparent, and the investigator should reconsider the selection of controls.

The use of controls selected from the source population is another way of circumventing the problem of admission rate bias. Population-based controls are particularly useful when the list of cases represents essentially all cases in a defined population (such as all infected farms in a county) or all cases of a disease in a set of farms serviced by a veterinary practice. Within reason, when selecting controls from defined populations, attempt to maximize collaboration among potential controls or nonresponse may bias the results in a manner similar to different admission rates.

If genetic comparability between cases and controls is desirable for the study, relatives of the case may be selected as controls. However, since siblings tend to share similar environments, their selection will indirectly make the environment of cases and controls more comparable, and this is not always desirable. In selecting siblings as controls it is important to select a fixed number of controls per case and to exclude those cases where this ratio can not be obtained. Otherwise large sibling groups may bias the results. Usually one would not select relatives of cases if the factor of interest is related to genotype (e.g., if the factor was phenotype).

If environmental comparability is required, controls may be selected from the same original source as the cases (i.e., from the same farm or kennel). Again, cases and controls should be selected in a fixed ratio to ensure that larger farms or kennels do not bias the results. (This was also noted when the example of ureaplasma and infertility was introduced.)

6.4.2 Comparability of Cases and Controls

Theoretically, the cases and controls should be similar in all respects except for the disease (dependent variable) being investigated. Of course, they would also differ with respect to the exposure factor if it were associated with the disease. One indication of comparability of groups is a similar response (collaboration) rate in both groups. Very different response rates should lead to skepticism about the validity of results, particularly if the overall response rate is low (less than 75–80%). In practice, the cases and controls may differ in many ways as described in 5.4, and two commonly used methods to increase the comparability of groups are analytic control and matching. Restricted selection (e.g., only selecting cows between 4 and 7 years of age) also tends to make the groups more similar, since the restriction applies to both the cases and controls.

In analytic control, data on ancillary factors are obtained and appropriate statistical methods (such as the Mantel-Haenszel technique) are used to prevent distortion of results from extraneous factors. Host factors are frequently confounding variables and should be included in the list of ancillary factors if it is known that the risk of disease is influenced by them. If the list of ancillary factors is long, complex analytic methods beyond the scope of this text (such as logistic regression) may be required for analysis of the data.

Matching may be used to increase the similarity of cases and controls. The characteristics of each case with regard to potential confounding factors are noted, and a control is sought with the same characteristics. In most studies the number of factors that can be matched is small (perhaps two or three); otherwise it becomes difficult to identify controls with the required characteristics. In case-control studies, only factors known to be associated with the risk of disease should be included as matching factors. It is a peculiarity of case-control studies that overmatching (matching for noncausal factors) may reduce the ability (power) to detect true associations between the factor and disease. If one wishes to study the effect of an extraneous factor, it is necessary to use analytic control rather than matching, since the effects of matched factors cannot be studied.

As an example, matching was used in a study of factors related to mycoplasma mastitis in dairy herds. Two sources of control herds were used, one matching on size of herd, the other on level of milk production (Thomas et al. 1981). See Table 6.5.

6.4.3 Obtaining Information about Factor of Interest

A major objective in case-control studies is to collect accurate, unbiased information about the factor of interest. To assist in this, data should be obtained in the same manner and with the same rigor from both cases and controls. One way of ensuring equal rigor is to keep the investigator blind to the disease status and/or to keep the respondent unaware of the exact reason for the study. To test its validity, the information collected may be compared with the data in other records or the results of selected tests. As was previously mentioned, this is very similar to evaluating a screening test. If the sensitivity and specificity of the question are equal in both cases and controls, although errors may reduce the apparent strength of the association, they will not falsely inflate it.

Table 6.5.   Means for selected production variables for mycoplasma case-herd and control-herd groups in California dairy herds

Herd group	Herd size	Percentage dry	Percentage culled	Milk (kg/yr)
Case				
1–49 colonies[a]	598	14	32	7470
50+ colonies	661	15	35	7607
Control				
Production matched	316	15	26	7535
Herd size matched	615	14	29	7746

Source: Thomas et al. 1981, with permission from Am. J. Vet. Res.

[a]Number of pathogenic mycoplasma colonies per ml of bulk-tank milk.

Note: Control herds with the same production as case herds are smaller and cull a smaller percentage of cows. Control herds of the same size as the case herds have higher production and lower culling rates. These suggest that infection is more common in larger herds, that milk production is lowered, and that culling is increased by mycoplasma infection.

6.4.4 Analysis

The proportions being compared (the proportion of cases that are exposed and the proportion of noncases that are exposed) in the case-control study should be calculated and displayed together with the results of statistical analysis and the appropriate epidemiologic measures of association (see Table 5.6 and Table 6.6).

If the factor has more than two levels on the nominal scale (e.g., breeds), the level of factor that makes the most biologic or practical sense should be chosen as the reference group. If the factor is ordinal in type, the nonexposed or least exposed group may be used as the reference group

Table 6.6.   **The relationship between level of crude fiber in the ration and the occurrence of left displaced abomasum in dairy herds**

Crude fiber $<16\%$	Case herds	Control herds	Chi-square	Odds-ratio
Yes	20	6	5.13	10
No	2	6		1
	22	12		
Proportion $<16\%$	0.91	0.50		

Source: Grymer et al. 1981, with permission.

(odds ratio = 1). A series of 2 × 2 tables each containing the referent group is constructed, and the strength of association assessed in the usual manner. As an example, the referent group in a study of the association between breed and hip dysplasia in dogs was "other breeds." This group consisted of a number of crossbred dogs and a number of breeds having only a few dogs each (see Table 6.7) (Martin et al. 1980).

Table 6.7.   **Rate of canine hip dysplasia (CHD) for breeds represented by twenty or more dogs radiographed at OVC, 1970–1978**

Breed	No. of dogs	Percent of CHD	Risk[a]	Significance of risk[b]
Afghan hound	46	10.9	0.49	NS
Alaskan malamute	66	37.9	1.38	NS
Bouvier des Flandres	55	36.4	1.21	NS
German shepherd	402	46.8	1.85	S
Great Dane	118	16.1	0.48	S
Great Pyrenees	29	20.7	0.76	NS
Irish wolfhound	36	22.2	0.77	NS
Newfoundland	116	63.8	3.66	S
Norwegian elkhound	29	34.5	1.42	NS
Old English sheepdog	119	47.1	1.88	S
Miniature poodle	48	25.0	0.94	NS
Standard poodle	33	30.3	1.10	NS
Golden retriever	140	55.7	2.75	S
Labrador retriever	211	37.4	1.27	NS
Rottweiler	26	30.8	1.10	NS
Saint Bernard	131	73.3	5.14	S
Samoyed	64	34.4	1.12	NS
English setter	38	39.5	1.53	NS
Irish setter	77	33.8	1.28	NS
Siberian husky	151	5.3	0.25	S
"Other breeds"	354	30.7	1.00	...

Source: Martin et al. 1980, with permission.
[a]Measured by odds ratio. This statistic compares the rate of CHD in each breed to the rate in "other breeds." Odds ratios significantly greater than one imply increased rates. Odds ratios significantly less than one imply decreased rates.
[b]The significance of the odds ratio is tested with a chi-square statistic. NS = not significant. S = significant at $p < 0.05$.

6.5 Cohort Study Design

In cohort studies, separate samples of exposed and unexposed units are selected. The groups are observed for a predetermined period, and the rate of disease in each is compared. In the ureaplasma example, the investigator might obtain an arbitrary number of ureaplasma infected cows and select a similar number of noninfected cows, perhaps matching for herd and age. Any cows known to be infertile would be excluded at the start of the study. (In a practical situation, one might have to settle for excluding all cows with obvious reproductive tract abnormalities unrelated to ureaplasma, within 60 days of parturition.) All cows would be observed for a defined period of time (say 90 days after breeding commenced), and the subsequent rate of infertility in each group identified.

Although bias is less of a problem in cohort than case-control studies, key items to ensure validity are the criteria for and selection of the exposed and unexposed groups, equality of follow-up in both groups, and accurate diagnosis of disease.

6.5.1 Selection of Exposed and Unexposed Groups

In most cohort studies, special exposure groups are purposively selected for comparison. This could include comparing rates of disease(s) in different breeds; comparing rates of pneumonia in animals on different rations; comparing rates of disease in animals with and without serum antibodies to selected antigens; or comparing disease rates and production levels in herds on preventive medicine programs to similar herds not on these programs. As mentioned previously, the sampling units are frequently obtained through purposive sampling, not probability samples from a defined sampling frame. Because of this and in order to extrapolate results beyond the study groups, some indication of how representative the study groups are of exposed and unexposed segments of the population should be obtained.

A further concern in selecting the cohorts is that they should be comparable (i.e., not differ in ways other than the exposure). This may require the measurement of ancillary variables so that analytic control can be used to adjust for known differences between the groups, although matching may be used to increase the similarity of the groups as it was in case-control studies. More than one unexposed group may be selected as the referent if the information provided will be useful. For example, in a study of the effects (benefits) of preventive medicine programs, the comparison group might include two groups: the first composed of herds using veterinary service regularly, but not a formal prophylactic program; and the second composed of herds using veterinary service only irregularly. Obviously, a clear and practical set of definitions of the different types of veterinary service would be required.

Although the exposure status of selected units may seem obvious, the probability of misclassification of exposure status can be reduced by clear, concise descriptions of what constitutes exposure (possession of the factor). Specific tests may be used to help assess exposure status in a manner similar to their usage as diagnostic aids. When feasible it is useful to classify the cohorts according to a gradient of exposure, allowing investigation of a potential dose-response relationship.

If prerecorded data on exposure history are used to define the cohorts, investigations into the meaning, validity, and completeness of the data should be performed. Certainly one should not interpret "no recorded history" of exposure as meaning no exposure, unless the records are known to be complete.

In prospective studies, the collaboration of a number of people will be required. Hence, it is important that a high percentage of selected individuals cooperate in the study, and failing this, the study design should increase the likelihood of equal cooperation rates in the exposed and nonexposed groups. If these rates are very different, lack of cooperation can distort the results of the study in the same manner as differential admission rates in case-control studies. In general, it is informative to elucidate reasons for lack of cooperation.

Whenever possible, all the sampling units entering the study should be examined for the presence of the disease(s) of interest at the start of the study. By starting the study with disease-free units, the investigator can determine incidence rates, and this also establishes a clear temporal relationship between the factor and disease. Sometimes such an examination is very difficult; thus the sampling units are assumed to be disease-free at the start of the study. This is frequently true in retrospective cohort studies.

6.5.2 Follow-Up Period

The cohorts should be observed for the occurrence of disease(s) at regular periods throughout the study; both groups should be followed with equal rigor; and the withdrawal of sampling units from the study should be minimized. Withdrawals can bias the results if the losses are related to both exposure and disease status. Obviously, this problem is more severe in studies spanning many years. If a high percentage (e.g., 95%) complete the study, potential biases from withdrawal will be minimized. Care is also required when cohorts are defined retrospectively, because many withdrawals (due to culling, sale, or death) will have occurred before the study begins. For example, if the weight gain and feed efficiency of a group of swine that received antimicrobial therapy were compared to that of an untreated group, one would have to note and adjust for death losses prior to slaughter. Such losses might not negate the results, but their potential significance should be borne in mind. Whenever possible, the reason(s) for withdrawal from a prospective cohort study should be recorded.

6.5.3 Determining Occurrence of Disease

The diagnostic criteria for the disease of interest must be clearly defined, and whenever possible those making the diagnosis should be unaware of exposure status of the units being examined. Since more than one disease may be of interest, the criteria for diagnosing a few important diseases should be specified in detail, with other diseases being diagnosed and recorded in a rigorous but ad hoc manner.

6.5.4 Analysis

If the duration of the study is relatively short, the average period of risk is equivalent in both cohorts, and the losses to follow up are minimal, the usual 2 × 2 table format may be used to display and analyze the data (see Table 6.8). The rates of disease in each cohort are calculated and compared directly, or the Mantel-Haenszel technique, or standardization of rates may be used to control the effects of extraneous qualitative variables.

Often the duration of the period at risk may differ greatly between cohorts. This is particularly likely when the cohorts are not completely formed at the start of the study. If the study is designed to last 3 years, the cohorts may be formed over this period as appropriate exposed and unexposed individuals are identified and placed under observation. A hypothetical example of this situation and the problems it creates is provided in Table 6.9.

Two analytic approaches are used to adjust for the differing periods of observation. The first method is based on the calculation of true rates and the concepts of unit-time (for example animal-years) of risk as introduced in Chapter 3. Each animal or sampling unit contributes 1 year each full year

Table 6.8. Feline leukemia (FL) incidence rate in cats with and without infectious anemia (FIA): a retrospective cohort study[a]

	FL +	FL −	Total	Incidence rate (risk) (%)	Relative risk
FIA +	6	291	297	2.02	11.9
FIA −	1	593	594	0.17	1
	7	884	891		
Chi-square = 8.71

Source: Priester and Hayes 1973, with permission.
[a]Called a prospective case-control study by the authors.

it is under observation (e.g., 1 unit observed for 3 years contributes 3 unit-years of observation, and 3 units observed for one year also contribute 3 unit-years). The total unit-time of risk in each group is used as the denominator for calculating true rates in the usual manner. Although these data may be summarized in a 2×2 table, the regular chi-square test should not be applied to these data. Thus, using true rates is useful for removing biases from differences in period of risk, but does not allow the evaluation of the

Table 6.9. Animal-years of observation in cohort or longitudinal studies

Suppose that in a cohort study the cohorts ($F+$ and $F-$) were not fully formed at the time the study began. In particular, assume the $F+$ group formed in the following manner. The number of cases of disease in each year of the study are shown also. (Assume also that an animal only gets the disease once.)

Calendar year of entry	Number entering	Disease incidence by year of study			
		1	2	3	Total
1	300	30	27	24	81
2	400		40	36	76
3	500			50	50
	1200				207

The $F-$ group and the number of cases formed in the following manner:

Calendar year of entry	Number entering	Disease incidence by year of study			
		1	2	3	Total
1	500	25	24	23	72
2	400		20	19	39
3	300			15	15
	1200				126

Had both groups been fully formed at the start of the study and been observed for 3 years, the usual 2×2 table format for calculating risk rates would be appropriate.

	$D+$	$D-$	Total animals	Rates/3 years (%)
$F+$	207	993	1200	17.3
$F-$	126	1074	1200	10.5

However, since these conditions were not met, the total period of observation for the cohorts may differ. In fact, the number of animal years of observation for the $F+$ group was

$$300 \times 3 + 400 \times 2 + 500 \times 1 = 2200$$

for a true rate of 9.41% per animal-year (207/2200).

The number of animal years of observation for the $F-$ group was

$$500 \times 3 + 400 \times 2 + 300 \times 1 = 2600.$$

for a true rate of 4.15% per animal-year (126/2600).

(These true rates are not exact because the diseased animals were not at risk after developing the disease—see Chapter 3.) After making this adjustment, the years of observation are 1969.5 and 2443 for the $F+$ and $F-$ cohorts, respectively.

role of chance by standard statistical methods. (Suggestions for analyses are included in Kleinbaum et al. 1982, pp 336–8.) If the groups are very large, sampling variation is not of great importance and may be ignored.

The second analytic approach is the follow-up life table method that allows the investigator to calculate risk rates. This is accomplished by taking into account the different periods of risk, and the technique also allows formal statistical evaluation of observed differences. This method is introduced in Table 6.10 as an extension of the problem presented in Table 6.9. An example of the application of follow-up life tables is shown in Table 6.11.

6.6 Choosing the Analytic Study Method

Often the choice of study method is influenced by the structure of the files or population to be sampled. For example, if the exposure and disease status of the units to be sampled are unknown, cross-sectional methods would be used. Case-control sampling may be a natural choice if records are filed or retrievable by diagnosis.

The choice of study type may also be influenced by the objective of the study and the amount of knowledge already known about the relationship between the factor(s) and disease(s) of interest. Case-control studies allow initial screening and identification of multiple risk factors for a given disease, whereas cohort studies are suited to the screening and identification of multiple effects from a single cause. Cross-sectional and longitudinal studies allow the simultaneous study of many factors and diseases, and in addition provide direct estimates of the frequency of these events in the source population.

Finally, one must be aware of general advantages and disadvantages specific to each design. Cross-sectional studies usually only provide estimates of prevalence; thus one can not differentiate factors associated with having disease from factors causing the disease. Cross-sectional and longitudinal studies are not well suited to studying rare diseases, whereas case-control methods (requiring the smallest total sample size of any study type) are ideal in this situation. Case-control studies are relatively easy and inexpensive to conduct, but suffer from many potential biases. Cohort and longitudinal studies provide direct estimates of incidence rates and the time sequence of events is well established. These studies are, however, the most difficult and expensive to conduct.

In summary, if the objective of the study is to screen for risk factors, use either cross-sectional or case-control studies, whereas if testing specific hypotheses use longitudinal or cohort methods. In some instances, field experiments are required as the ultimate evaluation of associations found in observational studies.

Table 6.10. Follow-up life table for analysis of data from cohort and longitudinal studies (data from Table 6.9)

	Exposed				Unexposed			
Years under observation	Number initially at risk	Number new cases	Number withdrawals	Probability of new case (P)	Number initially at risk	Number new cases	Number withdrawals	Probability of new case (P)
0 < 1	1200	120	450	.12	1200	60	428	.06
1 < 2	630[a]	63	324	.13	712	43	361	.08
2 < 3	243	24	219	.18	308	23	285	.14

This is a risk rate, and hence if animals are withdrawn or lost during the period, one half of the number withdrawn is subtracted from the number initially at risk before calculating the probability of becoming a case. Animals whose observation period is terminated by the end of the study are also considered as withdrawals.

The probability of not becoming a case during each period is found by subtracting P from 1. The cumulative probability of not becoming a case during the study period is the product of these probabilities. For the $F+$ cohort this is .88 × .87 × .82 = .63. Hence the probability of developing the disease in a three year period is $1 - 0.63 = 0.37$ or 37%. For the $F-$ cohort this is .94 × .92 × .86 = .74. Hence the probability of developing disease in the three year period for $F-$ animals is 0.26 or 26%.

[a]This is derived from the 700 animals starting the second year of observation, but subtracting the 30 + 40 cases that had already occurred in the first year of observation.

Table 6.11.   Survivorship of infant *Macaca mulatta* according to place of birth at the University of California Primate Center, 1968-1972

Age (days)	Cumulative probability (P) of surviving to specified age			
	Born inside		Born outside	
	P (%)	SE(P)	P (%)	SE(P)
< 8	97.8	0.91	91.5	2.71
8 < 15	95.9	1.22	83.9	3.58
15 < 22	94.1	1.19	82.9	3.66
22 < 29	93.7	1.24	80.1	3.89
29 < 60	91.5	1.50	76.2	4.15
60 < 91	89.6	1.68	74.3	4.27
91 < 122	89.3	1.71	72.4	4.49
122 < 153	88.5	1.78	70.4	4.47
153 < 184	86.7	1.93	67.4	4.60

Source: Hird 1975, with permission.

Note: The cumulative probability of surviving to a specified age for infants born inside can be compared to that for infants born outside; statistically, $P \mp 2SE(P)$ are approximate 95% confidence intervals. If the intervals do not overlap, the survivorship may be deemed different in the two groups (SE = standard error).

References

Dohoo, I. R., and S. W. Martin. 1984. Disease, production and culling in Holstein-Friesian cows. V. Survivorship. Prev. Vet. Med. 2:771–84.

Erb, H. N., and S. W. Martin. 1978. Age, breed and seasonal patterns in the occurrence of 10 dairy cow diseases: A case-control study. Can. J. Comp. Med. 42:1–5.

_____. 1980. Interrelationships between production and reproductive diseases in Holstein cows: Age and seasonal patterns. J. Dairy Sci. 63:1918–24.

Erb, H. N., S. W. Martin, N. Ison, and S. Swaminathan. 1981. Interrelationships between production and reproductive diseases in Holstein cows: Pathanalysis. J. Dairy Sci. 64:281–89.

Grymer, J., M. Hesselholt, and P. Willeberg. 1981. Feed composition and left abomasal displacement in dairy cattle: A case-control study. Nord. Vet. Med. 33:306–9.

Hird, D. W., R. V. Henrickson, and H. G. Hendrick. 1975. Infant mortality in *Macaca mulatta*: Neonatal and post-neonatal mortality at the University of California Primate Research Center, 1968–1972. A retrospective study. J. Med. Primatol. 4:8–22.

Hutchings, D. L., and S. W. Martin. 1983. A mail survey of factors associated with morbidity and mortality in feedlot calves in Southwestern Ontario. Can. J. Comp. Med. 47:101–7.

Kleinbaum, D. G., L. L. Kupper, and H. Morgenstern. 1982. Epidemiologic Research: Principles and Quantitative Methods. Belmont, Calif.: Wadsworth.

Leech, F. B. 1971. A critique of the methods and results of the British national surveys of disease in farm animals. II. Some general remarks on population surveys of farm animal disease. Br. Vet. J. 127:587–92.

Martin, S. W., K. Kirby, and P. W. Pennock. 1980. Canine hip dysplasia: Breed effects. Can. Vet. J. 21:293–96.

Pearl, R. 1929. Cancer and tuberculosis. Am. J. Hyg. 9:97–159.

Pearson, A. 1978. Left displaced abomasum. An epidemiologic study in Southwestern Ontario. Paper submitted as partial fulfillment of diploma in preventive medicine requirements, Univ. of Guelph, Ontario.

Priester, W. A., and H. H. Hayes. 1973. Feline leukemia after feline infectious anemia. J. Natl. Cancer Inst. 51:289–91.

Ruppanner, R. 1972. Measurement of disease in animal populations based on interviews. J. Am. Vet. Med. Assoc. 161:1033–38.

Ruppanner, R., and W. Goodger. 1979. Dairy cattle disease in California. Calif. Vet. 33:34–37.

Selby, L. A., L. D. Edmonds, D. W. Parke, R. W. Stewart, C. T. Marienfeld, and W. F. Heidlage. 1973. Use of mailed questionnaire data in a study of swine congenital malformations. Can. J. Comp. Med. 37:413–17.

Selby, L. A., L. D. Edmonds, and L. D. Hyde. 1976. Epidemiological field studies of animal populations. Can. J. Comp. Med. 40:135–41.

Sherman, J., W. R. Mitchell, S. W. Martin, J. Thorsen, and D. G. Ingram. 1979. Epidemiology of equine upper respiratory tract disease on standardbred racetracks. Can. J. Comp. Med. 43:1–9.

Thomas, C. B., P. Willeberg, and D. E. Jasper. 1981. Case-control study of bovine mycoplasmal mastitis in California. Am. J. Vet. Res. 42:511–15.

Woodward, C. A., and L. W. Chambers. 1980. Guide to questionnaire construction and question writing. Ottawa, Canada: Can. Pub. Health Assoc.

Woodward, C. A., L. W. Chambers, and K. D. Smith. 1982. Guide to improved data collection in health and health care surveys. Ottawa, Canada: Can. Pub. Health Assoc.

Design of
Field Trials

This chapter describes how to design and conduct prophylactic and therapeutic field trials. Acquiring such knowledge is particularly relevant today because there has recently been an increasing awareness of the need for such trials. Knowledge of the priniciples of field trial design allows veterinarians to better interpret the literature in applied as well as research journals. Also, many veterinarians are asked to collaborate in field trials with universities, drug companies, or government drug control and evaluation agencies. In addition, many practitioners utilize field trials to evaluate and improve the disease control regimes they offer their clients.

The essence of the experimental method is the planned comparison of the outcome in groups receiving different levels of a treatment. As an example, the treatment levels might be vaccine versus no vaccine, and the outcomes might be the rate of subsequent disease and the productivity of animals in each treatment group. In the context of this chapter, a treatment could be a therapeutic drug, a prophylactic biologic (e.g., a vaccine), or an entire program composed of many individual treatments (e.g., a preconditioning program for beef calves consisting of weaning, creep feeding, and vaccination). When designing a field trial, one attempts to ensure the comparability of the units receiving each level of the treatment and to reduce the experimental error so that practical treatment effects can be identified with the minimum number of experimental units. The comparability of the treatment groups depends chiefly on the method of allocating the experimental units to treatment groups and the management of the groups during the course of the trial. At the termination of the study, statistical tests are used to evaluate the likelihood that chance variation produced any observed differences in the outcome between treatment groups.

In a manipulative laboratory experiment, the investigator can control the allocation of experimental units to treatment groups and also the timing and nature of the challenge to treatment. In field experiments, the investigator can control the allocation of experimental units but usually has to depend on natural challenge of the treatment. However, careful selection of the experimental units can increase the probability that a sufficient challenge will occur. For ethical reasons, the only field experiments often possible (except for those conducted under artificial conditions such as at research stations) involve treatments having a high probability of being found valuable in preventing or treating the disease(s) of concern.

Frequently, field trials are used to test a specific hypothesis, but in addition they may be used to validate the findings of observational studies or laboratory experiments. Sometimes the results of field trials may provide an indirect evaluation of a causal hypothesis. For example, serologic evidence may incriminate an agent such as the bovine virus diarrhea (BVD) virus as a cause of respiratory disease in feedlot calves. Although it has not been possible to produce respiratory disease with BVD virus alone or in combination with other agents, ancillary findings from experiments and some observational studies give support to the hypothesis that BVD virus infection is a determinant of respiratory disease of feedlot calves. If a properly designed field trial of a BVD vaccine produced a decrease in the occurrence of respiratory disease, this evidence would indirectly support the hypothesis as well as provide a method of control of respiratory disease. If the vaccine did not produce a significant benefit, the hypothesis would not be rejected because the vaccination regime may have been ineffective. Finally, as will be discussed later, trials may be performed to estimate parameters for building computer models.

The important biometric features of field trial design are discussed elsewhere (Cochran and Cox 1957; Snedecor and Cochran 1980; Armitage 1971). In choosing a particular design, the investigator attempts to ensure the field trial results will be valid, the probability of type I and/or II errors is reduced, and the design is practical for the specific field conditions that exist. The application of these features to the design of experiments conducted on humans and/or on privately owned animals has been discussed from a number of viewpoints (Peto et al. 1976, 1977; Gilbert 1974; Byar et al. 1976; Martin 1978). An excellent introduction to clinical trials is provided by Colton (1974).

For a number of reasons, field trials have not been widely or well used in veterinary medicine, at least in terms of assessing the efficacy of vaccines against bovine respiratory disease (Martin 1983). Sir Austin Bradford Hill, a pioneer in the use of field trials in human medicine, concisely summarizes the need for clinical trials. Although directed toward medical doctors, the reader can extrapolate the following statements to therapeutic and prophylactic trials in veterinary medicine (Hill 1952):

Therapeutics is the branch of medicine that, by its very nature, should be experimental. For if we take a patient afflicted with a malady, and we alter his conditions of life, either by dieting him, or by putting him to bed, or by administering to him a drug, or by performing on him an operation, we are performing an experiment. And if we are scientifically minded we should record the results. Before concluding that the change for better or for worse in the patient is due to the specific treatment employed, we must ascertain whether the results can be repeated a significant number of times in similar patients, whether the result was merely due to the natural history of the disease or in other words to the lapse of time, or whether it was due to some other factor which was necessarily associated with the therapeutic measure in question. And if, as a result of these procedures, we learn that the therapeutic measure employed produces a significant, though not very pronounced, improvement, we would experiment with the method, altering dosage or other detail to see if it can be improved. This would seem the procedure to be expected of men with six years of scientific training behind them. But it has not been followed. Had it been done we should have gained a fairly precise knowledge of the place of individual methods of therapy in disease, and our efficiency as doctors would have been enormously enhanced.

Ethical considerations are an important feature of field trials also, and often influence whether an experiment can be performed. In this regard, Hill goes on to state:

In addition to asking whether it is ethical in the light of current knowledge to plan a randomized trial in which some. . . . will not be offered the new measure, it is also necessary to ask whether it is ethical not to plan a randomized trial, since failure to do so may subject the population as a whole to the perpetuation of an ineffective program.

The key items to be considered in the design and performance of a field trial are shown in Figure 7.1. The process of selecting the experimental group is of great importance because it may limit the generalization of the experimental results (i.e., the ability to extrapolate the results beyond the experimental units actually used in the trial). The follow-up period, which extends from the time of allocation to the end of the trial, can greatly influence the validity of the experimental results (i.e., the degree of certainty that the observed results are attributable to the treatment given). If one is forced to choose between validity and the ability to generalize, those issues concerned with validity should receive priority. The remainder of this chapter describes the major features of field trial design and performance in more detail.

7.1 Objective of the Experiment

The objectives should be clearly stated, and both major and minor objectives identified when appropriate. This description should identify the outcome (response variable) and allow the straightforward development of the required treatment contrasts; these are obvious with only two levels of treatment (e.g., new versus standard treatment) but less obvious if three or

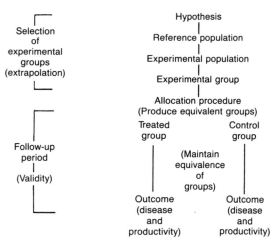

7.1. Key items in design and performance of field trial.

more treatment levels are present. In most studies the number of objectives should be restricted, perhaps to one or two; otherwise the design may become very complex and the performance of the trial jeopardized.

7.2 Reference and Experimental Populations

The population that will benefit if the treatment is effective is the reference population. In a prophylactic trial, the reference population consists of "healthy" individuals that are at risk of the disease, whereas in clinical trials it is those with a defined disease or syndrome. In both types of trial the experimental units are allocated to either the new treatment, the standard treatment, or the no treatment group. With due allowance for practical matters of convenience and cost, the population in which the trial is conducted (the experimental population) should be representative of the reference population. This allows the investigator to extrapolate the results of the trial to the larger reference population.

The collaborators in almost all field trials are volunteers. This may lead to concern about the validity of field trials since volunteers are known to differ in many respects from nonvolunteers. However, this fact should not invalidate the results of the trial provided the volunteers are allocated in a formal random manner to the treatment groups. When possible, it is useful to compare the characteristics of the volunteers to those of nonvolunteers as this information is valuable in guiding decisions concerning the extrapolation of results. Given that the treatment program is found to be beneficial, this information may prove useful in modifying the program to make it more acceptable when it is subsequently offered to members of the reference population.

7.3 Experimental Unit

The experimental unit is the smallest independent grouping of elements (i.e., individuals) that could receive a different treatment given the method of allocation; that is, providing the units are independent, the experimental unit is the smallest aggregate of individuals that is randomized to the treatment groups. Failure to identify the proper experimental unit is common and has serious consequences in terms of interpreting the results of an experiment. Suppose a new treatment was assigned to all animals in one herd with the standard treatment allocated to all animals in a different herd, using a formal random method such as a coin toss. Since a herd is the smallest grouping of animals allocated, such a scheme provides only one experimental unit per group; the number of animals per herd is of little importance. Since there is only one experimental unit per treatment, it is not possible to estimate the within-treatment variability (variance) and no formal statistical evaluation of observed differences is possible. Hence, the results can not be analyzed to establish the probability that chance variation produced the observed differences. Another example of the same mistake occurs when individuals are allocated to a certain treatment group and then housed together. Here the members of the same pen are not independent because extraneous factors (e.g., poor ventilation, infections) would tend to affect the entire pen and could produce a large difference in the outcome between treatment levels. In this situation, one could not separate a treatment effect from a pen effect. Thus the functional experimental unit is the pen. A similar mistake may occur when individuals are randomly assigned to a treatment level, and each individual is tested a number of times throughout the study. For purposes of statistically testing differences in outcome between treatments, individuals are the experimental unit, not the number of tests or samples.

In some experiments with more than one treatment, it may be desirable to have different experimental units in the same field trial. For example, the treatments of lesser importance may be assigned to herds or aggregates of animals, while the treatments of greater importance are assigned to individuals within the herd or group. These are called split-plot designs as described in 7.4.

7.3.1 Criteria for Entry to the Trial

The criteria that a unit must possess to enter the trial should be stated clearly. For example, only farms known to be infected with K99 *E. coli* would be included in vaccine trials against this organism. In clinical trials it is very important to specify the criteria used to diagnose the condition of interest (e.g., in a trial of alternative treatments of renal failure, it is essential to specify what constitutes renal failure). If these criteria are not valid or are not followed, the outcome can be severely biased. Adequately specifying the criteria for entry is particularly important when units with certain characteristics are to be excluded. For example, herds where pooled colostrum is fed would be excluded from a trial of an *E. coli* bacterin against neonatal diarrhea if individuals within the herd were to be allocated to vaccine or nonvaccine groups. If many investigators are involved, great care should be exercised to ensure the stated criteria for entry are understood and are followed.

7.3.2 Number of Experimental Units

Unless the study is designed as a sequential trial, the approximate number of units to be included in the trial should be determined before the study begins. In sequential trials, the number of units that eventually enter the trial depends on the results obtained during the trial. Sequential designs allow for frequent testing for significant differences between treatment groups so the trial can be stopped as soon as one treatment is found to be superior. These designs also have a maximum allowable sample size, allowing the trial to end if it becomes obvious the effects of the treatments do not differ by any practical amount. Sequential trials are of greatest value when the information about the response in one unit is available before the next unit enters the study (Armitage 1971).

In the field trials discussed here it is assumed that only treatments producing a sufficiently large true treatment effect to make them of practical importance are of interest; that is, the treatment effect must be sufficiently large to be of biologic and/or economic importance to members of the reference population. In a field trial, the observed treatment effect (the simple difference between the outcome in the treatment and control groups) is used to estimate the true treatment effect (the effect that would become known only after completing an infinite number of field trials). In making this inductive inference about the existence of a true treatment effect from the experiment results, there are two possible types of errors, usually designated as type I and type II. A type I error occurs when it is declared on the basis of the trial results that there is a true treatment effect when in fact there is not. A type II error occurs when it is declared on the basis of the trial results that no true treatment effect exists when in fact the treatment produces a worthwhile effect.

If the probability of a type II error (expressed as a proportion) is subtracted from 1, the result is referred to as the "power" of the experiment; the power being the likelihood that the trial will identify a true treatment effect correctly. Similarly, 1 minus the type I error is the confidence level. If the type I error is 5% (0.05) the confidence level is 95% (0.95). This latter value is the probability of the trial resulting in no significant difference when no real treatment effect exists.

Traditionally, there has been more concern about type I than type II errors, and the probability of committing this error is set by convention at or below the 5% level. In the absence of any knowledge about the relative seriousness of type I and II errors, the probability of committing a type II error is frequently set at four times that of the type I error (i.e., < 20%). However, when feasible, the magnitude of the two error rates should be based on the estimated costs — in biologic, humane and economic terms — of committing these errors.

The reason for discussing these error rates is that it is necessary to consider them when estimating the number of experimental units required for the trial. Too many units is expensive and may in a superficial analysis lead to declaring trivial treatment effects as significant. Too few units reduce the power of the trial (i.e., decreases the chance of detecting biologically significant effects).

Formulas appropriate for calculating the required number of experimental units are shown in Table 2.9. Tables of sample sizes are also available in standard statistical texts (Fleiss 1973). Usually it is best to view these determinations as ball park estimations rather than exact requirements. If the number of individuals required for the trial has been estimated using formulas appropriate for the random allocation of individuals, the total number of animals required when aggregates are randomized may need to be increased 4–5 times. For further discussion on this topic see Comstock (1978) and Cornfield (1978).

Although practitioners are encouraged to perform field trials, it should be recognized that it is much better to have one or two large scale investigations than numerous small ones. The reasons are twofold. First, in a trial with an insufficient number of units to give realistic power, the most frequent conclusion is "the differences between treatment groups were not significant"; thus, the trial produces no useful results. Second, if numerous small studies are conducted by different investigators, the probability that a significant difference will be observed in at least one study when no practical true treatment effect exists is considerably greater than 5%. One also needs to be aware of this problem when reviewing the literature because of the bias (called the publication bias) of many investigators to report differences found to be significant, but not to report "negative findings."

7.4 Allocation of Experimental Units to Treatment Groups

The use of a formal randomization procedure is desirable for the allocation of experimental units. Indeed, it is the use of formal random allocation that provides the primary advantage of field experiments over prospective cohort studies. In cohort studies the effects of known extraneous factors can be controlled by analysis, matching, or exclusion. Nonetheless, often it is not possible to account for the effects of all known extraneous factors, and the effects of unknown factors must be ignored. In experiments, random assignment is used to protect against any systematic differences in the treatment and control groups. In this way it prevents bias, balances any confounding variables (those factors related to the outcome and treatment), and guarantees the validity of the statistical test. The latter guarantee rests not on the assurance that the groups will be exactly the same with respect to known and unknown factors, but rather that the probability distribution of all possible outcomes of allocation is available. This allows the calculation of the probability (significance level) that differences in the outcome of interest equal to or more extreme than those observed might have arisen solely from the allocation procedure; these are viewed as chance differences.

Randomization can be achieved by flipping a coin, drawing numbers from a hat, through use of random number tables, or by using random number generators such as are available on some calculators and on most computers. Systematic allocation using a random starting point is an acceptable method of randomization under field conditions, but is less preferable than true randomization. To allocate 50 cattle to each of a vaccine and a control group, one could choose 50 random numbers between 1 and 100. The resulting numbers could relate to a tag number or to the sequence the animals follow in passing through a chute facility and would identify the animals to receive the vaccine. Vaccinating the first 50 animals caught and leaving the remainder as controls would not be an acceptable allocation procedure.

Often in a clinical setting, volunteers are sought and then the animals or units belonging to the volunteers are allocated to the treatment groups if they meet the criteria for treatment. It may be preferable to initially seek animals or units that meet the criteria for entry to the trial and then ask the owner to collaborate. Animals or units belonging to owners who refuse are given the treatment the investigator thinks is best; whereas those belonging to volunteers are allocated to the standard or new treatment group on a formal random basis. Subsequently, the outcome in all three groups (volunteer treatment, volunteer control, and nonvolunteer control group) is identified and used in the analysis. This procedure has advantages over initially seeking volunteers, but the investigator needs to take care lest "special clients" are discouraged from agreeing to enter the trial.

7.4.1 Allocation Methods

There are a number of different ways of allocating experimental units to treatment groups, each method being a different experimental design. In selecting a method one basically takes into account: the number and arrangement of treatments (whether an experimental unit can receive more than one treatment) including practical constraints in the delivery of a treatment (e.g., certain treatments can only be given to an aggregate of individuals, such as litters or pens); monetary constraints that tend to place an upper limit on the total number of experimental units; and maximizing the precision of the experiment (reducing the experimental error) given the previous limitations.

If no important predictors (covariates) of the outcome are identifiable, the units should be individually, randomly allocated. This is the simplest and most frequently used design and is called a completely randomized design. In large field trials ($n > 100$) with relatively homogeneous experimental units, a completely randomized design together with analytic control of potential confounding variables (covariates) is preferred. (Recall that randomization does not guarantee that all covariates will be equally distributed in the treatment groups.) The set of potential confounders must be listed beforehand so that the presence or level of those variables can be noted at the appropriate time during the field trial.

In some field trials, the variability within treatment groups can be decreased by grouping (blocking or matching) the units so they are similar with regard to important characteristics. The units within these blocks are then randomly allocated to treatment groups on a within-block basis; this constitutes a randomized block design. Each block constitutes a replication of the treatments. In clinical trials it may be advisable to "block" on one or two very important prognostic factors (e.g., severity or chronicity of disease, age of patient), ensuring equal distribution of these factors within the treatment groups. The determination of treatment effect is then done on a within-block (pair) basis. Whether to use blocking requires knowledge of the amount of precision gained by matching relative to the loss sustained by the reduction in the number of replications.

Sometimes the experimental unit may serve as its own control; these are called cross-over designs. In cross-over designs, the treatments are allocated to the same unit in random order over a series of periods. If treatments are likely to have a residual effect, the magnitude of the effect should be identified and accounted for prior to testing the significance of any treatment effect. Another strategy is to allow an adjustment period between treatments.

Factorial designs can be used if there are two or more treatments and each experimental unit can receive both treatments. With two different treatments, some units receive no treatment, others one treatment, and still others both treatments. There are two major advantages to factorial designs relative to the traditional method of studying only one factor at a time. First, two treatments can be studied with the same number of units required to assess one treatment. Second, the effects of combining the treatments (additive, synergistic, or antagonistic) can be evaluated. This latter feature is quite important in that many biologics (including vaccines) are given in combination, and their combined effects may differ from their singular effects. To keep the requirements for the trial practical under field conditions as well as to aid interpretation of results, most field trials should have a maximum of three factors.

Split-plot designs are a subtype of factorial designs; the difference is that the experimental unit for one factor (treatment) is different from that for the other factor (treatment). Often this design is chosen when one treatment can only be given to aggregates of individuals (e.g., antimicrobials in the water supply of a litter of pigs or a pen of cattle), whereas the other treatment can be allocated to individuals within the aggregate (e.g., assigning individual pigs or cattle to receive a vaccine). Split-plot designs have the same general advantages of factorial designs, particularly the ability to assess interaction between the treatments. If the whole-plot factor is not randomly assigned (e.g., perhaps the owner decided which litters would receive antimicrobials in the water), one cannot assess the effect of this treatment. However, any interaction between the two treatments can still be assessed. In other instances the split-plot design allows the actual field procedures to be performed with less hassle than if an ordinary factorial design were used (Martin et al. 1984). These five designs (completely randomized, randomized complete blocks, cross-over, factorial, and split-plot) are probably the most common designs used in field trials in veterinary medicine. However, there are a large number of other designs, and the advice of a statistician should be sought early in the planning phase of any field trial.

To avoid severe imbalance in the number of units receiving each treatment at any time throughout the study period, the randomization strategy should allow for equalizing the number in each group at fixed intervals (e.g., after every fourth or eighth unit has entered the trial). This procedure is called "balancing," and prevents temporal factors from biasing the outcome (e.g., severe weather at a time when the new treatment had been used most frequently).

7.4.2 Nonrandom Allocation Methods

Recently there has been much discussion about the ethics of randomized trials, and a number of articles describing alternatives to random allocation have appeared. Most of these methods use prior knowledge of treatment efficacy in addition to the ongoing results of the trial to decide the treatment given to the next experimental unit to enter the trial. Thus these techniques are restricted to trials where the units enter the study over an extended period of time, and the response of one unit can be assessed before the next unit is entered. Many clinical trials may fit this design.

One simple example of these designs known as adaptive allocation is called "play-the-winner." To utilize this method, at the start of the study a consensus is obtained about the treatment to be given to the first unit. If the response to this treatment is favorable, the same treatment is given to the second unit and each following unit until an unfavorable response occurs. When a failure is observed, the alternative treatment is used and continued until a treatment failure occurs, at which point the first treatment is used on the next unit to enter the trial. The process is repeated until the desired number of units has entered the study. This design ensures that the most efficacious treatment is given to the majority of animals in the trial, and this may reduce owner concerns related to the ethics of randomization. However, as the true difference between treatment effects decreases, the advantage of this method over the traditional random allocation is also reduced. Also, if adaptive allocation is used, it is extremely important to define what constitutes a failure. Otherwise, if the identity of the treatment is known, subjective bias in assessing the results may occur.

It should be noted that the use of historical controls (the before and after comparison) has virtually no place in field trials in veterinary medicine. The unpredictability of the outcome and the numerous possible differences between the before and after periods prevent the valid use of this design except in rare circumstances. This technique is particularly prone to bias if herds or flocks with a history of severe disease problems are given a treatment and the current disease status compared to the previous status. In addition to a host of possible differences between the periods that could influence the outcome (e.g., weather) the probability of problem herds getting worse is quite small, the probability of getting better rather large. Hence, almost any treatment may falsely appear to be effective (Acres and Radostits 1976).

7.4.3 Assigning Unequal Numbers of Units to Each Treatment

Assuming that only two treatments are being compared (in a completely randomized design) and in the absence of clear indications about the efficacy of the new treatment, the allocation of equal numbers to the treatment and control groups is preferable. But if evidence exists that the new treatment is likely to be better than the standard treatment, unequal allocation (not to exceed 2:1) can maximize the benefit to those in the trial. That is, 2 experimental units are assigned to the treatment group for each 1 experimental unit allocated to the control group. There is no value in proceeding beyond the 2:1 ratio, because in order to maintain the power of the field trial the total number of units may have to be increased to compensate for the unequal allocation.

7.4.4 Biologic Factors That May Affect Allocation

Certain factors have been described that may necessitate modifications in the design of vaccine and/or therapeutic trials. These factors usually involve an aspect of herd immunity, which allows groups of animals to stop or slow infection and/or minimize its effects, and may exist even when not all individuals within the herd are resistant. In this event, the vaccinated or treated majority may protect or otherwise reduce the challenge to the nontreated minority, minimizing differences in outcome between the treatment groups and leading to the conclusion the treatment was not effective. Also, if the treatment is applied to only a small proportion of the herd, the untreated animals present an unduly large source of infection or challenge, and the study again is biased toward accepting the null hypothesis of no treatment effect (Thurber et al. 1977). This can also happen in testing anthelmintics, since the untreated animals may seed the environment and increase the challenge to treated animals in the same area. The best way of circumventing these problems is to use experimental units that are or can be separated physically from each other (e.g., randomize herds rather than animals within a herd to treatment groups).

Another means of avoiding this problem is to use the herd as its own control in a cross-over design. In doing this, each herd is treated (or not treated) for a specified period of time, and at the end of each time period a decision is made (using a formal random process) whether to treat for the next period. A difficulty with this design is that the residual effects of spread of vaccine organisms and/or herd immunity may extend into adjacent treatment periods. Thus the duration of these periods would have to be carefully defined and/or the residual effects quantified and removed analytically. A further drawback to the cross-over design is the difficulty in ensuring equality of handling of each group if the treatments given in a period are known to the owner and/or the investigator.

7.5 Treatment Regimes

The different treatments (including their timing, method, and route of administration) and dosages should be clearly and completely specified. Besides providing clarity of purpose and performance to the study, it is the total program that is being evaluated, not just a specific treatment. If appropriate, the other treatments or manipulations that can or can not be given should be specified. Otherwise if the cointerventions are related to the treatment, the outcomes may be biased. In most field studies the program given to the comparison (reference) group must be the best treatment currently available. Only when no satisfactory treatment exists can field trials offering no treatment to the comparison group be justified. When a new treatment is being investigated, the highest recommended and safe dose should be used to increase the validity of negative findings. Where possible, more than one dosage level should be included so that any dose-response relationship can be identified.

7.6 Follow-Up Period

Management or other biases related to both conscious and unconscious beliefs about the value of the various interventions under study may give rise to differences developing between treatment groups. Most frequently, bias will be evidenced in the differential management of or assessment of outcome in members of the treatment and control groups. The simplest and most effective way of minimizing this bias is to prevent knowledge of the treatment status of individual experimental units by using blind techniques and placebos. Blind techniques may be used to keep one party (the owner) or the other (the investigator) or both ("double blind") unaware of the treatment status of any given experimental unit. In this manner, systematic differences between groups in the management of the animals or in assessing the outcome will be minimized.

To maintain blindness it frequently is necessary to use dummy treatments or placebos. Depending upon the situation, the placebo might be an innocuous look-alike antibiotic, a fake vaccine, or any substance or regime designed to mimic the real treatment. If two very different appearing drugs are to be compared, the syringe can be filled and the barrel taped to hide the identity of the drug. In some instances, no amount of camouflage can hide the identity of the treatment regime; nonetheless, it is essential to maintain as much similarity in the management and assessment of both groups as possible.

The effects of other problems such as noncompliance and withdrawal from the trial tend to be reduced through the use of blind techniques. When possible, the extent of compliance should be noted and reasons for withdrawal recorded.

7.7 Measuring Outcome

The outcome or response should be of practical importance to the animal and/or its owner (Burns 1963). Thus, titer response, blood level of drug, or parasite egg count per gram of feces should not be used as substitutes for measuring protection against disease or decreased production, as one may not predict the other (e.g., titer response often is a poor predictor of protection against disease).

For trials performed in domestic animals, at least two outcomes (one concerned with productivity and the other with morbidity or mortality) should be used, because it is possible for a treatment to affect one outcome but not the other. A treatment may lower morbidity rates but have little effect on growth rate or feed efficiency. This appears to be the case with vaccination against atrophic rhinitis in swine.

In choosing a parameter to represent the outcome or response, preference should be given to those that can be measured objectively and quantitatively over those that must be measured on a subjective basis. However with a little ingenuity, scoring systems can be developed to help increase the precision involved in subjective assessments. In either event it is preferable to measure the outcome without knowledge of the treatment status by using some form of blind technique. Obviously this is most important when the outcome is judged subjectively.

7.8 Analyzing Treatment Effect

The actual effect of the treatment regime is found by comparing the outcome in those members of the treatment and control groups who complied fully with the regime. The effect anticipated if the same treatment were offered in the same manner to similar groups can be obtained by using the original group allocation when calculating the treatment effects. The latter evaluation includes any effects resulting from noncompliance, deviation from original treatment allocation, evaluation, etc.

It is not the intention here to discuss the statistical tests that can be used to analyze the results of field trials. Simple statistical tests such as the student's t-test or the chi-square test will suffice in trials with only two treatment groups. If matching is used, the test should be chosen accordingly. Suffice it to say that the design of the study dictates which statistical test to use. The reader is encouraged to consult an appropriate statistical text for details.

Finally a brief comment should be made on significance levels. Often the statement "significant at the 5% level" is taken as proof of a treatment effect. In fact, the above statement merely indicates that if the only cause of differences in the frequency or extent of outcome is the allocation of experimental units, the likelihood of differences equal to or larger than those observed is less than 5%. Other factors besides the treatment could have produced the differences. In addition, the actual meaning of the significance level is difficult to interpret, because the literature is biased by the tendency to report positive and withhold negative results. For this and other reasons (such as frequent snooping at the data for significant differences), one should be somewhat conservative in interpreting the level of significance reported in the literature.

After reading this chapter, there will still be individuals who believe that any and all experimentation on clients' animals is unethical or that field trials are too difficult to control. For these individuals the results of observational studies and, more frequently, experience or expert advice form the basis of treatment selection. Unfortunately experience is often a poor method for determining the truth about treatment efficacy. Hence, the randomized trial remains the best current method of assessing treatment efficacy to ensure that we do more good than harm for our clients and their animals.

7.9 Examples of Field Trials

Table 7.1 summarizes some of the data resulting from a field trial of an *E. coli* bacterin and a reo-like virus vaccine in beef cows and calves (Acres and Radostits 1976). This well-designed trial utilized a factorial design to examine the separate and joint effects of the bacterin and virus vaccine. Great effort was taken to obtain valid data, and a placebo was used to minimize management bias in the performance of the trial as well as to prevent potential bias in assessing the outcome. The various rates and calculations are explained well and the discussion section should prove informative to those contemplating field trials. Unfortunately, neither the bacterin nor the virus vaccine appeared to be effective in reducing morbidity or mortality. (The reader may verify this by applying the chi-square test to the data in Table 7.1. The Mantel-Haenszel method of analysis may also be used; for example, to test the calf vaccine effect controlling for the effect of the bacterin given to the cow.)

Table 7.2 summarizes the results of another field trial involving gonadotrophin-releasing hormone (GnRH) (given at day 15 postpartum) and prostaglandins (given at day 24 postpartum) in a 300-cow dairy herd (Etherington 1983). (That only one herd was used is in retrospect the only major drawback of note to the design of this trial.) Again, a factorial design was used and the occurrence of a number of diseases as well as an

Table 7.1. Morbidity and mortality rates in beef calves, classified by vaccine-bacterin status

	Vaccine[b] to calf	Status of calf[c]		Total calves	Morbidity rate (%)	Mortality rate (%)
		Diarrhea	Died			
Bacterin[a]	Yes	32	3	163	19.6	1.8
	No	41	7	172	23.8	4.1
Placebo	Yes	33	10	160	20.6	6.2
	No	34	3	187	19.2	1.6

Source: Acres and Radostits 1976, with permission.
[a]K99 *E. coli* bacterin.
[b]Reolike virus vaccine (now called Rotavirus).
[c]Within 30 days of birth.

Table 7.2. **Reproductive performance parameters of 305 Holstein-Friesian cows classified by treatment groups**

| | Treatment groups | | | |
| | (1) Placebo placebo $n = 79$ | (2) GnRH[a] placebo $n = 73$ | (3) Placebo prostaglandin $n = 76$ | (4) GnRH prostaglandin $n = 77$ |
Outcome parameter				
Days from calving to first observed estrus	60.0	86.4	55.4	61.3
Days from calving to first service	83.9	108.1	91.5	84.5
Days from calving to conception	121.2	135.9	109.9	116.5
Services per conception	1.79	1.65	1.74	1.80
Number of heats detected before first service	0.61	0.5	0.65	0.65
Percent culled for reproductive reasons	10.1	6.8	3.9	3.9
Percent developing pyometra	6.3	17.8	2.6	9.0

Source: Etherington 1983, with permission.
[a]Gonadotrophin releasing hormone.

important productivity measure (the calving-to-conception interval) were selected as outcomes. Plasma progesterone levels were measured at three different times (days 15, 24, and 28) postpartum to provide an additional and objective biologic indication of the treatment effects. Placebos were used to maintain double-blindness, preventing both differential management and biased assessment of results (e.g., rectal findings). Wherever possible, subjective findings (such as rectal examination results) were quantified (e.g., the actual size of the uterine horn or ovarian follicle was estimated rather than being reported as small, normal, or large). The results of this trial failed to indicate any practical beneficial effect of GnRH on reproductive parameters; in fact the drug appeared to produce adverse effects on the ability of treated cows to conceive, primarily due to an increased occurrence of pyometra. Prostaglandins appeared to produce a beneficial effect alone and also by counteracting the adverse effects of GnRH. The actual analysis used (factorial analysis of variance) is beyond the level of this text; however, the above results should be reasonably apparent after perusing the raw data in Table 7.2. Given that only one herd was used in this study, it makes it difficult to extrapolate results to all dairy cattle. Nonetheless, it points out that what appear to be biologically sensible interventions may not always produce the desired effects.

Neither of the above experiments should be interpreted as providing conclusive evidence about the efficacy of the biologics studied. They serve as examples of good experimental design that will hopefully benefit those interested in planning field trials or in evaluating the results of published trials. General comments about the design of field trials to investigate vaccines against bovine respiratory disease are available also (Martin 1983).

References

Acres, S. D., and O. M. Radostits. 1976. The efficacy of a modified live Reo-like virus vaccine and an *E. coli* bacterin for prevention of acute undifferentiated neonatal diarrhea of beef calves. Can. Vet. J. 17:197–212.

Armitage, P. 1971. Statistical Methods in Medical Research. New York, N. Y.: John Wiley & Sons.

Burns, K. N. 1963. A comparison of the glucogenic effects of some compounds used in the treatment of ketosis. Vet. Rec. 75:763–68.

Byar, D. P., R. M. Simon, W. T. Friedewald, T. T. Schlesselman, D. L. DeMets, J. H. Ellenberg, M. H. Gail, and J. H. Ware. 1976. Randomized clinical trials: Perspectives on some recent ideas. New Eng. J. Med. 295:74–80.

Cochran, W. G., and G. M. Cox. 1957. Experimental Design. New York, N. Y.: John Wiley & Sons.

Colton, T. 1974. Statistics in Medicine. Boston, Mass.: Little, Brown.

Comstock, G. W. 1978. Uncontrolled ruminations on modern controlled trials. Am. J. Epidemiol. 108:81–84.

Cornfield, J. 1978. Randomization by group: A formal analysis. Am. J. Epidemiol. 108:100–2.

Etherington, W. 1983. The effect of gonadotrophin releasing hormone and/or cloprostenol on reproductive performance in Holstein-Friesian dairy cows: A field trial. M.Sc. thesis, Univ. of Guelph, Ontario.

Fleiss, J. L. 1973. Statistical Methods for Rates and Proportions. Toronto, Canada: John Wiley & Sons.

Gilbert, J. P. 1974. Randomization of human subjects. New Eng. J. Med. 291:1305–6.

Hill, A. B. 1952. The clinical trial. New Eng. J. Med. 247:113–19.

Martin, S. W. 1978. The design of field trials. Proc. 2nd Int. Symp. on Neonatal Diarrhea. Univ. of Saskatchewan, Canada.

————. 1983. Vaccination: Is it effective in preventing respiratory disease or influencing weight gains in feedlot calves? Can. Vet. J. 24:10–19.

Martin, W., S. Acres, E. Janzen, P. Willson, and B. Allen. 1984. A field trial of preshipment vaccination of calves. Can. Vet. J. 25:145–47.

Peto, R., M. C. Pike, P. Armitage, N. E. Breslow, D. R. Cox, S. R. Howard, N. Mantel, K. McPherson, J. Peto, and P. G. Smith. 1976. Design and analysis of randomized clinical trials requiring prolonged observation of each patient. I. Introduction and design. Brit. J. Cancer. 34:585–612.

————. 1977. Design and analysis of randomized clinical trials requiring prolonged observation of each patient. II. Analysis and examples. Brit. J. Cancer. 35:1–39.

Snedecor, G. W., and W. G. Cochran. 1980. Statistical Methods. 7th ed. Ames: Iowa State Univ. Press.

Thurber, E. T., E. P. Bass, and W. H. Beckenhauer. 1977. Field trial evaluation of a Reo-Coronavirus calf diarrhea vaccine. Can. J. Comp. Med. 41:131–36.

C H A P T E R 8

Theoretical Epidemiology: Systems Analysis and Modeling

Animal agriculture is an activity primarily carried out to produce food and fiber by the deliberate and controlled use of plants and animals (Spedding 1979). In this context agriculture can be thought of as being manipulative ecology with its basic operational units being production systems.

Animal production systems are complex. They are composed of and influenced by complex interactions among biologic, climatic, economic, social, and cultural factors. The biologic component includes plants, animals, disease, and the association between disease and animal productivity. Because of the complexity of production systems, decisions based on simple analyses involving only a few factors may not be effective in improving the efficiency of the system. Rather, optimal decisions are likely to be those based on an objective and holistic analysis. How to conduct such an analysis as well as the necessary decision-making strategies are embodied in the systems approach.

8.1 Systems Approach

Biologic systems may be thought of conceptually and practically in a vertical manner beginning with the smallest systems (atoms) and progressing through cells, organs, body systems, individuals, and populations (e.g., farms). Although it is an oversimplification, research at levels below the individual may be deemed reductionistic, whereas research at levels above the individual is holistic. The systems approach is based on the recognition that a broad perspective is necessary when investigating any type of organized system. Since the various parts of the system are linked together in an interactive and interdependent manner, examination of isolated components can lead to erroneous conclusions because critical feedback within the system may be overlooked (Morley 1972).

As mentioned earlier, veterinarians are becoming increasingly concerned with ecologically-complex health-related problems. Disease per se is only part of the production system, but it needs to be investigated with consideration given to both the complex interactions between factors that influence disease levels and to the possible ramifications of control procedures. This has led to a realization that the approach to health care must be based on comprehensive information using continuously upgraded decision-making skills. While philosophically accepted, this holistic approach has been rarely adhered to in practice because no appropriate method of analysis was available for complex systems. Investigators attempting to consider all factors tended to become lost in a mass of details.

Modern computers have provided a partial solution to this impasse, and in recent years there has been a rapid expansion in research that has used the computer to perform the time-consuming work associated with analyzing and simulating the behavior of complex biological systems. The computer allows problems to be approached in new ways and it allows one to deal with whole problems, not just parts of them.

The systems approach using electronic devices is not new. Airline pilots practice for hours on flight simulators before taking on the responsibility of passengers' lives. These professionals use models to test various alternatives prior to implementation and the making of potentially costly errors.

Systems thinking is not new to veterinarians either. Rather than using computers and complex mathematical functions, veterinarians have relied on experience, judgment, and common sense. However, the tasks are becoming more complex as the scale of enterprises increases, as the depth and diversity of technology intensify, and as the array of production alternatives broadens. As this happens, it becomes unrealistic for an individual's mind to master and retain an understanding of all parts of the system and the consequences of interrelationships within the system.

Although systems thinking is not new to veterinary medicine, what is perhaps more recent is the selection of end points other than disease (e.g., health and productivity), and the growing concern with levels of organization above the individual animal.

One of the roles of the epidemiologist is to bring together data from the field and the laboratory. In doing this the epidemiologist creates at least a conceptual model of the system under consideration, including its state of health, and wherever possible attempts to quantify the role of each component in the system. This is not a simple task because very often little is known about the quantitative aspects of agent transmission or the association of disease with productivity. One major benefit of modeling is that in attempting to construct a model one becomes aware of key data that are missing; this in itself is instructive in terms of understanding complex problems. Once constructed, most models can be used to help decide between alternative control procedures under various situations (i.e., they can be used as a tool to aid decision making).

The purpose of this chapter is to present some basic modeling concepts and to illustrate several of the common types of models. Further applications of models will be presented in subsequent chapters.

8.1.1 Definitions

Systems analysts and "modelers" often use words in a specific context that is different from their everyday meaning. Hence a set of definitions is useful (Anderson 1974).

System—a group of interacting components operating together for a common purpose, capable of reacting as a whole to external stimuli; it is unaffected directly by its own outputs and has a specified boundary based on the inclusion of all significant feedback pathways (Spedding 1979).

Model—representation of a real system; it is not an exact representation, merely a simplification of one form or another.

Components—identifiable units within the system.

Relational or flow diagram—one that is used to show the interrelationships of the components in a system.

Driving variables—those variables that affect the system but are not affected by it (e.g., meteorologic factors).

System state variables—components of the system that may change state (e.g., from healthy to diseased) over time.

Experiment—the process of observing the performance of the system or its model under a specified set of conditions.

Model characteristics—referred to as "simular," their real-life counterparts referred to as "simuland."

8.2 Types of Models and Their Development

Models are used in an attempt to approximate or mimic real-world systems and as such there are a number of different types. For present purposes, agricultural models will be classified as illustrated in Figure 8.1.

8.2.1 Physical and Descriptive

Physical models have been used for many years and in many different areas of activity. Chemists construct models of molecules in an attempt to gain a better understanding of their structure and properties. Agricultural engineers build models of farm buildings and test the effects of building design and placement on local air movement (including the accumulation of

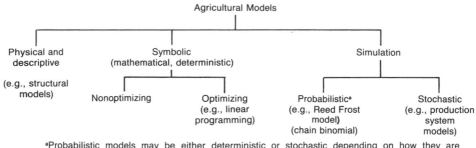

[a]Probabilistic models may be either deterministic or stochastic depending on how they are formulated.

8.1. Classification of agricultural models.

snow) in wind tunnels. The latter models allow for modifications to be made prior to large expenditures being committed to construct full-scale buildings.

Descriptive models include diagrams and charts designed to portray a real-world system or subsystem. These usually include the major inputs, outputs, and internal processes. Such relational diagrams can be used for a number of purposes including assisting with the organization of available information and identifying gaps in knowledge. An example of a relational diagram depicting events associated with reproduction in dairy cattle is presented in Figure 8.2 (Oltenacu et al. 1980). While they can help with the conceptualization of problems, such models do not yield information concerning how the system will perform under various conditions. To achieve this objective it is usually necessary to transform the model into mathematical form. One way of achieving this is through path models as was discussed in Chapter 5; other approaches are described here.

8.2.2 Symbolic

In general, symbolic models use mathematical symbols to describe the status of variables at a given time and to define the manner in which they change and interact (Emshoff and Sisson 1970). These models are usually deterministic in nature (i.e., they are concerned with average results). The output from deterministic models is controlled solely by the values of the parameters; there is no element of randomness, and hence output for a given set of inputs is always the same. Models of this type can be further subdivided into optimizing and nonoptimizing. An example of a symbolic nonoptimizing model would be the well-known law of physics $E = mc^2$. Models of this type will not be discussed further.

An optimization model is one that seeks the best mix of inputs to achieve an objective, and it usually consists of a mathematical function to

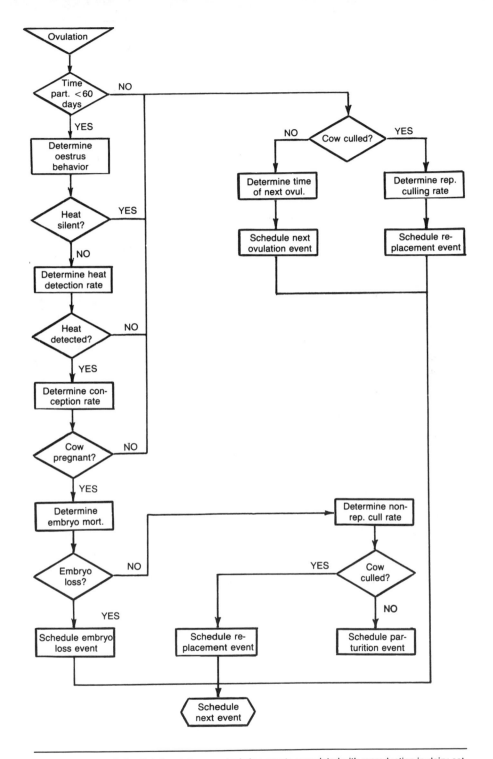

8.2. Relational diagram depicting events associated with reproduction in dairy cattle. (Source: Oltenacu et al. 1980, with permission)

be maximized or minimized and a series of constraints. Optimization models are frequently used in biometrics and economics, although perhaps the best known application of the technique is the use of linear programming (linear objective function) in least-cost feed formulation. An example of linear programming is presented in 8.3.1.

8.2.3   Simulation

A simulation model implies a dynamic process or representation of a system achieved by building a model and moving it through time.

In general, simulation models are designed to mimic the system under study as closely as possible. Hence, the model builder tries to achieve a substantial degree of epidemiologic realism in the structure of the model, and the parameters used are chosen so they can be readily related to features in the system being modeled. Simulation models are built using combinations of arithmetic and logical processes and, in this sense, have features in common with symbolic models. They are generally used to search for the best alternative, often by a process of trial and error.

For present purposes, simulation models have been subdivided into probabilistic and stochastic (Fig. 8.1). As the name implies, probabilistic models include basic concepts of probability theory and may (depending on how they are formulated) be deterministic or stochastic.

8.2.3.1 CHAIN BINOMIAL.   Chain binomial models allow the investigation of patterns of binomial phenomena over time. A well-known deterministic probability model is the Reed-Frost model of a theoretical epidemic (Abbey 1952). The model allows for the calculation of the number of cases and susceptibles in the population in successive periods of time; hence a chain binomial model results. The latter model will be discussed in 8.3.2.

8.2.3.2 MARKOV CHAIN.   If a system can be represented by a discrete number of possible states, and at each time interval individuals can move between states according to some given probability, the system may be modeled using a process called a Markov chain. Specifically, if the vector representing the number of individuals in each of n states is known (state vector S_1, $S_2, \ldots, S_n$), the probabilities of moving from one state to another can be represented as a transition probability matrix (P) with the following format:

$$
\begin{array}{l}
P_{11}\ P_{12}\ \ldots\ P_{1n} \\
P_{21}\ P_{22}\ \ldots\ P_{2n} \\
\qquad \cdot \\
\qquad \cdot\, P_{ij} \\
\qquad \cdot \\
P_{n1}\ P_{n2}\ \ldots\ P_{nn}
\end{array}
$$

where P_{ij} is the probability of going from state i to state j.

When the state vector is multiplied by the transition probability matrix, the number of individuals in each state at the end of the time period (t) under consideration is:

$$(S_1, S_2, \ldots, S_n)_t \times P = (S_1, S_2, \ldots, S_n)_{t+1}$$

8.2.3.3 STOCHASTIC. Models of this type include an element of randomness. Hence, the outcome of the model for a given set of inputs can vary depending on the element of chance. It is generally believed the inclusion of chance variation (randomness) makes the model more biologically realistic than could be achieved by the corresponding deterministic model. Monte Carlo sampling is basic to the concept of simulation models containing stochastic elements.

Monte Carlo sampling is a method of allowing for the effects of chance. In the application of this technique, random numbers are produced by computer programs and are then used to either sample continuous distributions or to decide whether a change of state of a binomial variable occurs. In the former case, a number between 0 and 1 is randomly produced and then used to select a sample from the cumulative distribution function of the biological variable under consideration. For example, if the biological variable is approximately normally distributed, this process will result in values at and about the mean of the distribution being sampled more frequently than those at the extremes. In the latter case a random number is produced between 0 and 1, and its value is compared to the long term expected probability of the event occurring. If the generated number is less than or equal to the defined probability, the event is considered to occur. In this way individual events occur stochastically, while the long-term frequency of occurrence is determined by the specified parameter value. If the model included the event milk fever occurrence, and it had previously been determined that the probability (rate of occurrence) of the condition in the age and breed of cattle under consideration was 0.15, the generated values would be compared to 0.15 to decide whether the individual animal would or would not develop the disease at that point in the modeling process.

8.2.4 Stages in Model Development

The general sequence of steps followed in model development within an overall systems analysis is outlined in Figure 8.3.

8.2.4.1 MODEL FORMULATION. There must be a clear statement of objectives. Models developed as ends in themselves will probably not turn out to be useful. In general, one should start simply and only build a complex model if necessary. This process necessitates a thorough systems analysis, which

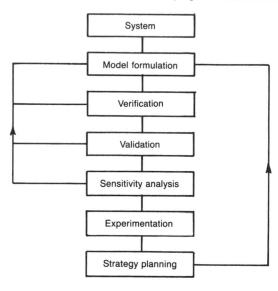

8.3.   Stages in model development.

consists of studying the system under consideration with a view to determining its principal components and their interrelationships. This usually culminates in a flow diagram. Boundaries for the system must be established, and the various driving and state variables and processes involved must be clearly outlined as well. Finally, the major features and relationships of the system are synthesized into a logical structure that may be implemented on a computer.

8.2.4.2 VERIFICATION.   After implementation the model must be verified. This is the process of ensuring that the model behaves in the manner that the modeler intended and assesses the adequacy of the equations and functions.

8.2.4.3 VALIDATION.   This is the process of assessing the accuracy of model output and of ensuring the usefulness and relevance of the model. Specifically, validation is an attempt to ensure that the model adequately mimics the simuland to justify proceeding. Ideally, subsections of the model should be validated as separate exercises prior to validation of the model as a whole, because errors in one section may be completely or partially compensated for by errors in another section. However, the most rigorous form of validation involves the detailed comparison of model output and historical or experimental measurements on the simuland when the driving forces for the model (e.g., meteorological data) are the same as those measured in the simuland.

8.2.4.4 SENSITIVITY ANALYSIS. This involves varying parameter values of the model in a systematic fashion and observing the resultant changes in model output (Anderson 1974). Sensitivity analysis may be conducted to demonstrate the degree to which conclusions based on initial parameter values remain valid if the values used are not accurate estimates of the true population value. Alternatively, it permits the simulator to evaluate the likely consequences of deliberately varying the parameter from the initial value as might be done in the assessment of alternative disease control strategies.

8.2.4.5 MODEL EXPERIMENTATION. If the model is epidemiologically realistic, and if the conclusions drawn from the validation testing and sensitivity analysis are correct, the model may be applied to the evaluation and comparison of alternative control strategies for the disease under study. All the considerations and criteria used in conventional experiments are more or less applicable to experiments with models.

8.2.4.6 STRATEGY PLANNING AND IMPLEMENTATION. The purpose of the above experiments is to guide the decision maker in establishing strategies (policy) as well as implementing them. This necessitates that the results of the model (perhaps a ranking of possible disease control options) be combined with other knowledge by the decision maker.

8.3 Example Applications

8.3.1 Linear Programming

As mentioned earlier, linear programming models are generally of the symbolic optimizing type (Fig. 8.1). As an example (Osburn and Schneeberger 1978), suppose a farmer wishes to grow hay or grain. He has 160 acres of cropland, $20,000 in operating capital, and 300 hours of labor available in each of the spring and summer periods. The requirements per acre for these resources are as follows:

	Grain	Hay
Spring labor (hr)	3.0	1.5
Summer labor (hr)	0.5	2.0
Operating capital	$100.0	$60.0

If hay returns $55 net per acre and grain returns $90 net per acre, what combination of hay and grain will maximize returns?

Stated mathematically, the problem is to:

maximize net returns, $Z = 90x_1 + 55x_2$
where $x_1 = $ acres of grain
$x_2 = $ acres of hay
subject to $x_1 + x_2 < 160$ acres of land
$3x_1 + 1.5x_2 < 300$ hours of spring labor
$0.5x_1 + 2x_2 < 300$ hours of summer labor
$100x_1 + 60x_2 < 20,000$ dollars

This problem can be solved in several ways. For this simple problem one can draw a graph and use it to find the desired solution (Fig. 8.4). In order to graph the inequalities, draw a straight line between the plotted positions reflecting the equality signs. For example, with regard to the land constraint, if x_1 is set to 0, x_2 becomes 160 and vice versa.

With regard to Figure 8.4, points on the feasible region surface ABCD may be viewed as the frontier of production possibilities, and some point on the line will satisfy the objective of maximum possible income. In this example, net returns are maximized with 40 acres of grain and 120 acres of hay [(40 × $90) + (120 × $55) = $10,200] given the linear constraints of the problem.

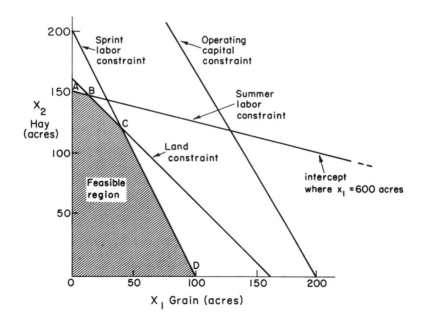

8.4. Plot of resource restrictions and region of feasible solutions for hypothetical 160-acre farm. (Adapted from Osburn and Schneeberger 1978)

For further reading, Carpenter and Howitt (1980) have applied this technique to determine the most economically optimal approach to the control or eradication of brucellosis in beef cattle in California.

8.3.2 Reed-Frost Model

Herd immunity can function to prevent the successful entry of an organism into a group or population of animals, and/or it can minimize the extent and rapidity of the spread of that organism once it becomes established. A simple model that describes major factors involved in herd immunity is known as the Reed-Frost model. As discussed earlier, the Reed-Frost model is of the chain binomial type. Although a number of the events and factors have been simplified somewhat to make the model workable, the model has proven useful in demonstrating those factors of paramount importance in herd immunity. The major assumptions in the model are: (1) infection is spread directly from infected individuals to others by "adequate contact" and in no other way; (2) once contacted, the individual (if susceptible) will develop the disease and be infectious in the next time period, following which it will be immune; (3) there is a fixed probability of adequate contact between any two individuals.

The number of immune and susceptible individuals and the number of cases (case as used here describes either a clinically diseased individual or an infected individual) are recorded at each time period after the introduction of the first infected individual. The single factor that carries the epidemic from one time period to the next is the probability of adequate contact. The latter is defined to be the likelihood in any time period that an infected individual will have contact with another individual sufficient to transmit the infection if the latter individual is susceptible.

The mathematical formulation of the Reed-Frost model is $C_{t+1} = S_t(1 - Q^{C_t})$, where C is the number of cases, S is the number of susceptibles, and Q is the probability of no adequate contact. (The probability of no adequate contact is found by subtracting the probability of adequate contact [P] from 1.) The subscript t serves as a time counter, and the length of the time period usually is set equal to the incubation or latent period of the disease. The time at which the first case enters the population is time 0 and each unit of time thereafter is numbered sequentially.

Specifically, the model equates the number of cases at any time to the number of susceptibles in the immediately preceding time period and the probability of contact of each individual with a case. Examples of output from the model under various conditions are presented in Table 8.1 and Figure 8.5.

This and other models together with studies of actual epidemics demonstrate that epidemics die out because of a combination of a low rate of adequate contact and a reduced number of susceptible individuals. Specifi-

Table 8.1.   An epidemic curve predicted by the Reed-Frost model[a]

Time interval (t)	Number of susceptibles (S_t)	Number of cases (C_t)	Number of immunes (I_t)
0	100	1	...
1	96	4	1
2	82	14	5
3	46	36	19
4	11	35	55
5	3	8	90
6	2	1	98
7	2	0	99

[a]The formula for the model is: $C_{t+1} = S_t(1 - Q^{C_t})$ given $P = 0.04$, $Q = 0.96$.
$C_1 = 100(1 - 0.96^1) = 4$; $S_1 = 100 - 4 = 96$.
$C_2 = 96(1 - 0.96^4) = 14$; $S_2 = 96 - 14 = 82$.

cally, if $P \times S$ is greater than 1, the epidemic can occur; whereas if $P \times S$ is less than 1, the epidemic will die out or not occur in the first instance. These constraints are much more instructive about the phenomenon of herd immunity than the simple statement that a specified percentage of the population must be immune to give the population protection. In fact, even if the percentage is high, if there are sufficient susceptibles that have contact with each other, and if the infection enters the population it will likely spread, since $P \times S$ is greater than 1. It must be remembered that the variable "the probability of adequate contact" is a complex variable and contains factors

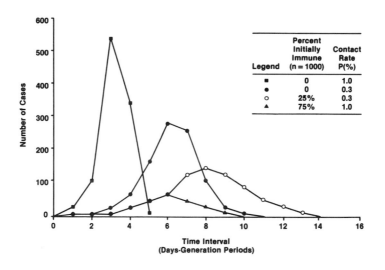

8.5.   Epidemic curves generated by Reed-Frost model.

specific to certain disease agents as well as to the social structure of the animal population. The actual probability of adequate contact can be estimated from observed epidemic curves by successively applying the following formula: $P = (C_{t+\text{incubation period}})/(S_t C_t)$.

If the number of susceptible animals in the population is decreased by increasing the proportion that is immune, the peak of the epidemic can be delayed and/or the magnitude and duration can be greatly reduced. Such an increase in immunity could come about because of a formal immunization process, or the resistance of the animals could be increased by more indirect means such as changes in husbandry and/or management practices. The latter may also be used to lower the probability of adequate contact.

8.3.3 Markov Chain Models

Carpenter and Riemann (1980) used a Markov chain model to conduct a benefit-cost analysis of a *Mycoplasma meleagridis* eradication program in turkeys in the United States.

Figure 8.6 presents a flow diagram depicting the various states of nature for both breeder and commercial meat birds. The transition between the various states represented by solid lines signifies a change in infection status or a bird being sent to market. Transitions represented by broken lines signify progeny or poult production. The probability values for each of these transitions are represented by their respective P_{ij} values and these are presented in Tables 8.2 (disease and marketing transition) and 8.3 (poult production). For example, the probability of moving from *M. meleagridis* free pedigree breeder status to a *M. meleagridis* infected pedigree breeder is signified as $P_{1,2}$ (Fig. 8.6) and the value for this is 0.05 (Table 8.2, row 1 column 2).

Once the structure of the model is defined and probabilities have been quantified, it is a reasonably simple matter to perform the actual simulation. However, since matrix algebra is used, the simulation is greatly facilitated if the model is implemented on a computer.

Table 8.2. Disease transition matrix for *Mycoplasma meleagridis*

	MM-free pedigree breeders	MM-infected pedigree breeders	MM-free pure-line breeders	MM-infected pure-line breeders	MM-free commercial breeders	MM-infected commercial breeders
MM-free pedigree breeders	0.95	0.05				
MM-infected pedigree breeders	0.00	1.00				
MM-free pure-line breeders			0.70	0.30		
MM-infected pure-line breeders			0.00	1.00		
MM-free commercial breeders					0.10	0.90
MM-infected commercial breeders					0.00	1.00

Source: Carpenter and Riemann 1980.

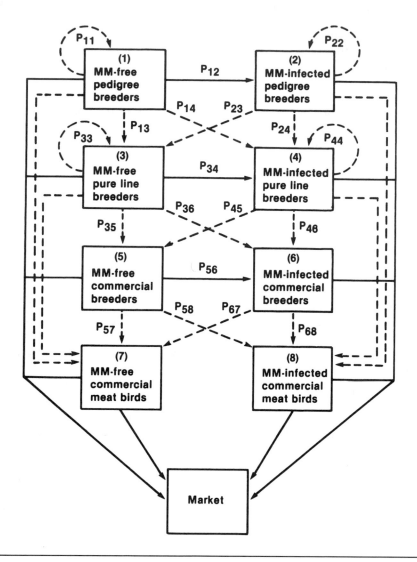

8.6. Flow chart between the generation levels and infection status (solid line) and poult production (broken lines). (Source: Carpenter and Riemann 1980)

Table 8.3. Turkey poult production transition matrix for *Mycoplasma meleagridis* (MM)

	MM-free pedigree poults	MM-infected pedigree poults	MM-free pure-line poults	MM-infected pure-line poults	MM-free commercial breeder poults	MM-infected commercial breeder poults	MM-free commercial meat poults	MM-infected commercial meat poults
MM-free pedigree breeders	.024	.000	.207	.011			.606	.152
MM-infected pedigree breeders	.023	.001	.196	.022			.076	.682
MM-free pure-line breeders			.018	.001	.226	.056	.559	.140
MM-infected pure-line breeders			.017	.002	.028	.254	.070	.629
MM-free commercial breeders							.800	.200
MM-infected commercial breeders							.100	.900

Source: Carpenter and Riemann 1980.

8.3.4   Stochastic Simulation Model of Ovine Fascioliasis

A simulation model of ovine fascioliasis (Meek and Morris 1981) will be described both to present the general process of building a model and to illustrate a stochastic simulation model. The overall objectives of this model were to investigate the factors influencing the epidemiology of ovine fascioliasis and to compare the economic value of various alternative control strategies for the disease.

8.3.4.1   MODEL FORMULATION.   Ovine fascioliasis (*Fasciola hepatica*) is a disease that can cause serious economic loss. The disease is biologically complex with interactions among a number of factors, including meteorologic factors, pasture growth, the disease agent (*F. hepatica*), the intermediate snail host (*Lymnaea tomentosa*), and the mammalian host(s). Hence, the process of choosing the best control strategy for particular circumstances can be difficult since it is not easy to take all relevant factors into account.

The general form of the model is illustrated in Figure 8.7. The model uses a combination of algebraic functions and Monte Carlo sampling from defined probability distributions to generate observations and changes of state. The model was designed to simulate the life cycle of *F. hepatica* and the dynamics of the usual intermediate snail host in Australia, *L. tomentosa*. It also simulates soil moisture, pasture production, sheep feed intake, and the resultant generation of marketable products. The life cycle of *F. hepatica* is greatly influenced by temperature and soil moisture. Temperature determines the rate of advancement through the life cycle and hence influences the timing of infection. Soil moisture acts as a limiting factor on the life cycle and hence influences both the timing of infection and its intensity.

The simular flock was composed of a maximum of 60 nonreproductive sheep. Animals are simulated individually with respect to such factors as intake (of both herbage and metacercariae), growth, and parasite burden, but are simulated as a flock with respect to grazing pattern and routine management practices.

In the model, sheep are shorn and culled at the end of each management year. The maximum percentage of sheep culled each year is assumed to be 20% of the initial flock size. The actual number culled decreases from this maximum if there has been a reduction in the number of sheep over the course of the management year (i.e., if simular deaths have occurred). All sheep that die or are culled are replaced at the end of the management year with shorn yearling wethers.

The simular pasture is defined to be 2 hectares in area and can be specified to be either irrigated or nonirrigated. The area is considered to be closed to external contamination by any stage of the *F. hepatica* life cycle. For purposes of simulation the area is subdivided into ten equal subareas.

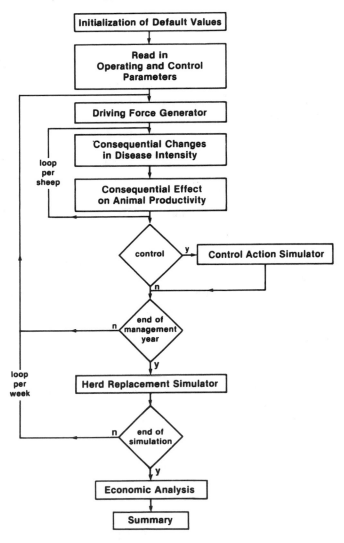

8.7. General form of liver fluke simulation model. (Source: Meek and Morris 1981, with permission)

Simular herbage can be regarded as a perennial species for which an annual cycle of sexual reproduction is not essential. Herbage growth rate is defined to be a function of day length, temperature, available soil moisture, and the quantity of herbage already present on the subarea.

The snail habitat is contained within the tenth subarea of the paddock. The maximum proportion of the subarea to be occupied by the habitat may be stipulated by the person conducting the simulation. The actual size of the habitat (within the defined limit) at any point in simular time is a function of temperature and moisture.

A schematic representation of the epidemiology of the disease (as modeled) is presented in Figure 8.8. The driving variables for the model are meteorologic factors, including maximum and minimum daily temperature and moisture (as either rainfall or irrigation).

The model simulates for the main part on a weekly basis. However, within the main cyclic pattern there are some daily cycles (such as the intake of metacercariae by sheep and the sheep/liver fluke interaction).

Egg contamination of the snail habitat is a function of the adult fluke burden of individual animals, the grazing pattern of sheep with respect to the snail habitat, and the size of the habitat. The rate at which the life cycle proceeds is a function of ambient temperature and the biologic state of the intermediate host snail.

Simulated sheep come in contact with encysted metacercariae if they graze contaminated herbage in subarea 10. The number of metacercariae consumed is a function of the animal's dry matter intake and grazing behavior and the concentration of metacercariae on the herbage.

A proportion of the consumed metacercariae develop to adult liver flukes. Parasitized sheep contaminate the paddock with eggs as long as the sheep survives or until the fluke burden is eliminated by a simular treatment.

Facility has been provided in the model for specifying the use of simular anthelmintics, molluscicides and management practices such as rotational grazing. These control methods can be simulated either singly or in combination.

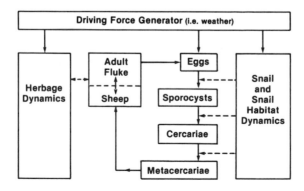

8.8. Schematic representation of interaction of major components involved in epidemiology of ovine fascioliasis, as represented in model. (Source: Meek and Morris 1981, with permission)

All financial items are calculated on the basis of a standard flock of 100 sheep. At the end of each management year an expected margin over variable costs is calculated. (The term variable strategy costs is used to include all expenses directly attributable to the control strategy being simulated.)

Because a control program for ovine fascioliasis can take up to 5 years to generate its full effects and because costs may vary over time, future costs and returns are discounted (see 9.5.2). To produce a more readily interpretable figure, the net present value for the chosen strategy is converted to an annual annuity. The evaluation and comparison of all control strategies are done on the basis of this annual annuity. For simplicity the annual annuity realized over a 5-year simulation is referred to as the financial return.

8.3.4.2 VERIFICATION AND VALIDATION. Once the model had been formulated and implemented, a series of verification and validation checks was performed, and modifications were made until the modelers were satisfied with the logical structure and operation of the model.

Whole model validation was conducted in two parts. First, the predictions of the model were compared with the result of a field investigation that utilized a resident flock and a series of groups of tracer sheep conducted on both irrigated and nonirrigated pastures near Melbourne, Australia (Meek and Morris 1979). Second, the predictions of the model were compared with the results of a field investigation conducted by an independent group of investigators in another part of Australia.

Validation was conducted using meteorologic data that had been recorded at the site of the field investigation. To do this, simular tracer sheep were allowed to grow throughout the year, but the model was adjusted so that the accumulating fluke burden did not affect the red blood cell volume of each sheep, nor did it decrease the animal's dry matter intake (i.e., equivalent to a series of tracer animals).

Simulations were conducted for each of an irrigated and nonirrigated simular area. The simular patterns of fluke acquisition by the tracer sheep for the 2 simular years that corresponded to the 2 field experimental years and for each of the irrigated and nonirrigated areas are presented along with the field results in Table 8.4. The simular and actual field-cumulative fluke burdens for both experimental years are in good agreement.

8.3.4.3 SENSITIVITY ANALYSIS. It was anticipated that model output would be sensitive to pasture egg contamination and the maximum proportion of the paddock that was defined to be snail habitat. Thus, simulations were conducted using various combinations of those two factors. Weekly pasture egg contamination remained constant at the stipulated level throughout each simulation. The proportion of the stipulated maximum snail habitat

Table 8.4. Comparison of the field[a] and simular fluke burdens

Experimental year	Date[b]	Irrigated		Nonirrigated	
		Field	Simular	Field	Simular
1974–1975	16 December 1974	6.4	3.7	0.2	0.0
	17 January 1975	61.6	62.2	0.0	0.0
	13 February 1975	85.2	41.4	0.0	0.0
	13 March 1975	80.8	98.8	0.0	0.0
	10 April 1975	75.0	230.2	0.0	0.0
	8 May 1975	36.5	19.4	0.0	0.0
	5 June 1975	77.2	20.2	0.0	0.0
	3 July 1975	17.2	13.8	0.0	0.0
	31 July 1975	28.8	10.5	0.2	0.0
	28 August 1975	4.0	7.9	0.0	0.0
	25 September 1975	0.8	4.1	0.0	4.6
	23 October 1975	2.0	0.2	0.0	4.2
	20 November 1975	8.0	9.0	3.2	5.0
	Total	483.5	521.4	3.6	13.8
1975–1976	18 December 1975	1.4	21.8	1.8	0.2
	15 January 1976	0.0	0.0	0.4	0.0
	12 February 1976	2.2	0.0	0.0	0.0
	11 March 1976	28.0	0.0	0.0	0.0
	8 April 1976	22.2	0.0	0.0	0.0
	6 May 1976	156.8	616.2	0.0	0.0
	3 June 1976	343.4	413.4	0.0	0.0
	1 July 1976	362.2	62.4	0.0	0.0
	29 July 1976	104.4	6.2	0.0	0.0
	26 August 1976	159.0	0.0	0.0	0.0
	23 September 1976	36.0	0.0	0.0	0.0
	23 October 1976	6.0	0.0	0.0	0.0
	18 November 1976	13.0	26.1	0.0	0.0
	Total	1234.6	1146.1	2.2	0.2

Source: Meek and Morris 1979, with permission.
[a]Mean for group of tracer sheep.
[b]Date at end of 28-day tracer interval. Field experiment commenced 11 November 1974.

size suitable for snail activity was allowed to vary as a function of the interaction between temperature and moisture, and the same meteorologic data file was used for all simulations. The results of this analysis are illustrated in Figure 8.9. Each horizontal surface is the mean yearly cumulative fluke burden for a 5-year simulation.

Simular fluke acquisition appeared to be approximately linearly related to snail habitat size, but resulted in a "logistic" curve with respect to increasing pasture egg contamination.

Under normal simuland conditions, pasture egg contamination is a function of the fluke burden of individual animals. It was therefore postulated that the acquisition of flukes would be sensitive to stocking rate and that both stocking rate and the proportion of the paddock that was snail habitat should be taken into consideration when assessing the effectiveness of any potential control strategy for the disease.

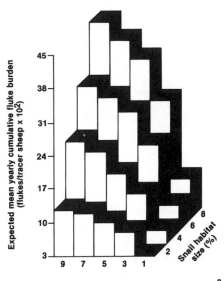

8.9. Expected mean yearly cumulative fluke burden of simular tracer sheep at various levels of total weekly fluke egg contamination and maximum snail habitat size. (Source: Meek and Morris 1981, with permission)

8.3.4.4 MODEL EXPERIMENTATION. At this stage, the model was applied to the evaluation and comparison of alternative control strategies for ovine fascioliasis. Although a number of experiments were conducted, only one will be described here: the use of simular anthelmintics.

Method. Five anthelmintic treatment strategies, selected as being representative of the range of possible strategies that might be employed in the field, were used for this analysis and are presented in Table 8.5. Strategy 1 involved salvage treatments only. Strategies 2–5 involved simular treatment of all sheep during the weeks of the calendar year specified. All treatment strategies were simulated for a 5-year period.

The model was used to estimate the expected financial return from each of the five strategies at each of a number of combinations of stocking rate and snail habitat size. For purposes of this analysis a range of stocking rates (varying from 20 to 30 sheep per hectare of irrigated pasture) and maximum snail habitat sizes (varying from 1 to 10% of the paddock) were used. The range of values used for the latter two factors was considered to be representative of most Australian field situations.

A multiple regression procedure was then used to produce a surface of best fit to the financial data generated by each of the five treatment regimes. By comparing the value of the dependent variable (financial return)

Table 8.5.   Simular anthelmintic treatment strategies

Strategy	Timing of treatments					
1	Salvage only					
2	3[a]	12	21	. . .	. . .	. . .
3	3	12	21	30	. . .	. . .
4	3	12	21	30	45	. . .
5	3	11	19	27	35	45

Source: Meek and Morris 1981, with permission from Elsevier Applied Science Publishers and the authors.

[a]Week of calendar year.

for the five regression surfaces, the treatment strategies were ranked at each of several thousand combinations of stocking rate and maximum snail habitat sizes. The five selected strategies were not compared with a "no treatment" strategy because of the extreme financial loss that occurred if no control or treatment measures were taken.

The four preplanned strategies were also ranked by percentage return on additional funds invested over and above the investment required for strategy 1 (salvage treatment).

Results. The result of ranking alternatives by highest financial return is presented as a decision chart in Figure 8.10. The contours delineate which of the five control strategies provides the highest net financial return at

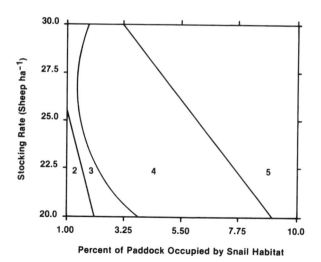

8.10. Decision chart for choice of treatment strategy (see Table 8.5) yielding highest margin over fluke control costs, at various stocking rates and maximum snail habitat sizes. (Source: Meek and Morris 1981, with permission)

each combination of grazing density and maximum snail habitat size.

A general trend across the surface is that as the stocking rate and/or the size of the snail habitat increases, the number of treatments per annum required for the most profitable strategy also increases. Strategies 4 and 5 are predicted by the model to yield the highest financial return over most of the surface, with the lower cost strategies (numbers 2 and 3) only being optimal at very low stocking rates (number 2) and/or snail habitat sizes (numbers 2 and 3). Note that strategy 1 (salvage treatments only) is not represented because it was not the most profitable strategy under any of the conditions presented.

The results of ranking alternatives by percentage return are presented in Table 8.6. The financial return realized from the use of strategy 4 is only marginally better than that of strategy 5 under the particular circumstances used. However, strategy 3 realized the highest percentage return under all price circumstances.

Table 8.6. Comparison of the financial return from each of the five control strategies

Item	Strategy[a]				
	1	2	3	4	5
Strategy costs ($)	16	21	29	37	44
Margin over variable strategy costs ($)	115	174	396	464	455
Margin over strategy 1 ($)	...	59	281	349	340
Return on funds invested in addition to strategy 1 (%)	...	1180	2162	1662	1214

Source: Meek and Morris 1981, with permission from Elsevier Applied Science Publishers and the authors.

[a]See text and Table 8.5 for details of control strategies and simular circumstances. All monetary values rounded to the nearest dollar.

Discussion. In general, if a farmer has unlimited funds, the strategy with the highest financial return would represent the most profitable option and should be chosen (Fig. 8.10). However, while a farmer would have knowledge of and control over the average stocking rate on a paddock, he may not appreciate the proportion of the paddock that is occupied by snail habitat. Therefore, the strategy chosen would depend to some extent on the farmer's risk aversion. The farmer who was risk averse would perhaps choose strategy 5.

If funds were limited, the decision on which strategy to use should be based on the principle of equimarginal returns, which states that the funds available should be invested progressively in uses that yield the highest marginal return as each successive dollar is invested. Although the percentage return on invested funds gives an imprecise assessment of marginal return, it does have value in facilitating comparison between alternative investments (Anderson et al. 1976). Therefore in situations where funds are very limited, strategy 3 may merit consideration (Table 8.6). The substantial return on funds invested in the use of anthelmintics is the result of the relatively low cost and high efficacy of the currently available products and the substantial gains in productivity that can be realized from their strategic use.

References

Abbey, H. 1952. An examination of the Reed-Frost theory of epidemics. Hum. Biol. 3:201.

Anderson, J. R. 1974. Simulation methodology and application in agricultural economics. Rev. Mark. Agric. Econ. 42:3–25.

Anderson, N., R. S. Morris, and I. K. McTaggart. 1976. An economic analysis of two schemes for the anthelmintic control of helminthiasis in weaned lambs. Aust. Vet. J. 52:174–80.

Carpenter, T. E., and R. Howitt. 1980. A linear programming model used in animal disease control. Proc. 2nd Int. Symp. Vet. Epidemiol. Econ., May 1979, Canberra, Australia.

Carpenter, T. E., and H. Riemann. 1980. Benefit-cost analysis of a disease eradication program in the United States: A case study of *Mycoplasma meleagridis* in turkeys. Proc. 2nd Int. Symp. Vet. Epidemiol. Econ., May 1979, Canberra, Australia.

Emshoff, J. R., and R. L. Sisson. 1970. Design and Use of Computer Simulation Models. London: Macmillan.

Meek, A. H., and R. S. Morris. 1979. An epidemiological investigation of ovine fascioliasis (*Fasciola hepatica*) on both irrigated and nonirrigated pastures in Northern Victoria. Aust. Vet. J. 55:365.

––––––. 1981. A computer simulation model of ovine fascioliasis. Agric. Syst. 7:49–77.

Morley, F. H. W. 1972. A systems approach to animal production: What is it about? Proc. Aust. Soc. Anim. Prod. 9:1.

Oltenacu, P. A., R. A. Milligan, T. R. Rousaville, and R. H. Foote. 1980. Modelling reproduction in a herd of dairy cattle. Agric. Syst. 5:193.

Osburn, D. D., and K. C. Schneeberger. 1978. Modern Agriculture Management. Reston Va.: Reston.

Spedding, C. R. W. 1979. An Introduction to Agricultural Systems. London: Applied Science.

Animal Health Economics

C H A P T E R 9

Animal Health Economics

The nature of the veterinary service provided to animal production, whether at the national or individual herd level, characteristically evolves with the stage of development of the community served. Thus, in the early part of this century, major emphasis was placed on the control of diseases that decimated animal populations over large geographic areas. Decisions on whether to control these diseases could usually be made without the aid of formal economic appraisal, because generally the losses greatly exceeded control costs. As epidemic diseases of this latter type were brought under control, emphasis increasingly shifted to the individual property and to the treatment of endemic, clinically-recognizable disease. While this latter approach met with a great deal of success, it suffered because it depended on the initial recognition of an abnormality by the farmer and was too heavily dependent on qualitative and subjective assessment.

In recent years a number of trends (including an increase in the scale of operation, intensification of resource utilization, and the substitution of labor with other usually capital-intensive resources) have typified animal production, particularly in those areas where intensive agricultural methods are practiced. These trends have resulted in those diseases or disease complexes that manifest themselves primarily through a decrease in productive efficiency and that in most cases are endemic becoming the most significant with respect to decreasing farm incomes (Morris 1975). These disease conditions often have a complex multifactor etiology that is intimately related to the production system. Also, since various intensities of control are often possible, it is necessary to determine the level of control that is economically optimal. In this regard, the feature of disease control that makes it such a valuable investment is that it generally increases the efficiency of the production process, and hence it is unlike most other goods and services the farmer may use that generally increase output without changing the nature of the process. This is one of the reasons why returns on funds invested in disease control are usually very high.

In a rapidly changing environment, decisions regarding animal health activities can rarely be made solely on biologic grounds. Rather, a dynamic integrated approach combining epidemiologic and economic analyses is required to determine the nature and scope of the health problem and the implications of intervention. As will be seen later, this is because economic appraisal is highly dependent upon the underlying technical appraisal. In general, economic analysis should be regarded as a tool providing additional information on which to base a decision, rather than a definitive method on which to base the final policy decision.

At the herd level, veterinarians are becoming increasingly aware that they work for farmers whose financial welfare is their interest. They are also realizing that whether their animals have a particular health problem (or have it at a particular level) is largely immaterial, unless it is economically advantageous to do something about it. Exceptions would include zoonotic diseases or the control of disease for humane reasons, where the intensity of control may be greater than that which would be economically optimal. Thus, the choice between the available control techniques is a function of their economic and biologic efficiency. Also, because farmers' participation is usually voluntary, they must be convinced that it is profitable to change their current management practices.

The above principles also apply at levels of organization beyond the farm, and most governments or agencies involved with disease control require that an economic analysis be completed so a rational choice can be made among alternatives competing for the same limited resources.

9.1 Value of Economic Analysis

The majority of the early reports utilizing economic techniques concerned themselves primarily with estimating the cost of a particular disease to an individual producer or a nation. However, this approach is undesirable because it incorrectly suggests that this amount of money is completely recoverable. In recent years the emphasis has moved to an evaluation of the economic benefits of control procedures. Not only is this approach more in accord with economic theory, but it also places a more positive orientation on the information by drawing attention to the benefits of action rather than the costs of inaction (Morris and Meek 1980).

The principal purpose of economic analysis is to aid decision making regarding limited resource allocation. Hence, it provides a basis for making rational choices from among alternative preventive or control actions under various circumstances. Monetary values are used only as a common denominator for the value of particular resources in society. Economists are aware of the limitations of this approach to valuation and have searched for a measure of satisfaction provided by a particular resource. The term "utility" is frequently used as a measure of this. A complete analysis should also indicate the confidence one can have in the monetary and/or utility ranking of the various strategies.

The objective of this chapter is to introduce some of the common methods that are used for the economic assessment of animal health activities and to place these in the context of the decision-making process, a schematic representation of which is presented in Figure 9.1. The first step in solving any disease control problem is to clearly define it and the criteria or goal(s) that will be used to choose between alternative control measures (including no action). One such criterion is economic efficiency. This implies that choices in health care should be made to result in the greatest average return or benefit from the resources available. At the farm level it is frequently assumed that this point is where profit is maximized; however, many other factors (such as risk aversion) may contribute to the final decision. The next steps in the decision-making process are data gathering and processing and the identification of alternative courses of action. To reach a decision as to which alternative to pursue, it is necessary to enumerate, measure, and value the benefits and costs for each alternative and to com-

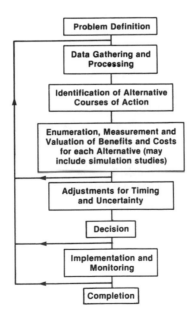

9.1. Schematic representation of decision-making process including economic appraisal.

pare these. As indicated in Figure 9.1, this may include simulation or optimization studies (see Chapter 8). At this stage it may be necessary to consider and account for uncertainty in the results and the timing of cash flow. The economic evaluation can then be completed using the appropriate technique, the results integrated with other pertinent data, and a decision made. The chosen alternative may then be implemented and monitored. The latter phase may again involve computer simulation studies.

The actual method of economic appraisal used in any given situation will depend upon a number of factors such as the type of health problem under consideration and the scope of the control program. A number of the common techniques are outlined in the remainder of this chapter.

9.2   Partial Farm Budgeting

In economic analyses, one must consider how variation in input to the animal production process influences the quantity and quality of output. If the intensity of control can be raised over a continuous spectrum so that a mathematical equation can be used to represent the data, this can be interpreted as a production function and the optimum level of control determined. It can be shown with the aid of such a production function that farmers should continue to increase inputs until reaching the point where marginal (additional unit) costs (i.e., expenses) equal marginal (additional unit) benefits (i.e., revenues). However, in health related matters, sufficient information is rarely available to produce a full production function and hence calculate values from it. Because of these difficulties, partial farm budget analysis may be used as it does not presuppose the estimation of a continuous function. It only requires the knowledge of two or more combinations of factors and their discrete input-output relationships.

While the partial farm budget technique can be applied to a number of different situations, a common application is to assess programs aimed at disease problems that can be assumed to occur on a farm with a high degree of certainty (e.g., bovine mastitis and internal parasitism) (Morris 1969).

The technique only considers those components of enterprise income and costs that are likely to be influenced by the proposed disease control procedure. In general, fixed costs (e.g., taxes) are largely ignored. The technique therefore differs from whole farm budgeting in that the latter is usually reserved for the assessment of a change that will affect the total farm operation (such as the purchase of additional property) whereas the former is usually reserved for assessment of small changes that do not affect total farm management.

A partial farm budget describes the economic consequences of a change in farm procedure. To achieve this, the budget items are categorized as: (1) additional monetary returns received due to adoption of the proposed control procedure (e.g., increased yield of product at possibly higher prices); (2) foregone returns (e.g., reduced numbers of culled animals); (3) additional costs incurred due to the control procedure (e.g., expenditure for drugs and management procedures); (4) costs no longer incurred if the program is implemented (e.g., salvage treatment procedures).

The change in net return is then calculated by summing the returns and costs, calculated under headings 1 and 4 above and subtracting from that the amounts calculated under headings 2 and 3. This net return is an estimate of the additional profit that will accrue to the producer as a result of adopting the disease control procedure and is usually expressed in terms of some basic unit (e.g., per hectare).

The virtue of this procedure is that it permits a realistic appraisal to be made of the consequences of various actions without necessitating the keeping of complete financial records for the farm. One of the inherent difficulties with the technique is that arbitrary decisions must be made about which items to include. The simplest solution is to include any item that may be affected, since if there is no effect it will not influence the outcome. Caution must be taken not to "double count"; that is, measure and include the same effect in two ways. Another limitation is that it allows comparisons to be made between the strategies tested but does not necessarily provide optimum solutions. When possible, it is also advisable to determine how sensitive the conclusions from the analysis are to changes in product price and biological response. (The subject of sensitivity analysis will be discussed later in this chapter, 9.4.)

An example of partial farm budgeting is presented in Table 9.1. The field trial from which these data were taken was designed to assess the economic benefits from two schemes, namely, traditional and critical strategies for helminth control in weaned lambs (Anderson et al. 1976). The traditional scheme was based on a survey of local control procedures, whereas the critical scheme was based on strategic treatments applied in the late spring and early summer period and was based on an objective appraisal. The latter schemes were also compared to no strategic treatment and bi-weekly drenching. The same information presented in the form of a partial budget and comparing the critical to the no strategic treatment schemes only would appear as:

1. Additional Returns
   Additional fleece wool shorn ($227 − $187) $40
   (see Table 9.1)
   Capital value of additional
   sheep surviving to March 1, 1971 ($263 − $222) $41
   Increased value of crutchings ($13 − $11) $ 2
                                                                  ────
                                                                  $83

2. Foregone Returns
   Difference in wool value from sheep which died ($5 − $5) $ 0
3. Additional Costs Incurred
   Extra anthelmintic and labor ($19 − $6) $13
4. Costs No Longer Incurred
   Nil $ 0
                                                                     ‾‾‾‾
Net return ($83 + $0) − ($0 + $13) $70

    In examining data such as that presented in Table 9.1 a question arises as to whether net return or percentage return on marginal invested funds most accurately reflects the most profitable option. In general, if the farmer has unlimited funds available, the scheme with the highest net return is the most profitable and should be adopted (the critical scheme in Table 9.1). If funds are limited, those available should be progressively invested in uses that yield the highest marginal return (Morris 1969). Here, the percentage return on invested funds gives an imprecise assessment of marginal returns; however, it does facilitate comparisons between the investment alternatives. In the example cited, the critical scheme is the option of choice regardless of the availability of funds. Very often this is not the case.

    Examination of the actual experimental results, from which these data were derived, revealed the factor that produced the main financial difference between the control strategies was the variation in mortality rate. The group of sheep receiving no strategic treatments suffered a 26% mor-

Table 9.1. A comparison of the returns from various control strategies for ovine helminthiasis (values adjusted to a flock of 100 sheep)

Item	(1) No strategic treatment	(2) Traditional scheme	(3) Critical scheme	(4) Biweekly drenching
Fleece wool shorn February 1971 ($)	187	199	227	268
Wool from dead sheep ($)	5	4	5	1
Crutched wool ($)	11	13	13	13
Capital value of surviving sheep 1 March 1971 ($)	222	233	263	342
Gross return ($)	425	449	508	625
Cost of labor and anthelmintic ($)	6	18	19	170
Marginal cost over strategy 1 ($)	...	12	13	164
Strategy net return ($)	419	432	489	455
Marginal return over strategy 1 ($)	...	13	70	36
Percentage return[a] on marginal invested funds	...	108	538	22

Source: Anderson et al. 1976, with permission.
  [a]Calculated as marginal return divided by marginal cost and expressed as a percentage (e.g., 13/12 × 100 = 108%).

tality rate compared to 12% in the critical scheme group. The mortality rate in the no treatment group would need to be as low as 13% before the benefit from adopting the critical scheme would be reduced to zero (i.e., the break-even point). The individual farmers could assess how plausible this would be under their own particular situations when making their final decisions.

9.3 Gross Margins Analysis

In attempting to determine whether a farmer has benefited or will benefit from an improvement in herd health, the analysis may be carried out by means of a partial farm budget, particularly if only one health problem is under consideration, or by assessing the change in some economic index of performance with time. One such index is the gross margin, usually expressed relative to some unit of production (e.g., gross margin per cow, per hectare, or per person). Gross margin analysis is the most practical method for assessing enterprise profitability, and it is widely used in farm management economics. It can also be used for comparing the profitability of different enterprises on a farm and for estimating the effect of changes within the limits of fixed assets and other resources available to the farmer (Ellis and James 1979b). With regard to animal health activities, gross margin analysis perhaps finds its greatest application in assessing the effectiveness of integrated health management programs. The general format for calculating the gross margin of an animal related activity is presented in Table 9.2.

Table 9.2. General format for calculating the gross margin of a food animal activity

Stock inventory value + cost of animals + cost of:			= total of beginning
beginning of year	bought	feed husbandry marketing breeding and replacements (where not raised on farm) health care, etc.	value and all costs
(1) +	(2) +	(3) =	(4)
Value of stock at + sales of animals and + sale of by-products			= total of end of year
end of year	animal products		value and all sales
(5) +	(6) +	(7) =	(8)

Total of (8) minus total of (4) = gross margin

In gross margin analysis, all actual income from the enterprise in question is totaled, and all variable costs directly attributable to operating that enterprise are subtracted. The resultant figure is known as the "enterprise gross margin" or "profit before fixed costs". Variable costs, as the name implies, vary as the size and/or level of an activity varies. If cattle numbers are doubled, variable costs such as feed, husbandry, and marketing costs will also increase. (Purchases of animals can be either a variable or capital cost. Annual purchase of stock to maintain a flock or herd at a constant level is a variable cost, but purchase of stock to increase the permanent numbers is treated as a capital investment.)

As well as being directly associated with the level of intensity of each activity, many variable input costs determine the yield or level of output of the activity. With crops, the amount and kind of fertilizer, seed, or sprays influence crop yield. Similarly, with animal activities, the level and type of feed, drenches, and vaccines used may have a major effect on animal production. Very little output would occur on farms unless money was spent on variable cost items. Fixed costs in the short run are incurred regardless of the level of output and include such things as taxes, insurance, and depreciation. Figure 9.2 illustrates in simplified linear form the relationship between fixed and variable costs and income.

Identifying the variable costs of an activity gives the farmer an idea of the size of the change in costs that would occur if one or more activities expands or contracts. For example, if the farmer decides to decrease the area of oats and increase the area of wheat, the variable costs will change, but the fixed costs are likely to remain about the same. Knowing the likely variable costs and gross income, the farm operator is in a position to assess the merit of making a change in activities. Operating profit can be calculated by subtracting fixed costs from the total gross margin.

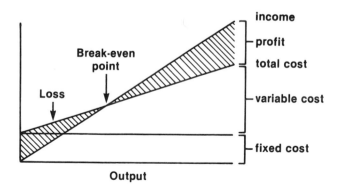

9.2. Hypothetical example relating fixed and variable costs to income.

Gross margin analysis was used to assess the results of a 4-year controlled study designed to investigate the impact of a dairy herd health and management program on dairy farms (Williamson 1980). The analysis involved 59 program farms and 47 surveillance farms. The gross margin consisted of three main parts: a livestock inventory, a section for dairy enterprise income (milk sales, livestock sales, and the value of milk or livestock transferred to other enterprises), and a cost section including supplementary feeds, livestock purchases, artificial insemination, and veterinary costs. Other benefits or costs directly attributable to the study were also included for the program group of herds. On a mean whole-farm basis, the program resulted in an improvement (as measured by gross margin) of $23.58, $65.56, and $90.30 per hectare respectively, in the second, third, and fourth year when compared to year one.

As previously mentioned, partial farm budgeting and gross margin analysis find their principal application in the assessment of control procedures for endemic diseases (such as bovine mastitis) and integrated health management programs. Difficulties arise when consideration is given to sporadic diseases (such as hypomagnesemia or enterotoxemia). Diseases of this latter type must be viewed for planning purposes as not certain to occur within the immediate planning period; there is a strong chance or risk component. One technique that can be applied to decision making about disease control under such conditions of risk is the payoff table.

9.4 Payoff Table

The use of the payoff table entails the calculation of the payoff (returns minus costs) for each of the strategies under consideration, given that an outbreak of the disease does or does not occur. An expected monetary value for each strategy is then calculated by multiplying each payoff by its probability, and summing these values over all possible outcomes for that strategy. The general form of the payoff table is presented in Table 9.3. The assigned probability of disease occurrence is best based on objective data, but subjective estimates frequently must be used. The usual decision criterion is to choose the strategy with the highest expected monetary value.

Table 9.3. General format for a payoff table

Possible outcomes	Probability of occurrence	Economic result of alternative strategies	
		1	2
Disease occurs	X	a	b
Disease does not occur	Y	c	d
Expected monetary value (strategy 1) = $(a \times X) + (c \times Y)$			
(strategy 2) = $(b \times X) + (d \times Y)$			

However, veterinarians should remember that not withstanding the above calculations, the final decision on what strategy to implement rests with the farmer, because the decision is made under risk of financial loss if incorrect (Morris 1969).

A practical example of the use of the technique for decision making regarding control strategies for thromboembolic meningoencephalitis (TEME) is shown in Table 9.4 (Davidson et al. 1981). The calculations are based on a feedlot situation where: the price of cattle is $1.32/kg; average weight of cattle is 300 kg; number of cattle per pen is 350; number of pens per year is 67; and the probability of a pen becoming infected with TEME is 15%. The alternatives investigated were: (1) no action, assumed to result in a 3% mortality rate if TEME occurred; (2) vaccination of all cattle, assumed to give perfect protection at a cost of $2 per head; and (3) mass treatment of all cattle at a cost of $114 per pen if a case occurs. In the last case an overall mortality rate of 1% is assumed. The dollar values presented in Table 9.4 are gross returns under each circumstance minus any vaccine or treatment costs. In this case and given the above assumptions, strategy 3 resulted in the highest expected monetary value and hence would be the option of choice.

The same data can be presented in the form of a decision tree (Fig. 9.3) in which choices (decision nodes) are represented by squares, probability events by circles, and outcomes are given at the right of the tree. Tree diagrams can become much more complex in nature as other dimensions (such as time) are added to the problem. Another example of the use of decision analysis relates to the treatment of ovarian cysts in dairy cattle (White and Erb 1980).

The importance of uncertainty as a factor influencing decisions about disease control has been underestimated. The environment in which practi-

Table 9.4.   Payoff table for various action-outcome combinations for thromboembolic meningoencephalitis (TEME)[a]

		TEME control alternatives		
Possible states	Probability of TEME	(1) No action ($)	(2) Vaccinate all cattle ($)	(3) Treat after first case of TEME ($)
No infection	.85	9,286,200	9,239,300	9,286,200
TEME infection	.15	9,007,614	9,239,300	9,185,700

EMV[b] (1) = (0.85)(9,286,200) + (0.15)(9,007,614) = $9,244,412.10
EMV (2) = (0.85)(9,239,300) + (0.15)(9,239,300) = $9,239,300.00
EMV (3) = (0.85)(9,286,200) + (0.15)(9,185,700) = $9,271,125.00

Source: Modified from Davidson et al. 1981, with permission.
[a]See text for explanation and derivation of financial returns.
[b]Expected monetary value.

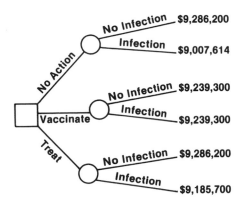

9.3. Decision tree representation of data presented in Table 9.4.

cal decisions are made is usually uncertain and involves complex relationships among many factors. In fact, farmers usually tend not to invest large sums of money purely on the basis of expected return when they are uncertain of the outcome (Anderson 1976).

There are a number of methods for dealing with uncertainty, one of which is to conduct a sensitivity analysis. In such an analysis, the sensitivity of the outcome to variation over the likely range of the items used in the calculations (e.g., costs, prices, probabilities, etc.) is assessed. The decision maker can then integrate these outcomes with one's own personal aversion to risk and subjective assessment of the likelihood of various combinations (such as extremes of price or mortality) in making a final decision.

Another dimension that can be used when making decisions under uncertainty is the concept of utility. If the decision maker has no risk preference (indifferent to risk), the expected monetary value approach and the expected utility approach are the same. (Fig. 9.4a.) However, if the decision maker has preference or aversion to risk as illustrated in Figure 9.4b, maximization of expected utility may be the appropriate approach. The approach is based on the fact that monetary amounts may not provide a measure of the relative value a person attaches to different sized gains or losses. The risk-aversion curve illustrated in Figure 9.4b implies that its owner values an extra $1000 at two-thirds the value of an extra $4000; whereas the individual with no risk preference (Fig. 9.4a) values a $4000 gain at 4 times a $1000 gain. The latter case is not characteristic of many people, especially when large sums of money (gains or losses) are involved.

As an example, suppose one has a choice between two costless alternatives: (1) tossing a fair coin for $100,000 if a head appears or $0 if a tail appears; or (2) a certain gift of $50,000. Which alternative would you

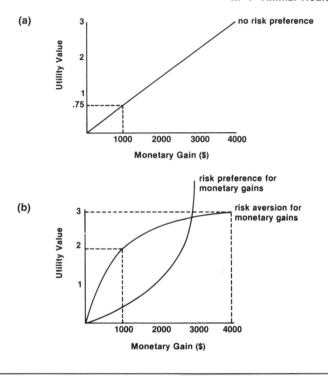

9.4. Example of utility curves for monetary gains.

choose? (Note that both have the same expected monetary value of $50,000.) Most people would accept the sure alternative; the value they attach to the 50% chance of $100,000 is more than offset by the 50% chance of receiving $0. People differ in their utility because of things such as their past experience or psychological makeup. As circumstances change over time (e.g., if a person becomes rich playing the stock market) the shape of their utility curve may also change.

In the expected utility approach, utility values are derived from the utility function. The latter values are then multiplied by the probability values to calculate the expected utility value, as opposed to the expected monetary value.

The same approach can be used without the consideration of economic values. In this approach the decision maker assigns a subjective assessment to the value of each possible outcome — for example, death (0), spontaneous resolution (100), and various other outcomes (e.g., surgery with serious complications, scaled appropriately between these extremes).

9.5   Benefit-Cost Analysis

If a control program involves substantial initial investment and the benefits gradually accumulate subsequently, it is necessary to weight annual costs and benefits by a factor making immediate costs and benefits more valuable than those occurring in the future. Benefit-cost analysis is a technique directly applicable to long-term investment in disease control and finds its principal application in the assessment of public disease-control programs, where a government or other agency will contribute to a large-scale program. In deciding whether to initiate a large scale animal disease-control program, governments or leaders must consider whether society as a whole will benefit from the action, whether transfers of financial or nonfinancial benefit between sections of the community may result, whether the project should receive priority over other projects, and how heavily economic and social achievements of the project should be weighted. An analysis of this type is termed benefit-cost analysis when measurable economic costs and benefits are considered and may include a tabulation of nonfinancial consequences as well. A related technique, cost-effectiveness analysis (9.5.4), is appropriate when only costs are being considered.

Once the alternative control strategies have been identified, there is a natural sequence to be followed so a decision can be made. For each alternative the steps include: the enumeration, measurement, and valuation of the benefits and costs for each time period; adjustment of these values to account for the effect of different cash flow patterns over time; and evaluation and strategy comparison.

9.5.1   Assessing Benefits and Costs

Benefit-cost analysis rests on the premise that a policy should only be implemented if the discounted benefits outweigh the discounted costs. To assess this, the benefits and costs over time must be identified and expressed in monetary terms.

In essence, benefit-cost analysis is a form of forward budgeting that includes methods of adjusting cash flow. Most of the benefits and costs of a program are received or incurred within its own budgets, whereas some benefits that may affect others are known as externalities. The former need to be included in all analyses, whereas the inclusion of externalities will depend to a great extent on the scope of the project (James and Ellis 1980).

In general, the costs of a particular program are related to the resources consumed. Once these physical resources have been determined, it is usually not difficult to assign a monetary value to them. Such costs generally include manpower and operating costs plus resources used by the program (such as vaccines).

To assess the benefits of a control program, it is necessary to know the effect of the disease in the absence of control, and to estimate the likely consequences of the program on these. In this way, many of the benefits are the result of the avoidance of losses; that is, the difference between the losses experienced under "no control" or under the current program and each of the alternatives being investigated. For example, many of the benefits of a foot-and-mouth disease (FMD) control program accrued from the avoidance of production losses such as mortality, the indirect and direct effects of FMD on meat and milk production, the losses associated with lameness in draught animals, and from restrictions on international trade (James and Ellis 1978). An alternative approach to estimating benefits is to determine how much less of each of the various production input resources would be used, as a result of implementing a program, to produce the existing volume of animal product.

In practice, the benefits of animal disease-control programs fall into three categories, the relative significance of each depending on the disease under consideration.

1. Readily quantifiable economic benefits (e.g., increased live births and milk production resulting from bovine brucellosis control).

2. Economic benefits that exist but are not so readily quantifiable in financial terms, either because market values are not clear or are not susceptible to accurate calculation, or because the biological consequences of a control program are uncertain (e.g., the effects of brucellosis eradication on the export price of beef).

3. Benefits not suitable for any form of economic evaluation, such as the psychological benefit to farmers and others that results from the removal of the fear of contracting brucellosis. Benefits of this sort would be included under intangibles.

A scheme depicting the conceptual approach used to calculate the estimated benefits and costs in each year of a planned project is presented in Figure 9.5. The benefits are the difference between the losses under the proposed new control strategy versus "no control" or the current program, where losses within each control option are a function of the level of disease in the population, the effect of disease on each productive unit (e.g., kg of milk production lost/cow affected), and the value of the product (e.g., the price of milk/kg).

While Figure 9.5 presents the basic approach, it is an oversimplification in that it implies that the economic benefits might be calculated based on current market prices (i.e., the existing price prior to implementation of the control program). This situation may suffice at the individual farm

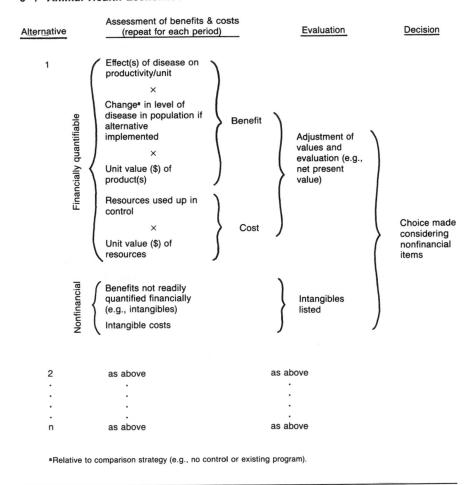

9.5. Schematic representation of conceptual approach to benefit/cost analysis.

level, but at the aggregate social level a number of complexities are introduced.

One of these complexities relates to the fact that the consumer is not likely to buy more product at current market prices simply because it is available unless demand is perfectly elastic. (Elasticity of demand is the slope of the demand curve and is defined as the percent change in quantity divided by the percent change in price. In the case of perfect elasticity the slope will be zero.) Usually, given that the demand curve is inelastic, consumers will demand a drop in price if they are to purchase the increased quantity available. If the elasticity of demand for swine was -0.5 at the farm level, a 1% increase in the quantity of swine produced would result in a 2% decline in prices.

The above discussion raises the concept of consumer and producer surplus. Consumer surplus represents the area of benefits under the demand curve that consumers receive in addition to what they pay through the market. Producer surplus represents the value that producers receive over and above their costs of supply. At the equilibrium price P_e (Fig. 9.6a) consumers and producers exchange the quantity Q for the total cost represented by the area OP_eEQ. However, consumers gain all the benefits under the demand curve up to E, thereby receiving the surplus represented by A. Producer costs are represented by the area under the supply curve up to E and therefore they receive a surplus of area B.

The consumer/producer surplus approach measures benefits as gains (or losses) in the sum of these two economic surpluses created by shifts in the supply curve under the assumption that society is indifferent to any resulting redistribution of income. Such shifts are generally the result of technological advances resulting from research and improved supporting services (e.g., veterinary care). For present purposes and by way of example, assume that the supply curve has been shifted due to a technological advance that allows the implementation of a new disease control program. By shifting the supply curve to the right, consumer surpluses are usually

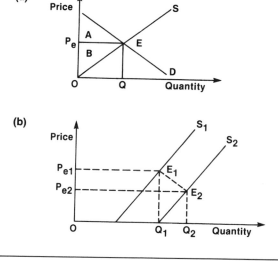

9.6. Consumer and producer surpluses. A = consumer surplus; B = producer surplus; S = supply; D = demand; P = price; Q = quantity; E = equilibrium.

increased whereas producer surpluses may or may not be depending on the elasticity of supply and demand. Figure 9.6b illustrates the impact of a shift in supply from S_1 to S_2 on consumer surplus and, for the sake of simplicity, assumes no change in producer surplus. In this example and as a result of the disease control program, the quantity of product available to be sold has increased from Q_1 to Q_2, and a new equilibrium between supply and demand is achieved at price P_{e2}. The change in consumer surplus is represented by the area $P_{e2} E_2 E_1 P_{e1}$, and in this case would represent a benefit to the consumer because of a lowering of the price. Two points arise from this. First, the slope (elasticity) of the demand curve should be considered when computing the benefits of a disease control program. Second, if as the result of a control program producers simply produce more, the benefits in the long term may accrue to the consumer, not the producer. Producers might collectively benefit by producing the same amount but using the improvement in technology to produce it more efficiently.

An in-depth discussion of these and other complexities (e.g., international markets) goes beyond the scope of this book. Many important judgments have to be made by professionals when valuing future benefits and costs. These have been briefly mentioned here in an attempt to establish the basic concepts and to bring out a number of important points. Interested readers may wish to refer to more advanced books such as those by Drummond (1980) and Sugden and Williams (1978).

9.5.2   Adjustment of Values

The time that a cost or benefit occurs has an effect on its value. Even in the absence of inflation, an individual places a higher value on one dollar received now than on one dollar received a year from now. There are at least two reasons for this. First, the goods and services the dollar will purchase may be desired now, and hence one is willing to pay a premium. Second, the dollar could be invested and earn interest, either in the bank or in some other alternative, and hence be worth more at the end of the year. The economic value of the estimated costs and benefits must therefore be adjusted to take account of the time they occur. The adjusted value of a benefit or cost is called its present value. The procedure used for the adjustment is called discounting and is the reverse of compound interest calculation (see below). Before applying these techniques it is necessary to establish several formulas. The following symbols will be used: i — the relevant annual interest rate expressed as a decimal; r — the relevant annual discount rate expressed as a decimal; n — the number of years; PV — the present value; FV_n — the future sum accruing at the end of n years; and A_1, A_2, A_3, ..., A_n — a series of n annual payments made at the end of each respective year. Note that the quantities PV, FV, and A may be either costs or revenues.

Compounding. In compounding, the time movement is from the present to the future. If the sum P is invested now at an annual interest rate of i, it will be worth $P(1 + i)$ 1 year from now. Two years from now it will have grown to $P(1 + i)^2$, assuming i does not change. In n years it will have grown to $P(1 + i)^n$. Hence the general compounding formula is:

$$FV_n = P(1 + i)^n$$

where FV_n is the terminal value after n years of the sum P invested now.

Discounting. In discounting, the time movement is from the future back to the present. The present value of the future sum FV_n is that sum P that if invested now would grow to FV_n by the end of the nth year. This can be calculated from the compounding equation:

$$PV = FV_n/(1 + r)^n$$

Present Value of a Series of Unequal Payments. If the sums A_1, A_2, A_3...A_n arise at the end of years 1, 2, 3 . . ., n respectively, the basic discounting formula can be applied to each payment, and the present value of the payment series is:

$$PV = A_1/(1 + r) + A_2/(1 + r)^2 + \ldots + A_n/(1 + r)^n$$
$$= \sum_{t=1}^{n} A_t/(1 + r)^t$$

The general formulas are presented in the form of a benefit-cost analysis in Table 9.5.

Table 9.5. General formulas for the calculation of project present values for benefits and costs

Year (1)	Present value of $1 (2)	Benefits		Costs	
		Actual (3)	Present value (4) = (2) × (3)	Actual (5)	Present value (6) = (2) × (5)
1	$\dfrac{1}{(1+r)}$	X_1	$X_1 \dfrac{1}{(1+r)}$	Y_1	$Y_1 \dfrac{1}{(1+r)}$
2	$\dfrac{1}{(1+r)^2}$	X_2	$X_2 \dfrac{1}{(1+r)^2}$	Y_2	$Y_2 \dfrac{1}{(1+r)^2}$
3	$\dfrac{1}{(1+r)^3}$	X_3	$X_3 \dfrac{1}{(1+r)^3}$	Y_3	$Y_3 \dfrac{1}{(1+r)^3}$
n	$\dfrac{1}{(1+r)^n}$	X_n	$X_n \dfrac{1}{(1+r)^n}$	Y_n	$Y_n \dfrac{1}{(1+r)^n}$
Total		$\sum_{t=1}^{n} X_t$	$\sum_{t=1}^{n} \dfrac{X_t}{(1+r)^t}$	$\sum_{t=1}^{n} Y_t$	$\sum_{t=1}^{n} \dfrac{Y_t}{(1+r)^t}$

Present Value of a Series of Equal Payments. If the payments A_1, A_2, $A_3 \ldots$, A_n are equal, this is called an annuity. The present value of an annuity is given by:

$$PV = A \left[(1 + r)^n - 1 \right] / \left[r(1 + r)^n \right]$$

When n tends toward infinity, this equation reduces to $PV = A/r$, the capitalization formula.

For purposes of demonstration and using the above discounting formulas, the present value of $1 at the end of various periods of time and at several discount rates is presented in Table 9.6. Just as the interest rate received affects the size of the dividend paid at the end of a period, so the discount rate affects present values. This raises the question of which rate should be used. In general, the discount rate should represent the opportunity cost of capital; and this will vary depending on the scope and nature of the given situation. For government sponsored projects, the rate should reflect the social value of capital, while for a wealthy producer it might represent the rate received on other investments, such as money in the bank (James and Ellis 1980). In general, one should choose a rate that reflects the environment in which the decision is being made, work through the calculation, and then rework the calculation using rates that represent the likely range of possible rates (i.e., one should assess the sensitivity of the decision over the likely range of discounting values).

Another frequent question is how to deal with the effects of inflation. In general, inflation can be ignored since all benefits and costs are being standardized to present values; interest is in the real value of a good or service, not its artificially inflated value. However, if the relative value of different items is expected to change with time, the values can be adjusted to reflect this prior to the discounting procedure (Ellis and James 1979a).

Table 9.6. Present value of one dollar at the end of various future periods of time and at various discount rates

Year	Discount rate (%)		
	8	10	12
1	.9259	.9091	.8929
2	.8573	.8264	.7972
3	.7938	.7513	.7118
5	.6806	.6209	.5674
10	.4632	.3855	.3220
15	.3152	.2394	.1827
20	.2145	.1486	.1037

9.5.3 Evaluation and Strategy Comparison

Having determined the benefits and costs, and having adjusted them to account for timing, they can now be compared. The decision criterion used for this is usually one or a combination of the following three measures of economic efficiency or investment worth: net present value, benefit-cost ratio, or internal rate of return.

Net Present Value. The net present value (NPV) criterion is defined as the present value of benefits (B) less the present value of the costs (C) incurred. The formula to calculate NPV is:

$$NPV = \sum_{t=1}^{n} [(B_t - C_t)/(1 + r)^t]$$

A positive NPV indicates that the control strategy is economically feasible and an alternative with a higher positive NPV is preferred. This measure is often affected by the scale of the project, and while it gives some idea of the value of implementing the project, it does not indicate how much the benefits may outweigh the costs in percentage terms.

Benefit-cost Ratio. The benefit-cost ratio (B/C) is defined as the present value of benefits divided by the present value of costs. The formula for its calculation is:

$$B/C = \sum_{t=1}^{n} [B_t/(1 + r)^t]/\sum_{t=1}^{n} [C_t/(1 + r)^t]$$

The costs incurred and the benefits received during each period of the project are stated as present values and totaled; the present value benefit total is then divided by the cost total. If the ratio is greater than 1, the investment is economically feasible. An alternative with a higher B/C is preferred.

Internal Rate of Return. The internal rate of return (IRR) criterion expresses the return to investment in terms analogous to an interest or discount rate. Specifically, it is defined as that rate of discount that makes the total of the discounted benefits equal to the total of the discounted costs (i.e., the rate of discount such that NPV = 0).

The main advantage of the IRR method is that there is no need to specify a discount rate before the calculation. One of its major drawbacks is that there is no simple formula to determine the rate, and hence it must be determined by an iterative procedure.

The higher the internal rate of return of an alternative, the more likely it is to be preferred. Specifically, the IRRs calculated for all the strategies under consideration are ranked and compared to the opportunity cost of capital, such as the borrowing rate of interest.

Each of the above indices can be deceptive under some circumstances and must be interpreted with care. In general, it is a good idea to calculate and take all three into consideration when making a decision.

Table 9.7 presents a hypothetical example of the use of benefit-cost analysis to choose between two potential investments (A and B). In the example the actual estimated future benefits and costs of each project are equal. However, because of the different cash flow patterns of the two projects, Project A would be the best investment as indicated by all three previously discussed criteria.

A practical example of a benefit-cost analysis to assess alternative programs for bovine brucellosis was conducted by Agriculture Canada (1979). A planning horizon of 20 years was used with the base year being 1977. The spread of brucellosis was estimated by means of a computer simulation model. The benefits of a particular control program were assessed as being the difference between the losses incurred without a control program and the losses incurred under each alternative control strategy. The benefits and costs for each of the four programs investigated are presented in Table 9.8.

Table 9.7. Use of benefit-cost analysis to choose between two potential investments, A and B (discounted at 10%)

Year	Present value of $1	Potential Investment			
		A		B	
		Benefits	Costs	Benefits	Costs
1	.9091	$ 250	$ 500	$ 0	$ 500
2	.8264	250	1000	100	500
3	.7513	500	500	100	500
4	.6830	500	0	250	500
5	.6209	500	0	500	0
6	.5645	500	0	500	0
7	.5132	500	0	500	0
8	.4665	500	0	500	0
9	.4241	500	0	1025	0
10	.3855	500	0	1025	0
Total		$4500	$2000	$4500	$2000
Total present value		$2638.38	$1656.60	$2240.91	$1584.90
Net present value (NPV)		$981.78		$656.01	
Benefit-cost ratio (B/C)		1.59		1.41	
Internal rate of return (IRR,%)		30.07		18.73	

Table 9.8.   Benefit-cost analysis of alternative programs for brucellosis

	Program[a]							
	1		2		3		4	
Year	Benefits[b]	Costs	Benefits	Costs	Benefits	Costs	Benefits	Costs
	(millions)							
1	1.79	17.09	2.11	16.06	2.00	15.02	1.99	14.81
2	2.50	17.09	3.01	16.06	3.06	15.02	3.81	13.76
3	3.87	17.09	4.70	16.06	4.66	15.02	5.20	13.76
4	6.38	17.09	7.31	16.06	7.31	15.02	7.64	13.76
5	11.08	17.09	11.93	16.06	12.02	15.02	12.20	13.76
6	19.06	17.09	19.85	16.06	19.98	15.02	20.11	13.76
7	31.54	17.09	32.31	16.06	32.46	15.02	32.55	13.76
8	48.98	17.09	49.75	16.06	49.90	15.02	49.96	13.76
9	69.93	17.09	70.73	16.06	70.88	15.02	70.93	13.76
10	90.87	17.09	91.71	16.06	91.87	15.02	91.91	13.76
11	108.19	17.09	109.12	16.06	109.28	15.02	109.31	13.76
12	120.33	17.09	121.35	16.06	121.53	15.02	121.55	10.59
13	127.83	17.09	128.98	16.06	129.18	15.02	129.19	10.59
14	132.18	17.09	133.46	16.06	133.68	13.54	133.69	10.59
15	134.70	17.09	136.16	16.06	136.39	13.54	136.40	10.59
16	136.30	17.09	137.94	16.06	138.18	13.54	138.19	10.59
17	137.37	17.09	139.21	16.06	139.46	13.54	139.47	10.59
18	138.15	17.09	140.21	16.06	140.47	13.54	140.48	6.50
19	138.73	17.09	141.01	16.06	141.29	13.54	141.30	6.50
20	139.17	17.09	141.71	16.06	142.00	13.54	142.01	6.50
Present value	437.71	145.50	445.60	136.73	446.42	125.78	448.00	109.69
Net present value	292.21		308.87		320.64		338.31	
Benefit-cost ratio 1[b]	3.0		3.3		3.6		4.1	
Benefit-cost ratio 2[c]	3.5		3.8		4.1		4.7	

Source: Agriculture Canada 1979, with permission.
[a]Programs described in text. Dollar values rounded to nearest $100,000.
[b]Includes only benefits to producer.
[c]Includes producer benefits plus benefits due to undulant fever and export trade.

A discount rate of 10% was used. The four programs investigated were: (1) test and slaughter, (2) test and slaughter plus adult vaccination, (3) test and slaughter with some depopulation, and (4) herd depopulation. Benefits to the producer involved milk yield, value of animals, calf crop, and conception rates. Other benefits examined included the effect of undulant fever on the human population and the effect of brucellosis on export trade. Costs included personnel, operation, and capital costs plus compensation payments.

As can be seen from Table 9.8, and as judged by the benefit-cost ratio and net present value, all programs were feasible with herd depopulation providing the greatest economic return on investment. Benefit-cost ratios for producer benefits only and for all benefits considered are presented separately.

In the past few years benefit-cost analyses have been used to investigate control activities for a number of animal diseases including foot-and-mouth disease (James and Ellis 1978; Powers and Harris 1973), swine fever (Ellis 1972), cattle tick (Johnston 1975), bovine trypanosomiasis (Habtemariam et al. 1982/1983), and bovine leukosis (Hūgoson and Wold-Troell 1983).

9.5.4 Cost-effectiveness Analysis

A technique that overcomes some of the difficulties involved in putting a dollar figure on all the benefits of a disease control program is cost-effectiveness analysis. This approach is appropriate where the benefits are difficult to quantify (e.g., the benefits to the human population of rabies control), when production losses under each control strategy are equal, or when the activity has been defined as essential for one reason or another. In such instances the requirement is for a method of analysis that determines how the desired result can be achieved at minimum (discounted) cost. In fact, the procedure is the cost part of a benefit-cost analysis carried out on its own. The question of whether the benefit is sufficiently worthwhile to justify the expenditure may, for example, be strictly a political one.

Thus, the benefit-cost group of techniques available range from benefit-cost analysis at one end of the spectrum, which deals only with financially quantifiable benefits and costs, through to cost-effectiveness analysis at the other end, where all benefits are considered unquantifiable, equal, or are otherwise ignored, and only the costs are calculated. In most cases the actual technique will be a hybrid of the two, in which monetary and non-monetary benefits are quantified and the nature of unquantifiable benefits for each strategy is stated.

References

Agriculture Canada. 1979. Evaluation of alternative brucellosis programs by benefit-cost analysis. Systems and Consulting Division Tech. Report.

Anderson, J. R. 1976. On making decisions. Span. 19:120–22.

Anderson, N., R. S. Morris, and I. K. McTaggart. 1976. An economic analysis of two schemes for the anthelmintic control of helminthiasis in weaned lambs. Aust. Vet. J. 52:174–80.

Davidson, J. N., T. E. Carpenter, and C. A. Hjerpe. 1981. An example of an economic decision analysis approach to the problem of thromboembolic meningoencephalitis (TEME) in feedlot cattle. Cornell Vet. 71:383–90.

Drummond, M. F. 1980. Principles of Economic Appraisal in Health Care. Toronto: Oxford Univ. Press.

Ellis, P. R. 1972. An economic evaluation of the swine fever eradication programme in Great Britain, using cost-benefit analysis techniques. Univ. of Reading, Dept. of Agric. Study No. 77.

Ellis, P. R., and A. D. James. 1979a. The economics of animal health. I. Major disease control programs. Vet. Rec. 105:504–6.

———. 1979b. The economics of animal health. II. Economics in farm practice. Vet. Rec. 105:523–26.

Habtemariam, T., R. E. Howitt, R. Ruppanner, and H. P. Riemann. 1982/1983. The benefit-cost analysis of alternative strategies for the control of bovine trypanosomiasis in Ethiopia. Prev. Vet. Med. 1:157–68.

Hūgoson, G., and M. Wold-Troell. 1983. Benefit-cost aspects on voluntary control of bovine leukosis. Nord. Vet. Med. 35:1–17.

James, A. D., and P. R. Ellis. 1978. Benefit-cost analysis in foot-and-mouth disease control programmes. Br. Vet. J. 134:47–52.

———. 1980. The evaluation of production and effects of disease. Proc. 2nd Int. Symp. Vet. Epidemiol. Econ., May 1979, Canberra, Australia.

Johnston, J. H. 1975. Public policy on cattle tick control in New South Wales. Rev. Mark. Agric. Econ. 43:3–39.

Morris, R. S. 1969. Assessing the economic value of veterinary services to primary industries. Aust. Vet. J. 45:295–300.

———. 1975. The economics of animal disease control. Proc. 19th Annu. Conf. Aust. Agric. Econ. Soc.

Morris, R. S., and A. H. Meek. 1980. Measurement and evaluation of the economic effects of parasitic disease. Vet. Parasit. 6:165–84.

Powers, A. P., and S. A. Harris. 1973. A cost-benefit evaluation of alternative control policies for foot-and-mouth disease in Great Britain. J. Agric. Econ. 24:573–79.

Sugden, R., and A. Williams. 1978. The Principles of Practical Cost-Benefit Analysis. Toronto: Oxford Univ. Press.

White, M. E., and H. Erb. 1980. Treatment of ovarian cysts in dairy cattle: A decision analysis. Cornell Vet. 70:247–57.

Williamson, N. B. 1980. The economic efficiency of a veterinary preventive medicine and management program in Victorian dairy herds. Aust. Vet. J. 56:1–9.

PART IV

Applied Epidemiology

CHAPTER 10

Rationale, Strategies, and Concepts of Animal Disease Control

The primary objective of epidemiologic studies is to provide data on which rational decisions for the prevention and control of disease in animal populations can be based. To this end, a number of concepts and specific methods have been presented for the investigation and understanding of disease in animal populations. In this chapter, examples of the application of these concepts and methods of disease control planning and evaluation will be described.

In pursuing these applications, the reader should be aware that only recently have quantitative epidemiologic methods been used, in a formal, explicit sense, by veterinarians outside government or research agencies. Nonetheless, with the increasing emphasis on preventive population medicine, particularly in the areas of veterinary public health and domestic animal practice, all veterinarians will require increased training in epidemiology. Certainly the authors of this text agree with the editor of the *American Journal of Public Health* and believe that, "Without epidemiology, there can be no scientific basis for public health practice, and without public health practice, the science of epidemiology becomes a meaningless academic practice" (Rosen 1972). It is hoped the readers can excerpt, from the applications presented, those ideas and methods necessary to enhance and elevate their abilities as preventive health care specialists.

10.1 Influence of Disease on Animal and Human Populations

In general terms, veterinarians are interested in the control of animal disease because they have a concern for the welfare of both animal and human populations. In fact, as Schwabe (1984) indicates, the major unifying feature of many diverse veterinary activities is their central and ultimate concern for human health. A complete assessment of the value of disease control measures necessitates an understanding of the ways that disease influences animal welfare, animal productivity, and its direct and indirect impact on humans. Without such information, the benefits of a control program cannot be readily determined. Therefore, before proceeding with a discussion of disease control strategies, a brief overview of the effects of disease is warranted.

10.1.1 Mortality

Premature death of animals is an obvious result of disease and has a pronounced effect on the productivity of animal populations. In intensive agriculture, the costs of mortality are greatest when animals of high genetic potential die during their peak reproductive years. Less concern has been evidenced about the cost of death in older animals; this is particularly true in domestic animals since the majority of these animals are culled to make room for more productive younger animals long before the human equivalent of old age occurs. In many third world countries where animals are depended on for transportation and agricultural power as well as food, mortality can have devastating effects both for individual families and for entire countries (Schwabe 1984, pp 17–22). In North America, considerable losses in young animals have been tolerated by animal owners for a number of years (witness the 20% death loss in female dairy calves in California), although it is hoped neonatal death losses can be reduced as more effective (biologically and economically) prophylaxis becomes available (Martin et al. 1975). Indicating the magnitude of the economic losses caused by mortality may provide sufficient incentive for the producer to more rigorously institute effective procedures to reduce mortality (Martin and Wiggins 1973).

10.1.2 Reduction in Yield and Quality of Product

The negative effects of ill health on the welfare of animals should be obvious to all. In addition, a number of studies have been conducted to quantify the influence of various diseases on the efficiency of production and the yield and quality of products derived from various animal species. Where intensive agriculture is practiced, decreases in one or more of these three aspects of animal "output" are now regularly used as indicators that one or more diseases or production problems may be present (Kaneene and Mather 1982). In fact, except in companion animals, these negative effects of disease on productivity are often the primary motivation for preventing and/or treating disease. Beyond these impacts of disease, it must be appreciated that the health of animals, particularly if they are pets, can have significant impact on the mental and physical health of man. Unfortunately, in many developing countries, losses from disease are often accepted as fixed costs of production, and neither individuals nor governments may be motivated to initiate adequate control measures.

For many diseases, the effects on quality are reflected in a lower market price for the animal or its product(s). In other cases the effect is not detected by the marketing process, although the consumer suffers a real loss. For example, bovine mastitis reduces both the amount of milk produced per animal and its quality (i.e., composition of the final product) (Philpot 1967). This results in less efficient production, a shortened productive life for the cow, and a reduced income for the producer. As a further example, the impact of trematode infection in sheep has been studied in some detail in recent years (Hawkins and Morris 1978) and a substantial depression in weight gain and wool growth, as well as in the quality of wool, has been demonstrated.

Increased knowledge has been gained regarding the underlying mechanisms by which disease reduces the productivity of the host (Roseby 1973). Disease may result in decreased feed intake, either as a direct result of decreased appetite or indirectly because of a reluctance of animals to forage (e.g., because of discomfort associated with movement, including prehension) and/or reduced feeding time (e.g., because of time spent rubbing to relieve itching). Other reductions in productive efficiency may be the result of a lowered efficiency of feed conversion due to depressed nutrient absorption or altered physiological processes resulting in lowered nutrient utilization.

A number of diseases also result in a reduced value of animals or their products at market (e.g., abscessed livers in swine and feedlot cattle, condemned carcasses because of septicemias, or decreased value of hides due to *Hypoderma bovis* infection). Other diseases influence the reproductive performance of animals; some dramatically (e.g., abortion resulting from *Brucella abortus*), whereas others have more subtle effects (e.g., delayed conception and increased health care costs due to postparturient reproductive diseases).

10.1.3 Herd Structure and Productivity

In addition to the cumulative effects of lowered individual animal productivity, there are a number of ramifications of disease that can be assessed only at the herd level. These effects generally relate to the demography (particularly the age structure) of the population. If, as the result of disease, there is a high rate of premature death or involuntary culling, the herd will often have a lower than average age. In the case of a dairy herd this may have a negative effect on productivity, because the diseased animals will not remain in the herd long enough to achieve their full genetic production potential (this occurs at approximately the fifth lactation). Another effect of the high rate of culling is the increased demand for, and hence cost of, replacement animals. The latter cost includes not only the purchase price but the increased risk of introducing disease with replacement stock. Coupled to these effects is the lowered ability to recognize and select animals of superior genetic merit (i.e., animals in the herd may not be able to express their full potential). Others could argue this is a form of natural selection in that although these animals may not be able to express their full productive potential, they may be expressing their lack of resistance to disease. Unfortunately this may be a very inefficient way of increasing the resistance of animal populations, and it also tends to reduce rather than increase productivity. In any event, production and disease should not be studied in isolation. It is encouraging to see studies being initiated by animal geneticists and veterinarians to evaluate genetic resistance to disease in concert with production potential.

10.1.4 Human and Animal Welfare

Zoonotic disease can and does directly affect human health (Schwabe 1984). Such diseases lead to human hunger, pain, and suffering, particularly in areas where medical care is not well developed. As well, animal disease can lead to decreased availability of animal products, decreased availability of animals for transportation, farm power, clothing and shelter, and even dung for fuel. In addition, using various chemicals to combat animal disease can result in residues in animal products or the environment that may directly affect human health (e.g., anaphylactic reaction to antimicrobial residues) or indirectly influence it via changed (usually increased) antibiotic resistance patterns. For further discussion of this, refer to Schwabe and Ruppanner (1972), Derbyshire (1982), and Schwabe (1984).

10.2 Methods of Disease Transmission

An examination of the methods by which disease transmission may most frequently occur is basic to an understanding of disease control. In this context, the terms "carrier" and "reservoir" require clarification.

A carrier is an infected animal that sheds pathogenic or potentially pathogenic organisms, yet remains clinically normal. Carriers have obvious epidemiologic significance as sources of infection, and they are more difficult to detect than the clinically diseased individual.

Reservoir is usually restricted to an animal species or inanimate substance upon which the organism depends for its survival. For example, the fox is a major reservoir of rabies in Canada and continental Europe; whereas the reservoir of *Histoplasma capsulatum* appears to be bird feces or soils enriched by bird feces. Many infectious agents have more than one reservoir. Other reservoir hosts of rabies in Canada include the skunk and certain species of bats. *Taenia saginata*, a cyclozoonosis, requires two reservoirs—man and cattle—to complete its life cycle.

The three common methods of transmission of infectious agents are contact, vehicle, and vector spread. Contact transmission includes direct and indirect means. Direct contact transmission denotes physical contact between the infected and susceptible individuals (e.g., venereal disease and rabies). Indirect contact transmission denotes contact between the infected and susceptible individual by means of fresh secretions (e.g., leptospiral organisms in urine), recently contaminated objects (e.g., water bowls), or by means of aerosol droplets resulting from coughing or sneezing. As mentioned earlier, contact with recently infected objects in the home, school, or workplace may be a more important means of transmitting human rhinovirus infection than aerosol transmission (Gwaltney and Hendley 1982). Knowledge that smallpox was spread primarily by direct contact was of great value in eradicating the disease. By complete traceback of a case's activities, it was possible to identify the initial source and to isolate and/or vaccinate potential cases.

Vehicle transmission of infectious agents involves inanimate substances (e.g., food, water, dust, and fomites). Vehicular transfer can be mechanical, the vehicle simply acting as a physical transfer mechanism (e.g., truck tires contaminated with foot-and-mouth disease virus and poultry feathers contaminated with Newcastle disease virus), or biological (multiplication or development of the agent takes place in the vehicle). An example of biological transfer would be the transmission of bacteria in milk. Vehicle transmission plays a significant role in the transmission of both endemic and exotic infectious agents, such as in *Mycoplasma gallisepticum* epidemics in poultry (Johnson et al. 1983).

Vector transmission denotes invertebrates that carry infectious agents between vertebrates. Again, such transmission can be purely mechanical (e.g., a "flying needle," such as mosquito transmission of equine encephalitis virus) or biological (e.g., the development of the larval stages of the dog heartworm, *Dirofilaria immitis*, usually in members of the Culex species of mosquitos; such development must occur for the larvae to become infectious to animals or man).

Two other terms applied to the transmission of disease are horizontal and vertical transmission. Horizontal transmission refers to the passage of infectious agents between animals of a similar generation and can occur by any of the methods previously discussed. Vertical transmission, on the other hand, means transmission from one generation to the next; this can be accomplished transovarially, in utero (e.g., *Toxocara canis* infection from the bitch to her pups), or via colostrum (e.g., bovine leukemia virus transfer from the cow to the calf). Often the distinction between methods of spread is arbitrary; nonetheless it is useful for descriptive purposes. For example, cows shedding salmonella in their feces or milk, or cows shedding parainfluenza viruses from their respiratory tract can vertically transmit these organisms to their offspring at or soon after birth. Such transmission could also be classified as contact transmission, if direct, or vehicular, if indirect.

10.3   Disease Control Strategies

Three terms are generally used in association with disease control activities: prevention, control, and eradication.

Prevention was discussed in a holistic sense in 1.2. In its restricted usage, it is generally applied to those measures designed to exclude disease from an unaffected population. This applies both to measures to exclude infectious agents from defined geographic areas (e.g., by quarantine), or to protect a given population in an infected area (e.g., by vaccination). Prevention can be applied at either the individual or the population level.

Control describes efforts directed toward reducing the frequency of existing disease to levels biologically and/or economically justifiable or otherwise of little consequence. Control implies activities conducted at the population level. With a number of endemic diseases (such as mastitis and enteritis), and assuming there are no welfare considerations, there may be a level of disease in the population below which the cost of further expenditure on control would be greater than the benefits derived.

Eradication describes efforts to eliminate selected organisms from a defined area. These efforts usually are directed toward interfering with the natural history of an infectious organism so as to make its perpetuation unlikely if not impossible. The scale of eradication can be local (e.g., farm level), national, or global. The general features of a disease that make it susceptible to eradication are discussed elsewhere (Yekutiel 1980). These features include: the disease must be of sufficient detriment that eradication is economically justifiable; the disease should have features that enhance case detection and surveillance; and there should be at least one tool that is effective in halting disease transmission.

Specific activities used in preventing, controlling, or eradicating disease may be used either singly or in combination.

10.3.1   Slaughter

This is the deliberate killing of infected, potentially infected, or contact animals in an attempt to "stamp out" disease and prevent it from spreading to a healthy population. This can be done selectively (on an individual animal basis) or by complete depopulation (on a herd/flock or area basis). Directed activity known as selective slaughter has been used in a number of campaigns against animal disease. This involves a method of case finding, usually by means of an immunologic screening test, and then the killing of test-positive animals; hence the name "test and slaughter." The characteristics of the screening test (3.7) play a major role in the effectiveness of this method, and there may be a need to reassess the efficacy (i.e., sensitivity and specificity) of the test as the prevalence of disease changes.

Selective slaughter may be used in early control efforts, particularly if the agent spreads very slowly. Selective slaughter was used extensively in the initial phases of many bovine brucellosis eradication programs. It is less disruptive than nonselective depopulation particularly if the disease is reasonably common. Depopulation is a more extreme situation, in which the whole population, including noninfected as well as infected individuals, is sacrificed. This may be applied to wild reservoir populations as well as domestic species. All swine were slaughtered during eradication efforts against African swine fever in the Dominican Republic (Chain and Rodriquez 1983). Depopulation tends to be favored over selective slaughter if the disease agent is exotic to the area or spreads rapidly, as well as in the terminal stages of eradication schemes. In North America, depopulation is often used when a herd is found to be infected with bovine tuberculosis. In this situation, it is most important that the surveillance program identify infected herds, the actual level of disease in the herd being of lesser importance.

10.3.2 Quarantine

Quarantine implies the enforced physical separation from the healthy population of infected or potentially infected individuals, their products, or items they may have contaminated. Such measures may be applied at the national, regional, or herd level, and they may be voluntary or required by legislation. For example, imported cattle are usually placed in quarantine stations for a defined period (usually the maximum incubation period) prior to being transferred to the property of the purchaser, to ensure (by clinical and/or serologic monitoring) that they are not infected with undesirable agents such as the virus of foot-and-mouth disease. Similarly, dogs are usually quarantined for a period to ensure they are free of rabies, before admitting them to rabies-free countries.

10.3.3 Reduction of Contact

As with quarantine measures, the objective here is to reduce or prevent contact (either physical or aerosol) between infected and noninfected animals. This can be done by separating animals in time (e.g., "all in–all out"

husbandry methods for poultry, swine, veal calves, and beef feedlot cattle),
by separating animals physically using barriers such as solid partitions between pens, or by building separate facilities (e.g., a separate calf barn so
that adult and young animals are physically separated; hence the calves
have a reduced risk of acquiring enzootic pneumonia). The installation of
adequate ventilation systems is necessary to reduce aerosol transmission in
intensively housed poultry, swine, and cattle (e.g., veal calf) systems.

10.3.4 Chemical Use

Chemicals may be used to reduce disease transmission in a number of
ways. Disinfectants may be used to reduce the risk of transmission of infectious agents (e.g., the use of formaldehyde between batches of eggs in
hatcheries, or the use of lime as a disinfectant subsequent to removal of
brucella infected cattle from a premise). Pesticides may be used to reduce
or eliminate vector populations (e.g., subsequent to a build up of mosquito
populations or the occurrence of equine encephalitis in horses) and hence
aid in the control of disease. An early example of the successful use of
chemicals was the use of arsenic dips in the southern United States during
the 1800s to free cattle from the tick vector of bovine piroplasmosis. As was
mentioned previously, this allowed control of the disease even before the
agent (*Babesia bigemina*) was identified. Today, antimicrobials often are
used for mass prophylaxis or treatment (e.g., sulfonamides in drinking
water for the control of coccidiosis in birds). Other applications of mass
treatment are the use of teat dips and dry cow therapy for the control of
bovine mastitis. Chemicals (such as in dry cow therapy) can also be used on
a selective basis, after culturing each cow, or on a herd-wide basis. In
general, because of resistance on the part of the vector and/or the agent,
and because of problems related to drug residues and other direct health
dangers to people handling these chemicals, it is important to focus on the
safe application of chemicals and, it is hoped, to reduce industry dependence on them. Decision analysis (9.4) and other econometric tools can be
extremely helpful in selecting the optimal time and place to use chemicals.
For example, applying mass antimicrobial therapy only in groups of cattle
experiencing disease outbreaks (such as thromboembolic meningoencephalitis) rather than unselective application of therapy to all groups of cattle.
Formal studies of the total antimicrobial usage and the resultant productivity of animals in mass prophylactic programs versus selective therapeutic
programs would provide useful data on this subject.

10.3.5 Modification of Host Resistance

A host's resistance to infection and/or disease may be modified by
increasing genetic resistance (e.g., by selecting strains of poultry resistant to
Marek's disease), by stimulating acquired resistance (e.g., mass immuniza-

tion), or by means of ensuring the transfer of passive immunity (e.g., assisting calves to nurse their dam and/or force feeding pooled colostrum).

Mass immunization programs have been successfully used in controlling many diseases of farm animals such as bovine brucellosis, and in diseases of companion animals such as canine distemper. In farm animals, vaccination is often used in an attempt to reduce the prevalence of endemic disease to levels such that selective slaughter and/or depopulation can be used. For example, vaccination against foot-and-mouth disease is practiced in many countries where the infection is meso- or hyperendemic. Identifying the appropriate time to eliminate vaccination as an element of an eradication program is difficult and has both scientific and social ramifications. If mass immunization is used, difficulties may arise with the ability of screening tests to distinguish between the natural and the vaccine induced immunological responses. This can cause particular difficulty for disease control programs and also for routine serological surveillance; if the vaccinal agent is capable of spreading, these difficulties are compounded. Mass vaccination is a frequent component of control programs directed against many exotic diseases, although the value of this practice is difficult to establish. Also, there is some concern about the spread of infection by vaccine crews in the early stages of eradication programs (Burridge et al. 1975).

Vaccination programs have usually been applied directly to protect the species of interest. However, recently there have been investigations in Europe and North America into vaccinating wildlife reservoirs against rabies by the use of oral vaccines (World Health Organization 1981). The intent of such programs is to control the disease in the reservoir population, and hence to reduce the risk of transmission to companion and farm animals and humans.

If there has been a drawback to mass immunization, perhaps it has been in the narrowing of our thinking and approach to the control of disease, as considerable emphasis has been placed on this single measure. Although many vaccines currently sold for the prevention of endemic diseases (such as respiratory and/or gastrointestinal disease) have never been shown to be effective, huge sums of money are spent advertising their potential benefit to professionals and lay people alike. The unfortunate aspect of this dependence on immunization is the potential for some of these vaccines to actually do more harm than good (Martin 1983).

10.3.6 Environment and/or Management Control

As discussed in Chapter 4, most disease results from an ecological imbalance between the host and its environment. If the environment can be altered to reduce the severity or likelihood of such imbalances, the result will be a reduced level of disease. Examples of such measures include improving the physical environment in barns by means of ventilation and lighting, the regular maintenance of milking equipment, and the use of single service paper towels as measures to aid in the control of bovine mastitis. This remains an area not fully investigated or utilized, although many practitioners are now stressing this aspect of disease control and placing less emphasis on the use of biologics. There is, however, a great need to formally evaluate the efficacy of any such disease control program.

Environmental hygiene also includes the physical cleaning of animals and their environment as well as management schemes such as pasture rotation and the use of portable calf pens. Environmental hygiene is essential during the slaughtering process both to prevent spread of infection to susceptible animals (e.g., preventing dogs and other animals from having access to offal) and to ensure a safe, wholesome product for the consumer. Despite the high level of slaughtering plant hygiene in developed countries, the consumer needs to be aware of hygienic food preparation methods at home, because agents such as salmonella are likely to remain on the final product.

10.3.7 Education

Programs to educate the public should be an integral part of disease control and eradication efforts. Unfortunately this often appears to be overlooked or becomes reduced to secondary importance relative to other more direct or dramatic measures such as mass vaccination. In veterinary medicine there are several classic examples where educational programs have been integral parts of a control program, such as the campaign to control hydatid disease in New Zealand (Schwabe 1984, pp 474–79) and Cyprus (Polydorou 1983), and recent efforts against African swine fever in the Carribean (Chain and Rodriquez 1983).

The requirement for veterinarians to educate themselves in a number of social areas where their activities have an impact is also related to this subject. This includes the human-animal bond (Schwabe 1984), how dairy farmers view veterinary services (Goodger and Ruppanner 1983), and how dairy farmers view themselves (Bigras-Poulin et al. 1983). Such understanding should greatly enhance the effectiveness of veterinary service.

10.3.8 Biological Control

This control method utilizes living things that humankind considers to be reasonably nondetrimental to its purposes to control other living things that have been judged to be harmful. Such measures may be aimed directly at agents of disease, or indirectly via control of vectors or reservoir populations. An example of the use of this method to control rabbits in Australia using myxomatosis virus was presented in 4.8.1. Another example involves the use of sterile male flies to control screwworm disease in cattle in the southern United States. Male flies are grown in large numbers in captivity, sterilized by radiation, and then released. The objective is to interfere with the reproductive cycle of the fly. Since the females mate only once, mating with an irradiated male leads to no offspring and hence a subsequent reduction in numbers of adult flies (Knipling 1960). Similar programs are now being mounted against the vector(s) of trypanosomiasis in Africa (Stephen 1975).

10.4 Integrated Disease Control Planning (A Conceptual Framework)

Disease control programs need to be well designed from both a biologic and economic point of view. They also need to be dynamic so they can evolve with the changing situation (i.e., the disease frequency and/or the biologic, economic, political, and/or social climate may change necessitating changes in the program) (Hanson and Hanson 1983).

When combating specific diseases, particularly if the objective is eradication, there are four general phases to the control program (Yekutiel 1980). In the first phase, personnel are trained, the population of concern is enumerated, the supply of local health services is assessed, and the required program administration is put into place. In the second phase, the area-wide directed activity against the disease commences. The nature of these activities will depend on the disease, the main method of attack (e.g., mass testing and slaughter versus vector control), and the social, political, geographic, and economic constraints of the area. This phase continues until the prevalence of disease is reduced to a level where continued transmission of the agent is unlikely to occur. The third phase is really a "mopping-up period" combined with intensive surveillance for remaining cases, and a traceback of all cases to ensure that the original source and all contacts of the case are detected and controlled. It is here the quality of disease detection activities is of paramount importance. The procedures used in the second phase may need to be reassessed for their accuracy since the relative importance of false negatives and false positives may change with disease prevalence. It is not unusual to find that the characteristics of the residual disease differ dramatically from the main features of disease when it was more prevalent; this feature was apparent in the terminal stages of the hog cholera eradication campaign in the United States (Hanson and Hanson 1983). The final phase of disease eradication programs involves vigilance in preventing the reintroduction of the disease and developing an early warning system for such introductions. This is of utmost importance if the time, effort, and money spent in the earlier phases is not to be wasted by allowing reentry of the disease. Most regional and national programs require an efficient local veterinary health-care delivery system, as well as good communication to those formally charged with the task of ongoing surveillance. Without an ongoing and appropriate veterinary infrastructure in the area, the early successes may be short lived.

As indicated, the process of disease control requires data that can be used to generate information on which to base and/or modify the control program. Much of the current gathering and processing of data on endemic disease is done to achieve an immediate perceived need (e.g., a particular research project or one particular disease), but does not have an ongoing or broad thrust. It would be extremely useful and informative to have a system to rationalize the current data collection systems so the overall effort can be more directed and effective.

For example, one could envisage a hierarchical data collection (monitoring/surveillance) system for endemic disease in which farms form the basic building blocks or foundation. Much data generated on a farm are of interest only to the individual manager; however, a portion is of direct value to the veterinarian. At the farm level, information of value to the manager would include action lists (e.g., cows due to calve in the next week, cows due in heat in the next week, etc.), and monitoring of production (e.g., the period from calving to first observed heat, milk production per day, etc.) so that problems can be identified early. Summaries of health problems and productivity are needed on a regular basis on each farm so that objectives can be compared to targets and health maintenance activities modified accordingly. The latter summary data could be put to good advantage at the veterinary practice level by integrating it with data from other clients (Stephens et al. 1982). This would allow a veterinarian to compare levels of disease and measures of reproductive and productive efficiency on an individual property with those of other clients, and also to continually monitor and quantify the health status of the population of animals in the area. Data on individual animals would also be of value to the veterinarian as a means of monitoring the response to therapy and/or the efficacy of prophylactic procedures directed at the individual. The veterinarian could prepare lists of problem cows and discuss alternative control measures with colleagues prior to visiting the farm.

In a similar manner, data from a number of veterinary practices could be combined with data from other sources (e.g., milk quality control laboratories, abattoirs, and diagnostic laboratories) at a Regional Epidemiology Center. These centers would use the integrated data for ongoing research dedicated to assist the veterinarians in that area solve problems related to disease control (the number of sampling units required and the complexity of the data sets would prohibit this at the individual veterinary practice level). In addition, such data could be used as a rational basis for establishing research priorities, monitoring disease, and for the signaling of problems requiring immediate follow up. Knowledge derived from such activities could then be fed back through the system by way of formal meetings, extension workers, research papers, shared information data bases, etc. Overall, such a system should result in a more efficient, directed, and harmonized thrust of the efforts of those involved with animal health maintenance.

If there was a desire to use the data from such a system for disease monitoring (see Chapter 11), then to ensure representativeness of these data, it would necessitate formal sampling of source farms. However, this should not be a major objective of the system, at least initially; rather, interested and capable farmers and veterinarians should serve as collaborators. Because almost all animal disease monitoring systems impact on or require the input of the individual animal owner, it seems logical that high levels of collaboration (hence representativeness) would be ensured if the system served the direct needs of animal owners and not just the needs of a governmental or other outside agency. Although no such overall system currently exists, there are a number of systems, for example, health management data systems for individual herds such as DAISY (Stephens et al. 1982), and others (Etherington et al. 1984). With appropriate nudging, modifications, and assistance, the current systems could form the basis of an overall hierarchical system.

References

Bigras-Poulin, M., A. H. Meek, S. W. Martin, I. McMillan, D. J. Blackburn, and D. G. Grieve. 1983. The influence of socio-psychological aspects of managers on disease occurrence and productivity of dairy herds. Proc. 3rd Int. Symp. Vet. Epidemiol. Econ., Sept. 1982, Arlington, Va.

Burridge, M. J., H. P. Riemann, W. W. Utterback, and E. C. Sharman. 1975. The Newcastle disease epidemic in southern California, 1971–1973: Descriptive epidemiology and effects of vaccination on the eradication program. Proc. 79th U.S. Anim. Health Assoc.

Chain, P., and I. Rodriguez. 1983. Communications aspects of the African swine fever eradication campaign in the Dominican Republic, 1978–1980. Proc. 3rd Int. Symp. Vet. Epidemiol. Econ., Sept. 1982, Arlington, Va.

Derbyshire, J. B. 1982. Microbial disease and animal productivity. In CRC Handbook of Agricultural Productivity. II. Animal Productivity. Boca Raton, Fla.: CRC Press.

Etherington, W. G., A. H. Meek, and B. W. Stahlbaum. 1984. Application of Microcomputers to Facilitate the Collection and Analysis of Health and Production Data on Dairy Farms. Ontario Veterinary College, Univ. of Guelph, Ontario.

Goodger, W. J., and R. Ruppanner. 1983. How large scale dairy operations view veterinary services. Proc. 3rd Int. Symp. Vet. Epidemiol. Econ., Sept. 1982, Arlington, Va.

Gwaltney, J. M., and J. O. Hendley. 1982. Transmission of experimental rhinovirus infection by contaminated surfaces. Am. J. Epidemiol. 116:828–33.

Hanson, R. P., and M. G. Hanson. 1983. Animal Disease Control: Regional Programs. Ames: Iowa State Univ. Press.

Hawkins, C. D., and R. S. Morris. 1978. Depression of productivity in sheep infected with *Fasciola hepatica*. Vet. Parasitol. 4:341–57.

Johnson, D. C., W. H. Emory, S. H. Kleven, and D. E. Stallknecht. 1983. The epidemiology and economic impact of a *Mycoplasma gallisepticum* epornitic in a major poultry producing area. Proc. 3rd Int. Symp. Vet. Epidemiol. Econ., Sept. 1982, Arlington, Va.

Kaneene, J. B., and E. C. Mather. 1982. Cost Benefits of Food Animal Health. East Lansing: Michigan State Univ. Press.

Knipling, E. F. 1960. The eradication of the screw-worm fly. Sci. Am. 203(4):54–61.

Martin, S. W. 1983. Vaccination: Is it effective in preventing respiratory disease or influencing weight gains in feedlot calves? Can. Vet. J. 24:10–19.

Martin, S. W., and A. D. Wiggins. 1973. A model of the economic costs of dairy calf mortality. Am. J. Vet. Res. 34:1027–31.

Martin, S. W., C. W. Schwabe, and C. E. Franti. 1975. Dairy calf mortality rate: Characteristics of calf mortality rates in Tulare County, California. Am. J. Vet. Res. 36:1099–1104.

Philpot, W. N. 1967. Influence of subclinical mastitis on milk production and milk composition. J. Dairy Sci. 50:978.

Polydorou, K. 1983. Disease control planning in Cypress. Proc. 3rd Int. Symp. Vet. Epidemiol. Econ., Sept. 1982, Arlington, Va.

Roseby, F. B. 1973. Effects of *Trichostrongylus colubriformis* (Nematoda) on the nutrition and metabolism of sheep. I. Feed intake, digestion and utilization. Aust. J. Agric. Res. 24:937–53.

Rosen, G. 1972. Editorial: The epidemiologic revolution. Am. J. Pub. Health. 62:1439–41.

Schwabe, C. W. 1984. Veterinary Medicine and Human Health. 3rd ed. Baltimore, Md.: Williams & Wilkins.

Schwabe, C. W., and R. Ruppanner. 1972. Animal diseases as contributors to human hunger. World Rev. Nutr. Diatetics. 15:185–224.

Stephen, L. E. 1975. African trypanosomiasis. *In* Diseases Transmitted from Animals to Man, 6th ed., ed. W. T. Hubbert, W. P. McCulloch, and P. R. Schnurrenberger. Springfield, Ill.: C. C. Thomas.

Stephens, A. J., R. J. Esslemont, and P. R. Ellis. 1982. DAISY: A dairy herd information system for small computers. *In* Cost Benefits of Food Animal Health, ed. J. B. Kaneene and E. C. Mather. East Lansing: Michigan State Univ. Press.

World Health Organization. 1981. Joint CNER-WHO scientific meeting on animal rabies on the occasion of the tenth anniversary of the Centre National d'Etudes sur la Rage. WHO/Rab. Res. 81.13.

Yekutiel, P. 1980. Eradication of infectious diseases: A critical study. *In* Contributions to Epidemiology and Biostatistics, vol. 2. Basel, Switzerland: S. Karger.

CHAPTER 11

Monitoring Disease and Production

11.1 Introduction and Overview

Animal disease monitoring describes ongoing efforts directed at assessing the health and disease status of a given population. This activity necessitates a system for collecting, processing, and summarizing data (e.g., tabulation and graphical presentation) and disseminating information to appropriate agencies as well as individuals. The term "disease surveillance" is used to describe a more active system and implies that some form of directed action will be taken if the data indicate a disease level above a certain threshold (e.g., surveillance systems for viral encephalitides). In either case, the primary purpose of such systems is to provide data on the occurrence of disease, its geographic and temporal patterns, and, in some instances in veterinary medicine, on the effect of disease on productivity. Monitoring systems can also provide data to aid decision making regarding the effectiveness of health programs and practices, and for the planning of new ones such as the retrospective studies on brucellosis control (Kellar et al. 1976; Gray and Martin 1980) or avian Newcastle disease control programs (Burridge et al. 1975).

Disease monitoring can be conducted on many axes; for example, it may be concerned with one disease or a number of diseases, and the system may cover one species or many species of animals. Disease monitoring may be conducted primarily for the benefit of the animals themselves, or primarily as an early warning system for potential human health hazards (Schwabe et al. 1971). Also, disease monitoring may be applied at different levels (e.g., regional, national, and international systems). In addition, data derived from herd health programs are closely related to disease surveillance systems operating at the farm level (see 10.4). The scope of most monitoring and surveillance systems reflects the nature of the disease(s) and requirements for its control. Farm level surveillance systems emphasize those diseases that are, at least theoretically, controllable by the individual farm owner. They tend also to stress the impact of disease on productivity as this, together with humane considerations, provides the incentive for disease control. Regional, national, and international systems usually emphasize diseases not controllable by the individual without at least some collective organized approach. Sometimes producer organizations form such cooperatives to control disease; however, in most instances, government veterinary agencies are intimately involved in coordinating and/or directing the system.

Each defined group of users will have different needs for disease monitoring, and one group may use the same information differently than another. For example, farmers and their veterinarians are likely to view the occurrence of a specific disease in their herd (e.g., cattle deaths due to salmonellosis) very differently than would a state veterinarian concerned with program (notifiable) diseases, or a public health veterinarian concerned with human health risks. Hence, no single monitoring system currently exists to meet the needs of such a broad range of individuals, and perhaps it is naive to think that such systems will exist in the foreseeable future. What is important, however, is that a particular monitoring system must meet the needs of those directly concerned with it. Whether the information is valid for other purposes, or can be extrapolated to the general population, will have to be assessed system by system. The most frequently cited specific uses of animal disease monitoring include:

1. estimating disease frequency (i.e., relative to other conditions and/or as actual incidence or prevalence rates). When sufficient data are available, seasonal, cyclical, and secular trends are searched for;

2. certifying that disease is absent (e.g., to certify that an animal herd or region is free from a specific disease such as brucellosis in cattle or hip dysplasia in dogs). The presence of a disease could affect the value of the animal/herd and restrict movement either into or out of these areas;

3. the early detection of foreign and/or emerging diseases (e.g., early detection of Newcastle disease in poultry and African swine fever virus in hogs, or detecting a significant increase in the frequency of diseases such as influenza in poultry, encephalitis in horses, or bovine leukemia); and

4. the making of management decisions based on the above (e.g., diagnostic laboratories need to consider their role as in 1 to 3 above and obtain equipment and staff accordingly, biologics companies can plan their production based on needs projected from current knowledge, and research organizations can allot monies based on clearly documented needs).

Before proceeding with a description of some existing systems, it is necessary to discuss various qualitative aspects of the data used in disease monitoring. Further discussions of this topic are available elsewhere (Hugh-Jones 1973; Anderson 1982; Beal 1983).

11.2 Qualitative Aspects of Data

11.2.1 Availability and Validity of Data

The availability and validity of data are of primary concern when using field data for disease monitoring. The collection of accurate and representative field data (i.e., active monitoring or surveillance) is expensive, and few systems designed solely for this purpose exist. To minimize the costs of operating ongoing disease monitoring systems, data on disease occurrence that is being recorded for another purpose is very often used (i.e., passive monitoring). The validity of the data for this secondary purpose requires careful evaluation. Although the data may be sufficiently accurate and complete for the intended primary purpose, they may be misleading if used for other purposes (Ray 1982).

Each monitoring system should tailor its principal objectives to its users, bearing in mind the political, social, economic, and cultural constraints of the area. As minimal criteria, the data must enumerate the occurrences of specific diseases and specify the time, location, and host characteristics of affected animals and of the population at risk. When possible, ancillary data on the biologic and/or economic impact of disease will prove useful in assigning priorities to disease control and will enable the decision makers (politicians, administrators, veterinary officials, and herd owners) to deal more effectively with the disease situation.

11.2.2 Specifying the Disease

Special attention needs to be given to defining what constitutes a case. Should only instances of clinical disease be included, or are subclinical cases to be counted as well? Is the isolation of the putative pathogen (e.g., salmonella) from a carrier enough to lead to an incident that will be recorded? What if the isolation is made from environmental samples, feed, or an intermediary host (e.g., bluetongue virus in an insect)? Does a positive seroreactor qualify as a case? Such decisions have to be made early by those planning the monitoring system and/or by those planning to use secondary data for the purpose of monitoring during the period of interest. New problems can arise if administrative and/or diagnostic changes are made. It should therefore be emphasized that rigorous definitions and procedures are needed to ensure valid compilations within the individual monitoring system. Where possible, it is advantageous if these definitions allow meaningful comparisons among different systems. However, starting a system with sufficiently restricted objectives and achievable goals is probably more important than designing a broadly useful system with goals that are ill defined and/or achievable only in the long term (Hugh-Jones 1975).

Another requirement for implementing an effective monitoring system is a standardized nomenclature containing a unique definition for each of the diseases (cases) involved. The reason for this is obvious when one considers that very often disease monitoring systems involve the pooling of data from several participating institutions (e.g., laboratories, abattoirs, or veterinary practices), each of which may have several diagnosticians. Although this may seem like a fairly simple requirement, experience has shown that it is very difficult to achieve. In most systems a unique numeric or alphabetical code is assigned to each member of a list of standard diagnoses. For example, the Standard Nomenclature of Veterinary Diseases and Operations (SNVDO) was the basis for the Veterinary Medical Data Program involving a number of colleges in North America (see Priester 1975 and 12.4.1 for details and examples of its usage). Although this results in the use of standard terms, it does not ensure that different people use the same code for similar disease problems, nor does it protect against the same code being used for different problems by different people (Erb and Martin 1978). In monitoring systems with limited scope, such problems may be quite easily overcome using ad hoc definitions and common instructions. However in larger, more generalized, and extended systems great effort is required to circumvent these problems.

11.2.3   Enumerating Disease Occurrence

The primary objective of any monitoring system is to provide, under the prevailing circumstances, a reasonably accurate estimate of the frequency of disease(s), usually but not always in a definable population(s). Each system should therefore be carefully evaluated for possible factors that in one way or another can introduce quantitative biases in the estimate. The main types of biasing factors include unrepresentative selection of cases, incomplete reporting, and poor sensitivity and specificity of the diagnostic procedures. The last two factors tend to result in an underestimate of the frequency of common disease problems, while the first factor may inflate the apparent occurrence of rare diseases. The apparent frequency of disease may exceed or be lower than the true frequency, depending on the sensitivity and the specificity of the test. A discussion of these factors in the context of monitoring zoonoses in the United States has been published by Schnurrenberger and Hubbert (1980). Specific examples of fallacies from inferences based on biased (unrepresentative and/or incompletely reported) data are given by McCallon and Beal (1982).

Another basic consideration in enumerating disease occurrence is to decide whether incidence, prevalence, or both types of data will be collected. Finally, one should consider the most appropriate unit of concern.

In some instances the animal is the most appropriate unit of concern; however in others, such as infectious disease control programs, the primary need is to ascertain whether a herd or flock is infected (Suther et al. 1974).

11.2.4 Temporal Aspects of Disease Occurrence

The approximate time of disease acquisition is of considerable value for developing causal hypotheses and monitoring as part of disease control programs. Thus, incidence data are preferable to prevalence data (the latter are nevertheless often used, because they are easier and less expensive to obtain). For the same reason, frequent reporting (days or weeks) to those who require the information is preferable to infrequent reporting.

Seasonal distribution and secular trends in disease occurrence are often presented as updated graphs of the number of new cases versus calendar time, on the assumption the population at risk is relatively constant throughout the period. For example, yearly summaries of salmonella infections are based on the number of cases from which these organisms were isolated (Centers for Disease Control 1982) (Fig. 11.1). A similar seasonal pattern is evident for *Salmonella dublin* isolations in cattle herds in Denmark (Husum 1984) (Fig. 11.2). Although the total population at risk in these examples may not change dramatically over the course of 1 year, the consistent increase in number of isolations during the early fall period would be more suggestive of environmental influences if the number of cases (samples) cultured were used as a denominator. This would allow one to assess whether the proportion of samples submitted for culture that were found positive for salmonella changed seasonally, or if the seasonal pattern was merely due to more samples being cultured in the presence of a con-

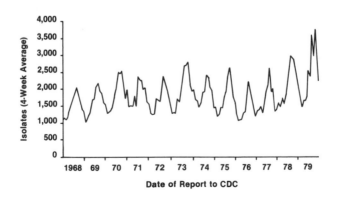

11.1. Reported human *Salmonella* isolations by 4-week average, United States, 1968–1979. (Source: Centers for Disease Control 1982)

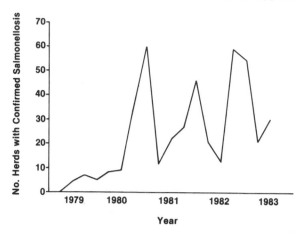

11.2. Number of cattle herds in a Danish county diagnosed with clinical *Salmonella* problems (calf mortality, diarrhea) as confirmed by laboratory isolations of particular *Salmonella dublin*. (Source: Husum 1984, with permission)

stant infection rate. Another example of the problem created by the lack of an appropriate denominator relates to the monitoring of hog cholera during the latter years of the eradication scheme in the United States. In this instance, the total number of confirmed cases of hog cholera was found to be a poor indicator of progress in that it reflected the amount of program activity as well as the level of infection. By expressing the confirmed cases as a ratio to the total number of suspicious cases, a much more useful measure was obtained; this ratio correlated closely with the prevalence of hog cholera in slaughtered swine (Beal 1983). Thus, whenever possible, the true population at risk or an appropriate surrogate denominator should be used, and the actual rates tabulated or plotted versus calendar time.

It should also be appreciated that a downward time trend in disease occurrence during the course of a control program can not be taken to prove a causal effect of the program per se, although it may suggest a causal hypothesis that might be tested using proper analytic investigations. Because of the numerous changes in the environment and populations that take place over time, it is generally impossible to attribute an observed change in disease occurrence over time to one particular factor such as a control program. This would be similar to using "historical controls" in an experiment or analytic study, a practice that is not recommended. For example, the observed attack rate of rinderpest in cattle in Great Britain during the 1860s has been used to justify the utility of predictive models (e.g., an early version of the Reed-Frost model) developed by William Farr

(Susser 1977). In this particular case, the downtrend in disease occurrence was predicted based on the observed number of cases, although the predicted decline was faster than the actual decrease in cases. Similar data have been used to demonstrate the impact of the Cattle Diseases Prevention Act that included the power to quarantine and slaughter cattle and was put into effect in February 1866. (This act compelled the slaughter of infected animals and the disinfection of infected premises and allowed the slaughter of healthy in-contact cattle where deemed desirable.) (Schwabe 1984, p 21; Hanson and Hanson 1983, pp 300–1). It is likely both reasons explain the disappearance of rinderpest and the success of the eradication campaign; however, the difficulty in establishing cause and effect based on one outbreak should be obvious.

A related, important temporal feature is that current data is usually of much more value than historical data. Thus, particularly in active surveillance systems, it is necessary to process the data in a timely fashion and distribute summaries to those who need to know as soon as possible thereafter. During the 1982 outbreak of foot-and-mouth disease in Denmark, practitioners and others were regularly informed about the occurrence of new infections and the progress of the eradication efforts.

11.2.5 Location of Disease

The data used in a monitoring system should contain sufficient detail to allow for a proper identification of the source of the animals in order to identify possible problem areas (herds, regions, etc.). Such data may be presented in the form of spot maps. Also, it is often advantageous to show changes in the geographic distribution of a disease with time (e.g., to illustrate the spread of the disease within a region). A spot map technique was used to portray the geographic distribution and movement of foot-and-mouth disease in Denmark in 1982 (Westergaard 1982) (Fig. 11.3). To an extent, valid interpretation of spot maps such as this demand some knowledge of the distribution of the population at risk. The actual temporal spread of infection is emphasized in the form of a histogram in Figure 11.4.

A major problem in locating diseased premises when monitoring at a central facility (e.g., from the slaughterhouse or marketplace) lies in tracing diseased animals to their herd of origin. In many instances, animal identification is not sufficiently advanced to allow easy traceback to the herd of origin. This is particularly true when animals can be bought and sold many times in a short period and concomitantly moved over vast distances. Recent studies on traceback of tuberculosis-positive animals in the United States revealed that a majority of infected premises were in a different state than the slaughtering plant where tuberculosis was detected (Roswurm 1972). Similar findings were noted when attempts were made to traceback sheep infected with *Echinococcus granulosus* to their herd of origin (Saw-

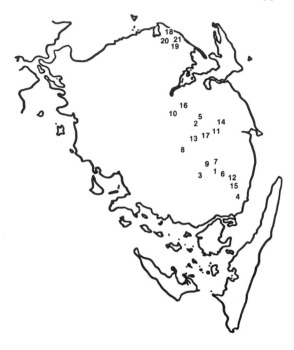

11.3. Location and sequence of the 17 herds on eastern part and 4 herds on northern part of island of Funen that were infected with foot-and-mouth disease in 1982. (Source: Westergaard 1982)

yer et al. 1969). Animal identification systems are numerous but many are designed only to identify the animal within the herd. New developments in electronic and other identification systems may improve this situation.

11.2.6 Characteristics of Diseased Animals

Species, breed, age, and sex of the animals, if recorded, make it possible to further specify the epidemiologic pattern of disease occurrence and help in the identification of particular risk groups. Such data may, however,

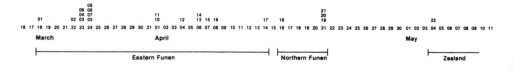

11.4. Temporal aspects of foot-and-mouth disease on island of Funen, March and April 1982. (Source: Westergaard 1982)

be difficult to obtain on a routine basis. In most slaughtering houses, it is not possible to accurately state the age of a particular animal, only to identify it as being mature or immature.

If differences in disease rates between farms, counties, or slaughterhouses might be attributable to differences in the composition of the underlying populations with respect to host characteristics, such rates should be calculated as host-factor-specific, or they should be standardized for any differences in the distribution of host characteristics between the units of concern (see 4.2).

11.2.7 The At-Risk Population

Basic information about the population at risk is important to any disease monitoring system. In herd-level systems this information usually is readily available, whereas at higher levels (e.g., provincial or national), its availability is more limited. In certain areas and countries, animal censuses are carried out at regular intervals. This information may be quite useful for general purposes; however, there are many situations where the data are not published in sufficient detail to make it suitable for disease monitoring purposes. The main problem is that, compared to the needs of the epidemiologist, the published statistics are rather crudely summarized (e.g., by year, geographical locality, species, age, or breed), but not by combined factors.

It is generally difficult to find accurate data on populations of nonfarm animals (i.e., companion animals and wildlife species). Census information is rare, but estimates may be based on insurance figures, questionnaire samples taken by industry (e.g., pet food manufacturers), vaccination sales figures, kennel club statistics, etc. (Canada Consulting Group Inc. 1983). An interesting method for estimating the canine population of an area is by counting dog scats (Anvik et al. 1974). However, all of these likely have various biases and should be used with caution. Formal sampling and/or a census often are the best procedures to accurately define the population at risk. Certainly, monitoring systems providing only numerator data are of less value than those also providing suitable population-at-risk data.

11.2.8 Monitoring Production Data

Monitoring production in relation to health and disease in farm animals is usually done on a within-herd basis, although there is a need for herd-level data. Dairy Herd Improvement Association (DHIA) type systems may yield the data needed by providing the sampling frame for a survey or an analytic or experimental study. Production recording schemes are currently undergoing extensive modifications to improve (reduce) the reporting time and also to incorporate data on selected diseases (Crandall 1982). As these systems become widespread and as the validity and comprehensiveness of the data included in them increase, they will provide an extremely useful data base for animal disease monitoring. In addition, it will be feasible to identify interrelationships between diseases, between genetic make up and disease, and the association between disease and level of productivity.

11.3 Monitoring Based on Incidence Data

Direct recording of new disease incidents as they occur in a population may require a significant effort, as in the case of continuous on-farm monitoring of common disease problems. Nonetheless, provided the benefits outweigh the costs, the farmer is quite likely to ensure completeness and accuracy of the data.

For selected disease problems, alternative sources of data may exist (e.g., when the disease is reportable to the veterinary authorities, or when diagnostic and/or therapeutic procedures require special assistance from veterinary hospitals or diagnostic laboratories). Records kept by these specialist institutions may then be used for estimating the occurrence of the disease as described in the following sections.

11.3.1 Disease Recording at Farm Level

The health-and-disease status of production animals is continuously monitored as part of the routine farm management practices, although the level of recording of disease incidents may vary greatly within and among different categories of herds.

In most traditional farm management systems, disease events, if recorded, are noted on the individual cow or sow card. This system provides an adequate recording basis for most decisions about individuals, but it is not well suited for monitoring the disease situation in the population (e.g., the herd). Abstracting such primary records is a tedious task, usually only performed in special situations (e.g., in the case of a retrospective evaluation of a developing disease problem in need of documentation or a retrospective analytic study) (Erb and Martin 1980). Farmers and/or their veterinarians rarely prepare formal herd summaries because of this. Systems for abstracting and summarizing these data are urgently needed, and it is important that computer software be more powerful than merely extending the individual animal card. Lack of conscientious recording may result in underestimation of some diseases and overestimation of others. In many current so-called herd health programs the emphasis is on reproductive tract health; hence, not surprisingly, diseases of the reproductive tract predominate (Williamson 1982). Some workers have indicated that data from such systems reflect self-fulfilling prophecies, and that this emphasis on reproductive disease is misdirected; other syndromes such as metabolic diseases may be more important production limiters (Heider 1980). Also, lay reporting of conditions limits the specificity of the diagnosis, although in initial investigations centering on common clinical entities this drawback may not be serious.

In modern industrialized animal-production units systematic recording of health and production related events is a necessity if the farm manager (the decision maker) is to have up-to-date, overall knowledge about the state of affairs in the animals contained in all sections of the unit.

Computerized herd health and production monitoring systems may simplify disease monitoring by including disease episodes among the events continuously recorded as part of the system input. This will make it possible to simultaneously update the individual animal record as well as the herd's disease-and-production status. Gould (1975) provides one overview of the uses of monitoring disease incidence within a dairy herd, and this aspect will be discussed further in 12.2. It is also important to reemphasize that disease incidents recorded at the herd level can have important applications outside the farm.

In a few countries (e.g., Norway) national production recording systems have recently been expanded to include disease events recorded by the herdsman and the veterinarian on the individual animal's card between production recording visits (Solbu 1983). As mentioned, this is also true of the DHIA computerized recording scheme centered in Provo, Utah (Crandall 1982).

In the United States, authorities have for many years discussed the establishment of a national animal disease reporting system that could provide accurate and up-to-date information on the incidence of the more common and economically important diseases occurring nationwide. The current interest seems to focus on a model developed in Minnesota in the early 1970s (Diesch 1982). The basic approach in this system is to collect information from a formally selected group of veterinarians and their clients; the major drawback is that since farmers use veterinarians to varying degrees and veterinarians often emphasize certain types of health problems more than others, it is not possible to extrapolate this information from the sample to the population. Nonetheless, this basic model may evolve into a unique system based on a formal random sample of herds, in which herd owners, practicing veterinarians, and other officials will record selected disease data on a strictly defined routine schedule (Beal 1983).

In most countries, however, only a few farms keep ongoing disease records (e.g., university or research institution farms where the ongoing research effort requires documentation). Table 11.1 is an example of the use of data from one such dairy herd where the incidence of left displaced abomasum (LDA) was found to increase dramatically between 1976 and 1978. The data further indicate that this followed an increase in average

Table 11.1. Average production figures and annual incidence rates of left displaced abomasum (LDA) during a 4-year period in a Danish university
dairy herd

Year	No. of 305-day lactation periods	Average production per lactation period			Incidence of LDA	
		Milk (kg)	Fat (%)	Butterfat (kg)	No. of cases[a]	Cow-years at risk[b] (%)
1975	304	4771	4.24	202	0	...
1976	281	4961	4.36	216	0	...
1977	270	5090	4.06	207	10	3.7
1978	272	5655	4.13	234	22	8.1

Source: Grymer et al. 1982, with permission.
[a]No LDA cases had ever been diagnosed in the herd prior to 1977.
[b]Approximately a 305-day lactation period.

milk yield as estimated from the DHIA system used for recording and monitoring of production data (Grymer et al. 1982). Whether milk production per se is the causal factor or merely a surrogate measure of other factors (e.g., change in the ration) is unknown.

11.3.2 Notifiable Disease Reporting

For many years, veterinary authorities have operated specific monitoring systems for many contagious animal diseases by declaring them "notifiable" (i.e., reportable). The associated regulations require farmers and veterinarians to inform authorities upon suspicion of an outbreak; the officials then proceed with clinical, pathological, and other diagnostic investigations. Laboratory tests are usually carried out to ensure a specific diagnosis, and control measures including tracing of contact and/or source herds are instituted following confirmation of the diagnosis. This approach has worked satisfactorily, especially with acute disease problems in well-established, intensive animal industries. Many successful eradication programs carried out in the past have relied totally or partially on this principle, and notification continues to be an important tool in the constant watch for introduction of exotic diseases into susceptible animal populations. Here again, one must be careful in using data for secondary purposes even within the same program. For example, those interested in detecting bovine brucellosis may test a number of "suspect herds," but because these herds are not necessarily representative of all herds, the resulting laboratory data on prevalence of infection can be misleading. Those interested in controlling brucellosis once it has been detected will regularly rebleed the herd and submit samples for testing. The results of these samples are usually combined into an overall diagnostic laboratory report and hence can bias these data if used as estimates of frequency of infection. On the other hand, the prevalence of brucellosis at slaughter might be an excellent indication of the level of brucellosis in the population, but these results are of little value for detecting brucellosis without an appropriate traceback system.

Underreporting may occur with notifiable diseases depending on the nature of the particular disease. In Vermont, in the 8 months prior to February 1968, only one case of chorioptic mange was reported. Subsequently, based on a thorough examination of cattle, over 1100 confirmed cases were detected in 3 months after examining only 17% of that state's cattle herds (McCallon and Beal 1982). Hence, underreporting is likely to be a problem if the disease is not considered serious because of lack of information, nomadism (in developing countries), distrust of governmental authorities, lack of appreciation of common responsibility, and/or shortage of compensation funds. A suggested way of improving reporting and overall compliance with disease prevention is to make the seller of an animal responsible for both on-site and off-site costs associated with selling an animal with a reportable disease. This would tend to make the marketplace a center for disease control rather than its spread (Hanson and Hanson 1983).

11.3.3 Routine Diagnostic Data

In many veterinary practices, records of cases are kept in sufficient detail to serve as a basis for billing the client. If each diagnosis is recorded, compilation of cases may be used as a substitute for true incidence recordings. Validity of the approximation depends on the proportion of cases in that area receiving veterinary care, and on the complete exclusion of prevalent cases (i.e., only new cases should be counted). (The latter is very difficult to achieve and hence data of this sort often reflect period prevalence more than incidence.) Conversion to rates also requires estimates of the population at risk from which the cases originate. In the absence of such estimates, disease frequencies are sometimes expressed as proportional morbidity rates (these should not be mistaken for nor referred to as incidence rates, 3.4). The denominator is not the true population at risk and may change independently of the numerator. Meaningful interpretation (e.g., of time trends) in proportional rates as indicators of similar changes in the corresponding incidence rates requires very rigorous assumptions about stability across time of several other factors, that influence the proportional distribution, and such assumptions are most often not justified.

In certain countries, all practicing veterinarians are required to report all diagnoses to a central office where countrywide statistics are compiled and published annually (Henricson 1975). Knowing the population figures for the entire country enables estimates of overall incidence rates of all reported diagnoses. Problems with large-scale monitoring systems such as this include nonuniform use of nomenclature and diagnostic criteria, underreporting due to nonveterinary attended cases, and insufficient details on animal characteristics.

In Denmark, an accounting system for practitioners computerizes client records, including coding of the diagnosis and treatment of each case seen by the veterinarian (Byager 1976). Recently, a study of foot rot in cattle was performed within a practice area to explore the possibility of using this source of information for epidemiologic purposes (Nylin 1980). The results of this study contain some interesting information on the temporal distribution of the disease occurrence as shown in Table 11.2. To what extent the estimated incidence rates shown accurately describe the occurrence of the disease in the population is at best uncertain, and one might argue that, because of a variety of biases likely to have influenced the data, the results presented may not be reliable.

Table 11.2. Incidence of foot rot in adult cows from 110 conventional dairy herds (i.e., with summer grazing on pasture and winter housing in tied stalls) and from loose-housed herds in a Danish veterinary practice area, 1974-1978

Type of herd	Year	Number of foot rot cases	Number of cows in the herds	Annual incidence rate (%)
Conventional herds	1974	31	2400	1.3
	1975	39	2400	1.6
	1976	37	2400	1.5
	1977	55	2300	2.4
	1978	96	2300	4.2
Loose-housed herds	1974	3	104	2.9
	1975	3	104	2.9
	1976	16	420	3.8
	1977[a]	55	420	13.1
	1978[a]	60	510	11.8

Source: Nylin 1980, with permission.

[a]The increase in the loose-housed herds during 1977–1978 was mainly due to many cases in two newly established herds.

Another example of the use of farm level data for disease monitoring is the Quebec Animal Health Insurance Plan in Canada (Leduc and Ruppaner 1975). This system pays a significant portion of the traveling and professional fees of large animal veterinarians in the province, the farmer being responsible for about 40% of the cost. To collect his fee, the veterinarian must complete a multipart form that describes the demographic characteristics of the animals examined, the diagnoses, drugs used, and costs. This form is signed by the farmer before the veterinarian submits his bill to the government. In the early years of the program (1972–74) only numerator data were available; however, data on the population at risk could easily be obtained and recorded to allow the calculation of meaningful rates. In Quebec, it is highly likely that the majority of clinical problems in domestic animals are seen by participating veterinarians, and thus the system provides a good overview of the magnitude of these problems.

Moving the locale for the monitoring of disease from the farm level to veterinary clinics, diagnostic laboratories, and referral hospitals can be a mixed blessing. It increases the validity of the diagnoses, but on the other hand it introduces a variety of possible selection biases, as well as often making the determination of the proper population at risk difficult. The importance of these more specialized institutions to disease monitoring lies more in their ability to detect new and emerging disease problems than in their contribution to a balanced overview of the general disease situation. In this regard, in Great Britain central computerized files of diagnoses made since 1975 at 34 Regional Veterinary Investigation Centers are maintained and used for annual reports and special retrievals in the Veterinary Investigation Diagnosis Analyses II system (VIDA II) (Davies 1979). Apropos of the previous discussion, the summary tables in the annual reports carry the following warnings with regard to interpretation of the data:

1. The specimens received represent a biased sample of the field problems of animal disease. Great caution must therefore be shown extrapolating these diagnostic data. The figures represent only the material which is submitted from practicing veterinary surgeons. They will not include those conditions which are easily diagnosed without recourse to a laboratory, and the number and type of submissions can be influenced by the economic climate. The statistics therefore do not bear any simple or direct relationship to the level of disease in the animal population.

2. Increases in the number of diagnoses for a condition may reflect a true increase in the number of incidents in the field, but may also be affected by such factors as increased awareness of a condition, or an improved diagnostic technique. Apparent trends, especially upward trends should be related to total incidents which in most species have also shown an upward trend over the past. (Author's note: this last statement relates to the proportional rate approach to describing relative frequency of disease.)

The unique feature of the VIDA II system is its list of conditions commonly accepted as "diagnoses." They may not be full descriptions of the syndrome identified; in some cases the diagnosis describes both the pathological change and the causative organism (e.g., mastitis due to *E. coli*), in others it refers only to the isolation of the presumed causative organism (e.g., rotavirus infection), and in yet others it refers to the lesions observed in an imperfectly described syndrome (e.g., fatty liver and kidney syndrome in poultry). The VIDA II diagnostic list currently extends to 399 diagnoses (cattle 101, pigs 72, sheep 96, birds 77, and miscellaneous 53) and it is in effect a written version of the verbal description commonly used by diagnostic officers and other pathologists. The diagnostic list is reviewed at regular intervals. No addition or other alteration is made until a steering group is satisfied that the new diagnosis represents a widely-recognized and reasonably well-defined entity (Davies 1979).

11.3.4 Special Surveys

There are a variety of ways that special surveys can supply useful data. These include a range of surveys of members of a particular industry about disease problems. Examples include interviewing people associated with the sheep industry (Ruppanner 1972), the collection of piglets to ascertain the extent of congenital lesions (Selby et al. 1976) and mail surveys of producers to estimate cow-calf reproductive efficiency and neonatal survival efficiency (Rogers et al. 1985). Special national disease surveys have been conducted in Great Britain and a summary of their results and comments on methodologic issues are available (Leech 1971a, b).

Other examples include special surveys to determine the cause of death in feedlot cattle. One such study based on postmortem examination of all dead cattle in a large feedlot confirmed previous suspicions and also validated the importance of some less frequent conditions such as atypical pneumonia (Jensen et al. 1976). A similar study was initiated as an integral part of a large field study of factors associated with morbidity and mortality in newly-arrived, stressed beef calves; summaries of these findings are available elsewhere (Martin et al. 1982a, b). In the latter study, approximately 80% of all dead calves were examined by pathologists using a formal protocol, and the cause(s) of death was established on this basis. However, during the first year of the study, farmers were hesitant to submit animals whose cause of death (e.g., accident or urolithiasis) was already known; thus the importance of these as causes of death was underestimated. A second problem is that the "cause of death" may not be a good indicator of the specific diseases that affect feedlot calves but only those diseases with a high case-fatality rate. For example, lameness is a common disease of feedlot cattle, but it rarely is given as the cause of death although it could be of importance indirectly (i.e., lame cattle don't eat and tend to develop pneumonia—the more direct cause of death—and die). Thus, the lesions (diseases) present at postmortem that are not thought to be immediately responsible for death may provide better insight into the types and levels of diseases in the feedlot.

Overall mortality rates and the incidence of certain fatal conditions also may be estimated where rendering plants (knackeries) are established. Outside of herd health systems, routine sources of mortality data in animals are very scarce, and although the disease conditions associated with the carcasses received at rendering plants are not routinely diagnosed, the total case load is often known and may in itself be of interest to monitor.

For example, the annual crude mortality rate in mature cattle and heifers in Denmark has more than doubled during the years 1960 to 1980 (Agger 1983), and explanations for this are being sought. Furthermore, random samples of the dead animals may be necropsied, and the resulting diagnoses used for monitoring purposes. Examination of wildlife found sick or dead can provide a valuable source of information on the occurrence, but not the rate, of certain transmissible diseases, including zoonoses and/or foreign diseases in an area (Hayes 1975; Geissler 1975).

As a final example of disease monitoring, a project designed to detect a disease in a specific population will be described. In such studies defined populations are followed over a period of years and the occurrence of disease and other untoward events recorded. This example, which is of particular interest to veterinarians, is the Animal Neoplasm Registry of Alameda and Contra Costa counties in California (Schneider 1975). All neoplasms from these counties, whether of human or animal origin were studied in great detail and their occurrence related to the population at risk. This procedure is not only useful for monitoring per se, but the geographic distribution of the neoplasms may signal environmental hazards. It is also possible to study the zoonotic potential of these neoplasms (e.g., is feline leukemia associated with human leukemia?) (Schneider 1983).

11.4 Monitoring Based on Prevalence Data

One of the main difficulties in recording incidence data is the necessity of maintaining a continuous watch over the population at risk to identify the occurrence of each new case. It is an easier task to investigate a population at a particular point in time and to record the prevailing cases. The information from prevalence studies may be considered a substitute for incidence data, or complementary to such data, depending on the circumstances and the disease in question. Prevalence is a poor substitute for incidence if the disease either results in a high mortality or because of immediate treatment or spontaneous resolution diseased animals quickly and frequently recover. In using prevalence data, attention should also be given to possible changes in the mean duration of the disease as this changes the relationship between prevalence and incidence. For certain conditions a prevalence survey is, however, the only realistic possibility (e.g., in serological identification of subclinical infections) and can provide useful information about the level and distribution of infection in the population.

11.4.1 Screening for Disease

A well-established procedure in regulatory medicine is systematic diagnostic testing (screening) of animal populations for infectious diseases such as tuberculosis and brucellosis. Provided the sampling units are randomly selected, the number of affected herds (animals) out of all herds (animals) tested in any single screening survey will yield valid prevalence estimates. In repeated national screening programs, identification of the proportion of newly infected herds (animals) may form the basis of national incidence estimates (see Table 11.3). However, if the testing is repeated on different samples of the population only prevalence estimates may be obtained directly. Indirect estimates of incidence rate per year (p) may be obtained using the following formula:

$$\log(q) = \frac{\log(1 - \text{prevalence proportion})}{y}$$

where $p = 1 - q$, and y is the age of the animal in years. This formula assumes a constant incidence rate in all ages, a susceptible population at birth, and little migration of animals or death/culling from the infection (Lilienfeld and Lilienfeld 1980, pp 358–59).

Special interest has been devoted to the development of tests applicable to animal products or by-products (milk, blood, tissue) that can be obtained at central destinations (e.g., creameries or salesyards) to avoid expensive and time consuming "down-the-road-testing." There are, however,

Table 11.3. Distribution of enzootic bovine leukosis (EBL)-positive herds in Denmark by year and region

Year	East-ern	West-ern	Total	Annual incidence rate/ 1000 herds in country[a]	No. of EBL-positive herds on 31 December each year[b]	Prevalence rate of EBL herds/ 1000 herds on 31 December each year[c]
1969	73	22	95	0.89	72	0.71
1970	80	35	115	1.19	100	1.08
1971	28	36	64	0.72	83	0.94
1972	19	26	45	0.54	46	0.57
1973	26	21	47	0.60	46	0.59
1974	10	10	20	0.26	35	0.47
1975	3	13	16	0.22	30	0.42
1976	16	8	24	0.35	37	0.55
1977	16	15	31	0.48	45	0.72
1978	3	8	11	0.18	41	0.71
	274	194	468	. . .	. . .	. . .

Source: Willeberg et al. 1982, with permission.

[a]The national number of herds used as denominators have been obtained from the published census data.

[b]Positive herds have been quarantined and subsidized, and voluntary depopulation carried out. "Duration" of positive EBL herd status of quarantined herds has therefore been widely variable.

[c]The national number of herds used as denominators have been obtained from the published census data to estimate the number of herds on December 31.

screening procedures (such as tuberculosis skin testing) for which no practical alternative methods exist. In national disease eradication campaigns (such as bovine tuberculosis eradication programs) when the frequency of disease becomes very low, the major effort shifts to case finding and away from monitoring per se. This is sensible from the point of view of eradicating the disease and from the fact that it, to an extent, obviates the problems associated with low predictive values of tests under these circumstances (Suther et al. 1974).

Testing of bulk milk samples for brucellosis (milk ring test) and mastitis (somatic cell counts and microbiological plating) still are extensively used in monitoring the prevalence of infectious diseases at the herd level (see Table 11.4). A discussion of how repeated prevalence surveys can be used to estimate incidence (using mastitis as an example) is available (Thurmond 1980). Innovative methods of monitoring populations (e.g., by culturing the milk filters used to filter milk as it is loaded from the bulk tank into the truck) are also being developed. One use of such methods is to monitor herds for organisms of potential zoonotic significance.

Table 11.4. Somatic cell counts (SCC) in bulk tank milk samples from the Danish dairy herds participating in the official mastitis control scheme, 1980–1982

Year	Number tested		Samples with SCC > 500,000 (%)	Arithmetic/geometric means ($\bar{x}$)	
	Samples	Herds		SCC × 1000 $\bar{x}$, all samples	Herds with SCC > 500,000 (%)
1980	433,856	35,015	21.4	390/310	19.6/12.8
1981	421,362	33,336	17.4	350/280	14.3/ 8.7
1982	401,937	31,984	16.8	340/280	13.2/ 7.8

Source: Schmidt-Madsen 1983, with permission.

11.4.2 Slaughterhouse Data

The collection of blood serum at slaughter for diseases such as brucellosis, enzootic bovine leukemia virus infection, and pseudorabies has been widely used as a seroepidemiologic method of case-finding and monitoring. Of course, identification of the herd of origin of a positive animal is crucial to the successful traceback needed to implement the disease control function.

The pre- and postmortem inspection of animals at slaughter is in itself an extensive disease monitoring process. This monitoring might be performed by publicly employed veterinarians to assist in case-finding (e.g., of bovine tuberculosis), or to ensure the wholesomeness of animal products (meat, milk, etc.), or by private veterinarians to assess the extent of selected diseases (atrophic rhinitis, enzootic pneumonia) in their client's animals (Backstrom 1981). The latter is useful to assist in identifying what diseases exist and their frequency, and as a means of monitoring the efficacy of changes in management and disease control (e.g., introduction of a vaccination program or modifying ventilation systems). Most of the lesions found during routine slaughter inspection are chronic and, although they may be limited in their diagnostic specificity, the prevalent and persistent lesions recorded at slaughter can indicate economically important problems. Many types of lesions that lead to total or partial condemnation are recorded mainly for monitoring purposes. It is well recognized that the extent of, and procedures used in, recording slaughter inspection findings may vary considerably from region to region and even among slaughterhouses within a region. A major challenge to increase the value of the inspection process for disease monitoring is to standardize these procedures and to describe lesions in a manner that will be informative to the animal owner and veterinarian. The potential value of slaughterhouse inspection findings is great; unfortunately, however, those in charge of ensuring wholesomeness of food may function more or less independently of those in charge of publicly funded disease control, who in turn may function independently of the needs of the animal owner and the private practitioner. Rationalization of the overall process would go a long way toward increasing the value of this system.

As one example of a rationalized system, the Danish slaughterhouse monitoring system has, since 1979–1980, developed into a national pig herd health scheme. Problem herds are identified on the basis of data from computer files containing the monthly kill and the slaughter inspection findings in the form of standard codes for each individual swine herd in the country. When retrieving a list of the potential problem herds, the data in the computer files are compiled, adjusted, and weighted according to possible confounding and biasing factors, such as the variation among slaughterhouses in mean rates of lesions and the size of the herd. Joint herd visits to the problem herds by a local practitioner and the regional swine extension specialist are arranged, and they are expected to pay special attention to environmental and managerial factors that might be causally involved in the herd's disease problems. This system provides a modern example of the close relationships among epidemiologic principles and methods, disease monitoring, and disease control (Willeberg 1980; Willeberg et al. 1984).

11.4.3 Serum Banks

A special, "artificial" source of prevalence data is the so-called "serum bank" (i.e., a collection of frozen serum samples collected over a number of years from the populations of interest) (Moorhouse and Hugh-Jones 1981;

Kellar 1982). The main objective of such banks is to provide a source for "retrospective monitoring" of the occurrence of seroreaction to disease agents, which subsequent to the time of sampling become of interest. As an example of the utility of serum banks, it was possible to date, within one month, the first occurrences of the 1978 canine parvovirus pandemic (Carmichael and Binn 1981). Retrospective studies of bovine leukemia virus infection have also been performed and recently reported (Hugh-Jones et al. 1984).

11.5 International Monitoring

In the previous sections various monitoring systems at the local, regional, and national levels have been used to illustrate common concepts and features of disease monitoring systems. As mentioned, monitoring of animal diseases also takes place at the international level (Willeberg 1975). The primary objective of international organizations involved in animal disease monitoring such as the International Office of Epizootics (OIE), the Food and Agriculture Organization (FAO), and the World Health Organization (WHO) of the United Nations is to promote the exchange of information on disease occurrence. This can help in the prevention and control of animal diseases, facilitate international trade of animal products, improve and safeguard economies, increase protein supplies, and decrease human suffering in underdeveloped countries of the world. These international organizations and their associated monitoring systems have primarily taken on functions as clearinghouses for the compilation and exchange of information about the animal disease situation in the participating countries (i.e., data from national disease monitoring systems). One of the most visible efforts of the three organizations in this connection is their publication *The Animal Health Yearbook*, which contains up-to-date information on the occurrence and control of some important animal diseases around the world. In this, as in other monitoring programs, a limiting feature of the compiled information is the basic validity and completeness of the source data—in this particular case the official disease information made available by governments of the individual countries. This information is supplemented by the recent publication of the Commonwealth Agricultural Bureau (see references in preface).

References

Agger, J. F. 1983. Production disease and mortality in dairy cows: Analysis of records from disposal plants 1960–1982. Proc. 5th Conf. on Prod. Dis. in Farm Animals, Aug. 1983, Uppsala, Sweden.

Anderson, R. K. 1982. Surveillance: Criteria for evaluation and design of epidemiologic surveillance systems for animal health and productivity. Proc. 86th Annu. U.S. Anim. Health Assoc.

Anvik, J. O., A. E. Hague, and A. Rahaman. 1974. A method of estimating dog populations and its application to the assessment of canine fecal pollution and endoparasitism in Saskatchewan. Can. Vet. J. 15:219–23.

Backstrom, L. 1981. Conducting slaughter checks for swine disease recordings. Proc. Swine Herd Health Programming Conf., Sept. 20–22, University of Minnesota.

Beal, V. J. Jr. 1983. Perspectives on animal disease surveillance. Proc. 87th U.S. Anim. Health Assoc.

Burridge, M. J., H. P. Riemann, W. W. Utterback, and E. C. Sharman. 1975. The Newcastle disease epidemic in southern California, 1971–1973: Descriptive epidemiology and effects of vaccination on the eradication program. Proc. 79th U.S. Anim. Health Assoc.

Byager, J. 1976. The computer accountancy system developed by the Accountancy Association of Practising Danish Veterinarians. Proc. Symp. New Techniques in Vet. Epidemiol. and Econ., July 1976, Reading, England.

Canada Consulting Group, Inc. 1983. Pets in Ontario. A report prepared for the Ontario Veterinary Association.

Carmichael, L. E., and L. N. Binn. 1981. New enteric viruses in the dog. Adv. Vet. Sci. Comp. Med. 25:1–37.

Centers for Disease Control. 1982. Salmonella surveillance annual summary, 1980.

Crandall, B. 1982. Computer capabilities through DHIA in the state of Utah. In Cost Benefits of Food Animal Health, ed. J. B. Kaneene and E. C. Mather. East Lansing: Michigan State Univ. Press.

Davies, G. 1979. Animal disease surveillance in Great Britain. Proc. Int. Symp. Anim. Health and Disease Data Banks, Dec. 1978, Wash. D.C. USDA misc. publ. 1381.

Diesch, S. L. 1982. Animal disease surveillance in Minnesota. In Cost Benefits of Food Animal Health, ed. J. B. Kaneene and E. C. Mather. East Lansing: Michigan State Univ. Press.

Erb, H. N., and S. W. Martin. 1978. Age, breed and seasonal patterns in the occurrence of 10 dairy cow diseases: A case-control study. Can. J. Comp. Med. 42:1–9.

————. 1980. Interrelationships between production and reproductive diseases in Holstein cows. Data. J. Dairy Sci. 63:1911–17.

Geissler, P. H. 1975. Storage, retrieval and statistical analysis of wildlife disease data. In Animal Disease Monitoring, ed. D. G. Ingram, W. R. Mitchell, and S. W. Martin. Springfield, Ill.: C. C. Thomas.

Gould, C. M. 1975. The veterinary practitioner in disease monitoring. In Animal Disease Monitoring, ed. D. G. Ingram, W. R. Mitchell, and S. W. Martin. Springfield, Ill.: C. C. Thomas.

Gray, M. D., and S. W. Martin. 1980. An evaluation of screening programs for the detection of Brucellosis in dairy herds. Can. J. Comp. Med. 44:52–60.

Grymer, J., P. Willeberg, and M. Hesselholt. 1982. Milk production and left displaced abomasum: Cause and effect relationships. Nord. Vet. Med. 34:412–15.

Hanson, R. P., and M. G. Hanson. 1983. Animal Disease Control: Regional Programs. Ames: Iowa State Univ. Press.

Hayes, F. A. 1975. Wildlife considerations as a prerequisite to combatting foreign diseases. In Animal Disease Monitoring, ed. D. G. Ingram, W. R. Mitchell, and S. W. Martin. Springfield, Ill.: C. C. Thomas.

Heider, L. E. 1980. What is being taught about cattle herd management related to disease prevention? Proc. Vet. Prev. Med. Epidemiol. Work Conf., Feb. 4–6, Fort Worth, Texas.

Henricson, B. 1975. Problems of government production and utilization of information on animal diseases. *In* Animal Disease Monitoring, ed. D. G. Ingram, W. R. Mitchell, and S. W. Martin. Springfield, Ill.: C. C. Thomas.

Hugh-Jones, M. E. 1973. The uses and limitations of animal disease surveillance. Vet. Rec. 92:11–15.

―――. 1975. Some pragmatic aspects of animal disease monitoring. *In* Animal Disease Monitoring, ed. D. G. Ingram, W. R. Mitchell, and S. W. Martin. Springfield, Ill.: C. C. Thomas.

Hugh-Jones, M. E., P. Moorhouse, and C. L. Seger. 1984. Serological study of the incidence and prevalence of antibodies to bovine leukemia virus in aged sera. Can. J. Comp. Med. 48:422–24.

Husum, P. 1984. Bovine salmonellosis viewed in the light of more than 3 years of epidemiologic experience. Dansk Vet. Tidsskr. 67:82–86.

Jensen, R., R. E. Pierson, P. M. Braddy, D. A. Saart, L. H. Lauerman, J. J. England, J. Keyvanfar, J.R. Collier, D. P. Horton, A. E. McChesney, A. Benitez, and R. M. Christie. 1976. Shipping fever in yearling feedlot cattle. J. Am. Vet. Med. Assoc. 169:500–6.

Kellar, J. A. 1982. Canada's bovine serum bank: A practical approach. Proc. 3rd Int. Symp. Vet. Epidemiol. Econ., Sept. 1982, Arlington, Va.

Kellar, J., R. Marra, and W. Martin. 1976. Brucellosis in Ontario: A case-control study. Can. J. Comp. Med. 40:119–28.

Leduc, R., and R. Ruppanner. 1975. Collection of data on animal disease using the Quebec Animal Health Insurance Program. *In* Animal Disease Monitoring, ed. D. G. Ingram, W. R. Mitchell, and S. W. Martin. Springfield, Ill.: C. C. Thomas.

Leech, F. B. 1971a. A critique of the methods and results of the British National Surveys of disease in farm animals. I. Discussions of the surveys. Br. Vet. J. 127:511–22.

―――. 1971b. A critique of the methods and results of the British National Surveys of disease in farm animals. II. Some general remarks on population surveys of farm animal disease. Br. Vet. J. 127:587–92.

Lilienfeld, A. M., and D. E. Lilienfeld. 1980. Foundations of Epidemiology. New York: Oxford Univ. Press.

Martin, S. W., A. H. Meek, D. G. Davis, J. A. Johnson, and R. A. Curtis. 1982a. Factors associated with mortality and treatment costs in feedlot calves: The Bruce County Beef Project, years 1978, 1979, 1980. Can. J. Comp. Med. 46:341–49.

Martin, S. W., J. D. Holt, and A. H. Meek. 1982b. The effect of risk factors as determined by logistic regression on health of beef feedlot cattle. Proc. 3rd Int. Symp. Vet. Epidemiol. Econ., Sept. 1982, Arlington, Va.

McCallon, W. R., and V. C. Beal, Jr. 1982. The fallacy of drawing inferences from biased data: Some case examples. Proc. 86th U.S. Anim. Health Assoc.

Moorhouse, P. D. and M. E. Hugh-Jones. 1981. Serum banks. Vet. Bull. 51:277–90.

Nylin, B. 1980. Foot rot: An epidemiological investigation based on data from accounting records in a veterinary practice. Dansk Vet. Tidsskr. 63:233–41.

Priester, W. A. 1975. Collecting and using veterinary clinical data. *In* Animal Disease Monitoring, ed. D. G. Ingram, W. R. Mitchell, and S. W. Martin. Springfield, Ill.: C. C. Thomas.

Ray, W. C. 1982. Problems in developing valid data for performing mathematical studies of bovine brucellosis eradication programs. Proc. 3rd Int. Symp. Vet. Epidemiol. Econ., Sept. 1982, Arlington, Va.

Rogers, R. W., S. W. Martin, and A. H. Meek. 1985. Reproductive efficiency and calf survivorship in Ontario beef cow-calf herds: A cross-sectional mail survey. Can. J. Comp. Med. 49:27–33.

Roswurm, J. D. 1972. The status of the state–federal tuberculosis eradication program. Proc. 76th U.S. Anim. Health Assoc.

Ruppanner, R. 1972. Measurement of disease in animal populations based on interviews. J. Am. Vet. Med. Assoc. 161:1033–38.

Sawyer, J. C., P. C. Schantz, C. W. Schwabe, and M. W. Newbold. 1969. Identification of transmission foci of hydatid disease in California. Public Health Rep. 84(6):531–41.

Schmidt-Madsen, P. 1983. Report on the Danish Mastitis Control Program, 1982. Copenhagen, Denmark: Veterinary Directorate.

Schneider, R. 1975. A population-based animal tumor registry. In Animal Disease Monitoring, ed. D. G. Ingram, W. R. Mitchell, and S. W. Martin. Springfield, Ill.: C. C. Thomas.

———. 1983. Comparison of age and sex-specific incidence rate patterns of leukemia complex in the cat and the dog. J. Natl. Cancer Inst. 70:971–77.

Schnurrenberger, P. R., and W. T. Hubbert. 1980. Reporting of zoonotic diseases. Am. J. Epidemiol. 112:23–31.

Schwabe, C. W. 1984. Veterinary Medicine and Human Health. 3rd ed. Baltimore, Md.: Williams & Wilkins.

Schwabe, C. W., J. Sawyer, and W. Martin. 1971. A pilot system for environmental monitoring through domestic animals. Joint Conference on Sensing of Environmental Pollutants. New York: Am. Inst. Aeronaut. Astronaut. Paper 71–1044.

Selby, L. A., L. D. Edmonds, and L. D. Hyde. 1976. Epidemiological field studies of animal populations. Can. J. Comp. Med. 40:135–41.

Solbu, H. 1983. Disease recording in Norwegian dairy cattle. I. Disease incidences and nongenetic effects on mastitis, ketosis and milk fever. Z. Tierz. Zuechtungsbiol. 100:139–57.

Susser, M. 1977. Judgement and causal inference: Criteria in epidemiologic studies. Am. J. Epidemiol. 105:1–15.

Suther, D. E., C. E. Franti, and H. H. Page. 1974. Evaluation of comparative intradermal tuberculin test in California dairy cattle. Am. J. Vet. Res. 35:379–87.

Thurmond, M. C. 1980. Determination of incidence rates for chronic mastitis using heifer prevalence data. Am. J. Vet. Res. 41:1682–85.

Westergaard, J. M. 1982. The epidemiology of foot-and-mouth disease outbreaks on the islands of Funen and Zeeland in Denmark. Proc. 16th Conf. of the FMD Comm., Sept. 1982, Paris.

Willeberg, P. 1975. International cooperation in animal disease monitoring. In Animal Disease Monitoring, ed. D. G. Ingram, W. R. Mitchell, and S. W. Martin. Springfield, Ill.: C. C. Thomas.

———. 1980. Abbatoir surveillance in Denmark. Proc. Pig Vet. Soc. 6:43–56.

Willeberg, P., C. E. Franti, A. Gottschau, J. Flensburg, and R. Hoff-Jorgensen. 1983. A preliminary evaluation of the Danish control program for enzootic bovine leukosis. Proc. 3rd Int. Symp. Vet. Epidemiol. Econ., Sept. 1982, Arlington, Va.

Willeberg, P., M. A. Gerbola, B. K. Petersen and J. B. Andersen. 1984. The Danish pig health scheme: Nationwide computer-based abattoir surveillance and follow-up at the herd level. Prev. Vet. Med. 3:79–91.

Williamson, N. B. 1982. Applied veterinary health and management programs for dairy herds in Australia. In Cost Benefits of Food Animal Health, ed. J. B. Kaneene and E. C. Mather. East Lansing: Michigan State Univ. Press.

CHAPTER 12

Field Investigations

12.1 Epidemic Diseases: Outbreak Investigation

Epidemic (as discussed in 4.8) refers to the unexpected increase in disease or death to a level clearly greater than normal. Thus, if ongoing monitoring programs exist, the level of disease or death may be referred to as an epidemic if it exceeds two standard deviations above the mean. In agriculture, however, the level of production often is the outcome of concern, not the presence or absence of disease. Hence, by extrapolation of the earlier definition, a production epidemic might be said to exist when the level of production decreases by two standard deviations below the mean, or when the production drop reaches a critical level that signals a potential problem; this level may differ from area to area and from one production unit (farm) to another. Also, it is entirely possible to have a production-based epidemic in the absence of an epidemic of clinical disease. (Although disease often is a production limiter, disease may be one of the less important factors limiting production on a specific farm.)

Veterinarians are frequently called to investigate outbreaks (i.e., epidemics) of disease or death. In general, the major objectives of such investigations are halting the progress of the disease, determining the reasons for the outbreak, instituting corrective measures, and recommending procedures to reduce the risk of future outbreaks. Although the methods used to accomplish these objectives will vary from situation to situation, there are two general approaches, each dictated by the rate of spread of the problem (i.e., suboptimal productivity, disease, or death). Specifically, disease and production outbreaks can be classified as being of the slowly spreading propagative type or of the rapidly spreading common source type. Thus, the first step in outbreak investigation is to note the temporal pattern of the outbreak (i.e., examine the epidemic curve) and ascertain whether it is likely a point (common source) or a propagated epidemic. Although the difference between these outbreaks is somewhat arbitrary, an extremely rapid increase in the number of cases is suggestive of a common source epidemic (i.e., all animals exposed to the source at about the same time), whereas a slower build up is suggestive of a propagated epidemic. As mentioned, the method of investigation will be influenced by the temporal features of the outbreak.

The features required for successful animal disease control programs have been described in a recent text (Hanson and Hanson 1983) and are beyond the scope of this book. The intent of this section is to present methods for elucidating the source of an epidemic that are broadly applicable in many settings. The specific program(s) required to affect control will depend on the nature and scope of the problem as well as the existing circumstances. Schwabe (1984, pp 411–19) presents two examples of propagative outbreak investigation (brucellosis and plague) and two of point epidemic investigation (botulism in humans and in mink).

12.1.1 Propagated Epidemics

A general outline of the sequence of steps involved in the investigation of a propagated epidemic on a given premise is shown in Figure 12.1. In propagated epidemics, the agent is either spread from animal to animal by contact, or animals are initially exposed to the agent via vehicles or vectors over a protracted period of time, hence explaining its slower development

IS IT A PROPAGATED EPIDEMIC? ⎯⎯→ NO ⎯⎯→ See point epidemic (see Fig. 12.2)

↓   YES

EXAMINE THE FIRST FEW ANIMALS THAT BECAME SICK
  (Does this explain the epidemic? i.e., Are they the source?)

↓   IF THE SOURCE IS NOT FOUND

EXAMINE RECENT ADDITIONS TO THE HERD/FLOCK
  (Does this explain the epidemic? i.e., Are they the source?)

↓   IF THE SOURCE IS NOT FOUND

NOTE RECENT CHANGES IN MANAGEMENT, HOUSING, RATION, ETC.
  (Use the method of agreement or method of difference.)

↓   IF THE SOURCE IS NOT FOUND

A MORE DETAILED STUDY, INCLUDING LABORATORY ANALYSIS OF APPROPRIATE SAMPLES, IS
↓   REQUIRED.

WHEN THE SOURCE IS FOUND, ONE SHOULD INSTITUTE TRACEBACK PROCEDURES TO IDEN-
  TIFY THE ORIGIN OF THE PROBLEM AND PREVENT FURTHER SPREAD OF THE PROB-
  LEM.

12.1. Steps in investigating a propagated epidemic.

relative to a common source epidemic. (It is important to emphasize that one should not assume the agent is infectious, as the frequency of chemical toxicities is likely to increase in the future.) Because of its relatively slow rate of spread, one can usually establish a diagnosis by clinical examination of affected animals and laboratory tests. This knowledge can simplify the investigation process; however, it is not an essential step and one should not devote undue time to establishing the diagnosis, at least initially.

Whether or not a diagnosis is established, one should attempt to identify the first few animals to become sick and note their characteristics (e.g., if they are recent purchases or if they have been in contact with other animals and/or premises). If the disease under investigation is identified and if the first few animals to become ill are the likely source of the agent in the current outbreak, then isolation, treatment, or removal of these animals may be appropriate. Traceback to their origin may be essential if the disease is serious, infectious, and/or if it is a disease for which government veterinarians have legislative responsibility (e.g., notifiable diseases). If no obvious clues are provided following an examination of the first few animals to become diseased, and if the disease appears to have an infectious etiology, it is important to inquire about recent animal acquisitions; many times these animals are carriers and may not develop clinical disease. Again, if the investigation implicates particular animals as the likely source(s) of the problem, isolation, treatment, removal, and/or traceback of these animals may be necessary. If no animals or other logical sources of the problem have been identified, data should be collected and analyzed on possible environmental sources of the agent, in a manner similar to that performed in the investigation of common source epidemics (see 12.1.2). If the problem is localized to one premise, note, for example, details about changes in management, husbandry, purchase of new feed, and ventilation. In this approach, one searches for a factor common to all affected animals (i.e., method of agreement), or a factor that differs between affected and normal animals (i.e., method of difference) on that premise. The latter methods would also be applicable if the problem involved more than one premise, thus, search for factors common to all affected farms and/or for factors whose presence differs between affected and nonaffected farms using a case-control approach.

12.1.2 Point Epidemics

The general sequence to be followed when investigating a point epidemic is presented in Figure 12.2. In this regard, standardized procedures for investigating common source outbreaks have been developed (Committee on Communicable Diseases Affecting Man 1976, 1979).

The private practitioner is usually called to investigate a point epidemic before it reaches its peak. As such, these are emergency situations and the

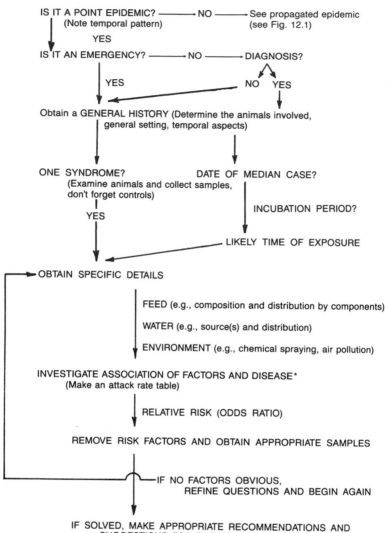

IS IT A POINT EPIDEMIC? ──────→ NO ──────→ See propagated epidemic
(Note temporal pattern)   (see Fig. 12.1)

YES

IS IT AN EMERGENCY? ──────→ NO ──────→ DIAGNOSIS?

YES   NO   YES

Obtain a GENERAL HISTORY (Determine the animals involved,
general setting, temporal aspects)

ONE SYNDROME?   DATE OF MEDIAN CASE?
(Examine animals and collect samples,
don't forget controls)

YES   INCUBATION PERIOD?

                         LIKELY TIME OF EXPOSURE

OBTAIN SPECIFIC DETAILS

FEED (e.g., composition and distribution by components)

WATER (e.g., source(s) and distribution)

ENVIRONMENT (e.g., chemical spraying, air pollution)

INVESTIGATE ASSOCIATION OF FACTORS AND DISEASE*
(Make an attack rate table)

RELATIVE RISK (ODDS RATIO)

REMOVE RISK FACTORS AND OBTAIN APPROPRIATE SAMPLES

IF NO FACTORS OBVIOUS,
REFINE QUESTIONS AND BEGIN AGAIN

IF SOLVED, MAKE APPROPRIATE RECOMMENDATIONS AND
SUGGESTIONS FOR FUTURE PREVENTION

*THINGS TO CONSIDER: UNIT OF CONCERN?
NATURE OF SAMPLE?
STATISTICAL ANALYSIS?

12.2. Steps in investigating a point epidemic.

veterinarian must act quickly to find the source and prevent the exposure of more animals. Less often, the epidemic has run its course prior to the time the veterinarian is called. In both cases, the task is the same, and although the sequence of the investigation will vary from situation to situation, it is very important to recognize a point epidemic early in its course, focusing attention toward finding the common source, be it air, food, or water. Again, it is important to emphasize that one ought not assume an infectious agent as the cause of the disease.

In an emergency situation, little time should be spent attempting to diagnose the disease condition, unless a diagnosis is obvious. Initially, one should obtain a general history, including data on host, husbandry, geographic, and environmental factors. Examine some of the affected animals clinically, and if appropriate at postmortem, to ascertain the main features of the syndrome and whether the outbreak is consistent with one syndrome. Clinical examination or postmortem examination can often pinpoint the nature of the disease and its likely source (Thomson and Barker 1979). In the absence of a diagnosis, and/or if more than one syndrome is involved (the rare case), the investigation procedure may need to differ for each syndrome. In either event, adequate tissue and other samples should be taken and either submitted for immediate laboratory processing or stored for future laboratory work as the situation dictates. This may entail sampling affected animals as well as clinically normal animals in the high risk area, or animals outside the high risk area (the latter "normals" provide necessary benchmark data in case the responsible agent proves difficult to identify).

Besides directly indicating the disease and/or its source, if a diagnosis can be made, it may assist indirectly in identifying the source and nature of the problem, because many agents have a strong association with specific sources (e.g., salmonella with poultry products and powdered milk). In addition, and of greater utility, for many diseases the average incubation period can be used to determine the most likely time(s) of exposure. (In foodborne outbreaks of disease in humans, information on the incubation period is often used to identify the most likely meal at which exposure occurred.) This can be done quite formally in retrospective investigations of outbreaks. To accomplish this, the midpoint of the epidemic (usually the date the 50th percentile — median — case occurred) is identified and then the average incubation period for the disease is subtracted from this to identify the most likely time and/or place of exposure.

At this point in the investigation, the investigator usually has sufficient information to formulate some theories about the reason(s) and source(s) for the outbreak. Based on this information, appropriate questions regarding the environment, food, and water are developed. If feedstuffs were suspected one would collect data on the composition of the ration and look for associations between each ration component and disease (e.g., in a feedlot outbreak, compare the distribution of roughages and concentrates to the distribution of disease). Usually, one or more suspect sources will be identified at this stage of the investigation. It is often a good idea to take some samples at this point. The samples may be submitted to a laboratory if a reasonably good diagnosis has been made; alternatively, they may simply be stored for possible future use. If no associations are found for air, water, or feed, the cycle should be repeated using more refined questions.

Although the investigation often is performed under less than ideal circumstances, it is advisable to record all collected data as neatly, completely, and in as orderly a manner as possible. Tabulation of data in the form of an attack rate table is useful (see Tables 12.1 and 12.2).

12.1.3 Attack Rate Table

In constructing an attack rate table, one must first decide whether the individual animal or a group (e.g., a litter or pen) is the correct unit of analysis. As a guideline, if the animals are housed, fed, or watered as a group the correct unit is the group. Initially, when the group is the unit of analysis, it will suffice to classify each group of animals as affected or not. The actual level (i.e., morbidity or mortality rate) of disease within a group may be required only for detailed studies or for final interpretations.

Second, it is important to consider whether data are available from a

Table 12.1.   Food-specific attack rate table, food poisoning outbreak at a sugar bush, Quebec, April 1984

Food	Ate foods listed			Did not eat foods listed			Difference between attack rates
	Ill	Total	Attack rate (%)	Ill	Total	Attack rate (%)	
Pea soup	59	255	23.13	2	24	8.33	14.80
Pork and beans	57	235	24.25	4	44	9.09	15.16
Ham	59	265	22.26	2	14	14.28	7.98
Salt pork	46	210	21.90	15	69	21.73	0.17
Omelette	56	223	25.11	5	56	8.92	16.19
Potatoes	44	199	22.11	17	80	21.25	0.86
Pancakes	47	186	25.26	15	93	16.12	9.14
Eggs in syrup	44	92	47.82	15	187	8.02	39.80
Milk	32	157	20.38	29	122	23.77	−3.39
Tea	11	41	26.82	49	238	20.58	6.24
Coffee	27	126	21.42	30	153	19.60	1.82
Water (surface well)	18	105	17.14	42	174	24.13	−6.99
Bread	49	220	22.27	13	59	22.03	0.24
Butter	43	208	20.67	18	71	25.35	−4.68
Pickles	31	122	25.40	28	157	17.83	.7.57
Maple syrup	49	207	23.67	12	72	16.66	7.01
Maple taffy	14	77	18.18	49	202	24.25	−6.07

Source: Marcoux et al. 1984, with permission.

Table 12.2.   Exposures of cases and controls and odds ratios for selected risk fac-
               tors, *Campylobacter jejuni* case-control study, Colorado, 1981

Risk factors	Cases exposed	Controls exposed	Crude odds ratio	Matched odds ratio
Raw milk	8/40	5/71	3.30	6.93
Raw water	7/40	4/71	3.55	10.74
Cats in household	18/40	15/71	3.05	3.21
Undercooked chicken	7/26	4/57	1.88	6.27

Source: Hopkins et al. 1984.

representative cross-section of the population at risk, or whether the data are obtained in a case-control fashion (i.e., data are obtained from some or all of the cases and from some of the unaffected population). In the former case, the risk (rate) of disease can be directly determined for each suspect factor (Table 12.1). In the latter case, direct estimates of attack rates are not possible and one must compare the proportion of cases that were exposed to a factor to the proportion of exposed noncases using the odds ratio (Table 12.2).

A third consideration is whether to use formal statistical tests to evaluate the probability of "chance variations" explaining the observed differences. In general, formal testing is required only in the final stages of the investigation and/or in nonemergency outbreak investigations.

Once the data are summarized and tabulated, the following guidelines are useful to determine if an item (e.g., a ration component) is the source of the agent. If exposure to a specific source (factor) is the cause of the outbreak: (1) there should be little or no disease in unexposed units (i.e., individuals or groups); (2) most of the affected units should be exposed to that item; and (3) as a result of 1 and 2, the relative risk (or odds ratio) and/or the attributable rate should be large for exposure to that item.

A general guideline is to ignore those items to which all the population at risk is exposed, unless it is possible to refine questions about these items and hence investigate the relationship between subitems and the disease. For example, all cattle in a feedlot might receive silage, yet rather than ignoring this item, one might inquire about different lots of silage before proceeding. On the other hand, if there is only one source of water for all animals and the distribution of the outbreak is not uniform throughout the population, water could be considered an unlikely source of the problem.

The data in Table 12.1 relate to an outbreak of food poisoning in people who had eaten at a maple sugar bush party in Quebec, Canada. The food items served at the bush party are listed and the number of people eating and not eating each food item noted, together with the number in each of these groups that became ill. After calculating the attack rates, the attributable rate is calculated for each food item; the food item with the largest attributable rate being the most likely source of the problem. (The relative risk or odds ratio could also have been used for this purpose.) In this instance, the eggs in syrup were the most likely source; culturing of these yielded a coagulase-positive staphylococcus. Later, this organism was demonstrated to be of the same phage type as was found in the stool and vomitus of the ill people.

The data in Table 12.2 relate to selected risk factors for cases of *Campylobacter jejuni* infection (only those factors producing an elevated odds ratio are shown). Since the total exposed population was unknown, the sampling of affected and nonaffected people was done in a case-control fashion. Cases were obtained from hospital and laboratory records. Two controls were chosen for each case and were matched for age and sex. One control was the nearest neighbor of the case, the other was a best friend of the case. Because of this selection procedure, disease rates by item cannot be calculated; hence odds ratios are used to measure the strength of association. Note that the odds ratios (Table 12.2) were larger when the analysis considered the matching; this would indicate that age and/or sex were related to both the risk factors and *C. jejuni* infection. The risk factors themselves were interrelated and the Mantel-Haenszel procedure was used to control for these (data not shown). Two of the risk factors for infection, raw water and raw milk, are also associated with large-scale outbreaks of *C. jejuni* intestinal disease in man.

At this stage of the investigation, sufficient information should be available to identify and remove (control) the most likely sources. Samples of the suspect items should be collected, if they haven't been, for future microbiologic or chemical analyses. In special circumstances, a feeding or exposure trial can be used to quickly evaluate suspect sources (e.g., using laboratory animals, or using "poor-doers" in a chronic-case pen in a feedlot or swine facility).

A final and important step is to recommend procedures to prevent recurrence of the problem. These might involve suggestions about using a different water source, different ration preparation and handling procedures, or ensuring appropriate ventilation when agitating slurry. A detailed written report outlining the investigation, its findings, and recommendations should be given to the client at the termination of the investigation.

If multiple premises are involved in an outbreak, the approach is similar to that outlined. If the temporal pattern of the outbreak suggests a point epidemic, and only one syndrome appears to be present (in the absence of a confirmed diagnosis), a formal search for the common source should commence. The unit of analysis is the premise (e.g., herd or flock). If the outbreak appears to resemble a propagated epidemic, the investigation may be more complex. Nonetheless, examining the first premise to report problems for recent additions (of animals, feedstuffs, equipment changes, fertilizers, insecticides, etc.) should be an early task as one is looking for a single factor common to all farms. In addition, a formal comparison of the characteristics of, and recent happenings on, affected farms to the characteristics of nearby nonaffected farms using the attack rate table approach should prove useful in identifying the source of the problem. Again, although a confirmed diagnosis is helpful in directing the investigation, one should not delay the collection of appropriate data by waiting for a diagnosis to be made. Such a delay may prove costly because the source (e.g., contaminated feed) may continue to spread and/or the source (e.g., contaminated feed or disinfectant) may be used before appropriate samples are collected. In the latter instance, it may never be possible to complete the investigation, leaving the client and the investigator with only circumstantial evidence.

12.2 Endemic Diseases

12.2.1 Epidemiology and Health Management

Health management, as the name implies, is the action of managing the health (including prevention and treatment of disease) of animal populations. In farm animals, the process represents an extension to what are currently called herd health programs (Botterell 1976). Some have coined the term planned animal health and production services (PAHAPS) for these activities (Blood 1979). Health management programs require knowledge from a number of areas, including traditional medicine (etiology, pathogenesis, diagnosis, and treatment of disease), animal behavior, nutrition, animal management, and housing, as well as epidemiology and economics. (One might also add selected skills from sociology and psychology, since an understanding of the owner/manager may prove vital to the introduction and continued success of health management programs.) In general, health management programs are targeted at animal populations; however, the actual delivery will likely involve different levels of organization from the individual (animal/animal owner) to larger groups (herds, kennels) as the units of concern.

The specific roles of epidemiology and economics in health management programs are still evolving (Martin 1982), but they tend to function as integrative disciplines in that they provide the concepts and tools to understand and investigate relationships among the factors contributing to the productivity of the animal population(s) of concern. Although the principles of health management apply to veterinary public health, private food animal and companion animal medicine, and regulatory (public) veterinary medicine, nowhere is the need for epidemiologic input greater than in the field of health management of farm animals, particularly those animals reared under intensive management conditions. Schwabe et al. (1977, p 276) indicate quite correctly that the current intensification of animal agriculture in North America has been made possible largely because of the efforts of publicly employed veterinarians who were able to control diseases such as Texas fever, *Trichinella spiralis*, contagious bovine pleuropneumonia, and more recently hog cholera. Today, the national veterinary service in most countries with intensive agricultural industries has the responsibility for the ongoing exclusion of many potentially devastating diseases such as foot-and-mouth disease and African swine fever, as well as pursuing the control and/or eradication of endemic diseases such as brucellosis and tuberculosis. All these activities are essential to provide an umbrella of protection over the intensive domestic animal industries.

Epidemiologic methods were essential to these early activities in domestic control and still play a central role in the programs of organized veterinary medicine. The major intent of this and the subsequent section is to demonstrate and reinforce the potential value of an epidemiologic approach to health management at the farm/veterinary practice level by private practitioners.

This section could begin with an exhaustive list of diseases for which the natural history remains unclear. This list would certainly include diseases such as bovine virus diarrhea, infectious bovine rhinotracheitis, avian mycoplasma infections, bluetongue, and Aujeszky's disease. However, such a listing might in itself suggest that an agent by agent or disease by disease approach to disease control is the best way of proceeding. Certainly past successes have shown that such an approach works; yet, the major problems confronting domestic animal industries today are multietiologic in nature. Hence, a manifestational rather than an etiologic classification of problems seems more appropriate. (Multietiologic implies that many agents and/or many factors in addition to specific agents are involved in causing that disease.) These multietiological manifestational syndromes include respiratory disease in the swine, beef, and poultry industries, neonatal mortality and reproductive inefficiencies in all species, and metabolic diseases and mastitis in dairy cows. By their very nature, these diseases are difficult to study under controlled laboratory conditions; hence, the real world (i.e., the feedlot, swine barn, or poultry house) will become an important "laboratory" for their investigation. It is here that the applied techniques of epidemiology, including analytic studies, field experiments, and simulation modeling, will prove extremely useful.

It would be false to suggest that well-designed field studies have appeared only recently, or that without formal epidemiologic training, good field studies and field investigations are not possible. Certainly, qualitative epidemiologic skills have been used for many years, often in conjunction with microbiologic and clinical skills. What is true, however, is that quantitative epidemiologic techniques have only recently been applied to investigations of problems in farm animal industries. For example, the first formal case-control study in farm animals was an investigation of the etiology of left displacement of the abomasum in dairy cows reported in 1968 (Robertson 1968).

In domestic animals, in addition to untangling the various diseases involved in these multietiologic syndromes, the major questions to be resolved are the impact of these syndromes on productivity, and identifying the factors causing the syndromes. As well as the obvious value to the animal owner, answers to these questions should provide a rational basis for establishing research priorities. To ensure that production is emphasized as the end point, it might be instructive to identify specific deficit areas of production and then identify the causes of these deficits. It is quite likely that management errors and subclinical problems as well as clinical disease per se will be identified in this manner. Identifying the causes of these production deficits will frequently lead to studying the interrelationships among diseases, identifying important host characteristics, and elucidating the more important environmental determinants of the problem. Just as infectious agents affect each other directly and indirectly, and the effects of multiple infections on the host may be additive or interactive, diseases also tend to be associated with each other and their combined effects on each other and on production may be additive or interactive.

New and more exacting epidemiologic techniques applicable to health management will be developed as studies at the individual animal level progress to studies at the herd level. For example, in 1975, epidemiologic studies at the Ontario Veterinary College (OVC) were initiated into the interrelationships among diseases and their effects on productivity in 18 dairy herds. The data base was assembled in a manual fashion by copying the information from individual cow cards, OVC hospital records, and Record of Performance production testing program records. Much data were discarded because of apparent errors, and the definitions of many of the disease syndromes had to be quite general. A number of clinicians had input data into the medical records or on the cow cards. Consequently the diagnoses, although probably of high quality, were based on nonstandardized terminology. Despite these difficulties much useful information was obtained from these initial studies (Erb and Martin 1980; Erb et al. 1981).

Subsequently, a prospective study was initiated that included more herds ($n = 32$) in a wider geographic area serviced by three different veterinary practices. In this study, dairy farmers were asked to maintain records specifically for the senior investigator. In most instances this only required increased vigilance on the part of the farmer because most already had a recordkeeping system; the new feature was that someone was going to formally analyze the data. Through regular farm visits by the senior investigator and with the help of the enthusiastic dairy farmers and their veterinarians, a large high quality data base was established. Again, however, many diagnostic categories had to remain general to take account of the variation in terminology and procedures among veterinary practices. Much useful research data were obtained in this study, and new epidemiologic techniques for case-control studies were developed to assist in its analysis. In addition, practical advice about the advisability of selected management practices (e.g., the effect of delaying the first breeding to approximately 90 days postpartum) based on formally analyzed field data was generated (Dohoo 1983). Also in this study, initial attempts at explaining herd-to-herd variation in production and disease rates were completed (Dohoo et al. 1984).

The most recent epidemiologic studies at the individual cow level were based on data resulting from a field trial designed to study the efficacy of two biologics on reproductive performance. The study took place in one large (300 cows) dairy herd, and the majority of observations were made and recorded by one veterinarian. Together with much attention to detail, this provided a high quality data base that in addition to meeting the field-trial objectives has been used to study interrelationships among diseases and their effects on productivity in dairy cows. Not only are the diagnostic criteria well defined, some of the diagnoses are supplemented by the results of laboratory tests (e.g., plasma progesterone levels) (Etherington et al. 1984a).

As the use of computers in the livestock industries increases, large, accurate data bases will become available on which to base research activities and from which invaluable data for extension activities can be drawn. As dairy farmers gain positive results by keeping and analyzing (in conjunction with the veterinarian and extension personnel) data on their animals, there will be a natural tendency to increase the quality and the quantity of the data recorded. Thus, future large-scale research projects may be based on data derived from recording systems primarily instigated to assist the farmer and the veterinarian to make better management decisions (see 10.4). With some concerted efforts toward standardization of diagnostic terminology, such a data base, when supplemented by well planned metabolic and microbiologic profiles, should allow a comprehensive picture of relationships among management factors, agents, disease, and production at the individual cow level. It should also prove useful for studies of the association between genotype and disease occurrence.

The health management area requiring increased study over the next few decades is at the herd level (i.e., the identification of factors that influence herd-to-herd variation in productivity and disease occurrence). Just as it is difficult to understand how individuals function by examining cells and organs, it is difficult to understand how herds or other aggregates of individuals function by studying only individuals. Until recently, however, the technology to study sufficiently large numbers of herds has not been available; the widespread use of computers and the increased availability of appropriate software has largely circumvented this limitation. For example, a further major epidemiologic project involving the dairy industry and workers at the OVC focused on a random sample of southwestern Ontario dairy herds. The 104 farms took part in a 3-year study designed to investigate associations among disease, drug usage, and productivity. Two-thirds of the farms provided farm-level data only (e.g., the number of cows with retained fetal membranes and/or metritis each month), whereas one-third provided both individual cow level and herd data (i.e., which cows had metritis) (Meek et al. 1986).

One recent example of a health study where an aggregate of individuals was the unit of concern is the Bruce County Beef Health Project conducted in Ontario, Canada (Martin et al. 1982a). This project commenced in 1978 and continued for 3 years. In each of the years, between 60 and 70 feedlot operators collaborated in the project by providing daily treatment and death loss records, weekly ration content descriptions, and a record of all processing (vaccinations, deworming, castration, etc.) for each identifiable group of calves. Each year there were approximately 110 groups of cattle, containing an average of 140 beef calves each. The demographic characteristics of each group of calves, their source, and method of transportation to the feedlot, as well as their housing and management were recorded by the investigators shortly after arrival. Approximately 80% of all animals that died were examined by pathologists, microbiologists, and parasitologists at the OVC.

The majority of the calves in this study were highly stressed; they were raised on open pastures in western Canada, weaned, trucked to salesyards, and shortly thereafter transported by truck or train for a period of 3–7 days (2000–3000 km) to Ontario. Some went directly to feedlots, others were sorted into homogenous groups and resold at salesyards in Ontario. Most of the calves had never eaten from a feed bunk or drunk water from a bowl or trough prior to this. Not surprisingly, because of these stresses and the often inclement weather during this time of the year, the calves were susceptible to many disease conditions; particularly respiratory disease, the main clinical condition being a respiratory syndrome associated with fibrinous pneumonia. However, because it is difficult to clinically distinguish among the respiratory diseases, the general syndrome is usually referred to as the shipping fever complex.

The findings of the pathologists reinforced the overall importance of respiratory disease with the proportional mortality rate for respiratory disease varying from 54% to 64%. Yet, the proportional mortality rate for fibrinous pneumonia decreased dramatically in the last year of the study from 43% to 29% in the face of a stable overall mortality rate. It was postulated that this decline was due to producers avoiding certain management practices that had been associated with fibrinous pneumonia in the previous years. Since it was not possible to derive accurate cause-specific morbidity data, in one series of analyses the groups of calves were categorized in a case-control manner into those having one or more deaths from a specific cause versus no deaths from that cause. Differences between these groups in terms of demographic characteristics, housing, feeding, and processing factors were studied. In general, the important factors were those associated with crude mortality rates (Martin et al. 1982b); this may have been due to the overwhelming importance of a few diseases, such as fibrinous pneumonia, bronchial pneumonia, interstitial pneumonia, infectious bovine rhinotracheitis, and infectious thromboembolic meningoencephalitis.

The major method of analysis used to sort through the large number of potential risk factors was multiple regression. This technique allows the investigator to examine the effects of one factor while other factors in the regression equation are held constant mathematically. In this regard, least squares multiple regression is analogous to the Mantel-Haenszel technique and is appropriate when the outcome (dependent variable) is a quantitative variable. Logistic regression, a powerful extension of the Mantel-Haenszel technique, also was used in one set of analyses (Martin et al. 1982b). (The basic limitation to the Mantel-Haenszel technique is that one must explicitly create a 2 × 2 table at each level of the confounding variable, or combination of confounding variables. With five binary variables, at least 32 tables are required, and if the data set contains only a few hundred sampling units—groups of calves in the case of the Bruce County Study—many of the cell entries will be zero. Logistic regression, in a manner similar to multiple least squares regression, allows one to obviate this problem.)

Detailed discussions of the results of the above project are available and are not germane to the objectives here. The major point to stress is that formal analyses at the group and/or farm level are extremely useful in providing information for rational decision making. However, no one study should be viewed in isolation. Results from all studies, be they observational, experimental, or theoretical, must be integrated with local experience and interpreted in combination. (Throughout this text, constraints have been mentioned in terms of one's ability to learn by experience. While it is true for manual skills that practice makes perfect, the same is not necessarily true when making management decisions. Although experience ought not be ignored, one needs to recognize its tendency to lead to authoritarian rather than authoritative discussions.)

During the past decade, a number of well-designed farm-level studies of dairy farms have been initiated or reported. If these studies have a drawback, it is that the number of herds involved was too few to allow formal analyses of factors that might have impacted on productivity or disease occurrence. Nonetheless, there is an excellent series of reports on the Australian experience with planned animal health programs (Blood et al. 1978; Cannon et al. 1978; Morris et al. 1978a, b; and Williamson et al. 1978). Recently, two reports on herd-level studies in Minnesota dairy herds have also been published (Hird and Robinson, 1982, 1983).

Investigations into calf survival have also been conducted at the herd level, although not many studies have formally analyzed differences in morbidity and mortality among herds for their relationship to management practices. Nonetheless, insight into how to conduct field studies of calf survival and the problems associated with them can be found in recent articles. A study of calf survival in Norway utilized data from a large number of herds; however, the emphasis appeared to be on individual calf survival and factors relating to this (the outcome was lived or died for each calf in the study). Herd-level and individual animal factors were used as predictor variables but did not appear to be important (Simensen 1983). The results of a recent study in Ohio suggest that management factors are more predictive of disease problems in calves than is the presence or absence of putative pathogens (Hancock 1983). Again, this was difficult to formally assess because of the small number of herds in the study.

Currently, a study of calf survival and factors influencing it is being conducted on 104 dairy farms in Ontario as part of a larger overall dairy farm study referred to previously (Meek et al. 1986). At the beginning of the study, each farm was visited and a calf management policy questionnaire was administered by personal interview. At that time, the physical calf rearing facilities were also evaluated. At the end of the first year, each farmer was mailed a "re-check" questionnaire containing a subset of questions from the original survey. At the end of the second year, all farms were visited and, where possible, fecal samples from the youngest one or two calves under 2 weeks of age were obtained for microbiologic screening. These samples were used to assess the relationships between pathogen status and disease. All farmers kept daily log sheets of all calf births, preventive and disease treatments, and deaths among preweaned calves, and these sheets were picked up during regular visits by the project field technicians. At the end of the survey, as part of a more general management questionnaire, the dairy farmers were asked to note any recently implemented calf management policy changes. It is anticipated that the results of this study will provide solid, scientifically valid evidence on the effect of a number of factors that are thought to impact on calf morbidity and mortality (Waltner-Toews 1985). A herd-level field trial of rota-corona virus vaccine and *E. coli* bacteria was conducted as part of this study (Waltner-Toews et al. 1985).

Although this section has emphasized bovine health management, the philosophy of health management at the herd level is perhaps more advanced in the swine industry, and examples of this will be presented in subsequent sections. Also, despite the overwhelming emphasis on and importance of the individual in companion animal medicine, there is a great need for the formal application of epidemiologic methods in this area. Studies dealing with such items as population disease control, population control, animal behavior, and the human-animal bond (Loew 1976; Schwabe 1984) are desperately needed.

12.2.2 Problem Resolution in Intensively Managed Units

Although disease outbreaks still occur, many of the diseases that have high case fatality rates, or pose a significant direct public health threat, or interfere with international trade have been brought under control in many countries. If these diseases still exist, they often do so at hypoendemic or sporadic levels. Since 1960, it has become apparent that endemic, often subclinical, diseases have a large impact on the productivity of intensively reared animals. As mentioned, control of many of the epidemic diseases allowed a fundamental change in the structure of agriculture toward larger monospecies farms. Thus, in the past few decades, veterinarians have begun to turn their attention toward the farm or flock as the unit of concern rather than the individual animal. This trend is particularly advanced in the poultry industry, commercial swine operations, and the beef feedlot industry. Even in the dairy industry, where individual purebred animals still have great economic value, the trend is away from the individual toward the herd. As part of this change in emphasis, veterinarians must acquire new skills to identify and deal with problems at the herd level; an extrapolation of skills appropriate to individual animals is not a satisfactory solution. Basic epidemiologic training can provide many of these skills, but veterinarians will have to modify and extend many of the current problem-solving techniques of epidemiology to make them more suitable for use in intensive animal industries. Today, there is only sparse information on the concepts and techniques of problem solving at the herd level in veterinary medicine. The following discussion should prove useful as an initial methodology in this regard, and it is hoped, will provide the stimulus for the required new developments in this area.

The discussion assumes that an adequate on-farm data recording and analysis system exists, because in the absence of such a system problem solving at the herd level becomes a difficult, often hit-and-miss operation. The record system need not be computerized, but it is likely most farms will utilize a computerized system in the future.

The development of both computer software and hardware products appropriate to veterinarians and their clients is an active and evolving area. It is not the intent to describe or evaluate these systems here, but rather to provide a sound basis for their introduction, adaptation, and usage (Meek et al. 1975). The evolution of one major system (DAISY) designed for the dairy industry is a useful study for those contemplating work in this area (Stephens et al. 1982). Programs for the swine industry are also appearing rapidly, particularly after descriptions of the design (Pepper et al. 1977) and use of (Pepper and Taylor 1977) a breeding records system in England were published. A recent comprehensive overview of swine recording systems in the United Kingdom (Davies 1983) and a formal evaluation of a number of dairy recording systems (Etherington et al. 1984b) are also available. A schematic outline of the steps involved in designing and using a health-oriented data base is shown in Figure 12.3. These include formulating a set of written production-based objectives, deciding on critical levels for a number of parameters that signal the need for investigation, preparing action lists to remind the client and the veterinarian of routine duties as well as identifying problem areas and/or problem animals, and monitoring the production response. If current objectives are not being met, the herd management and/or health maintenance program will require modification. If the current objectives are being met, steps may be required to safeguard the herd; in other cases production targets may be raised.

Two important features of a health management strategy are: First, it is unlikely that by helping to achieve production goals the veterinarian will

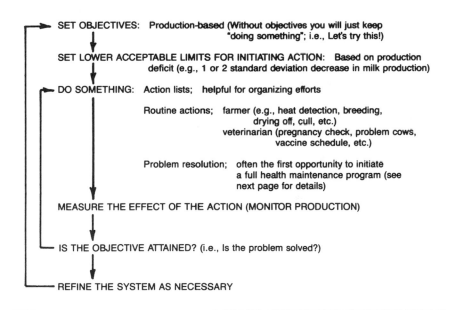

12.3. Schematic outline of a health management stragegy for individual production unit.

have no work. Rather, most clients will ask the veterinarian to remain as an integral component of the management of the production unit. Second, it is of paramount importance that the veterinarian and client learn from their activities, be they successes or failures. Otherwise there is a tendency to redouble efforts yet go nowhere, as if on a treadmill (Esslemont et al. 1981). If problems exist, be they production deficits or increased disease occurrence, an outline of procedures to resolve them is presented in Figures 12.4 and 12.5. In this outline it is assumed that a dairy herd is the unit of concern; however, similar charts could be drawn by analogy for poultry, swine (e.g., see Davies 1983, p 55), and beef units.

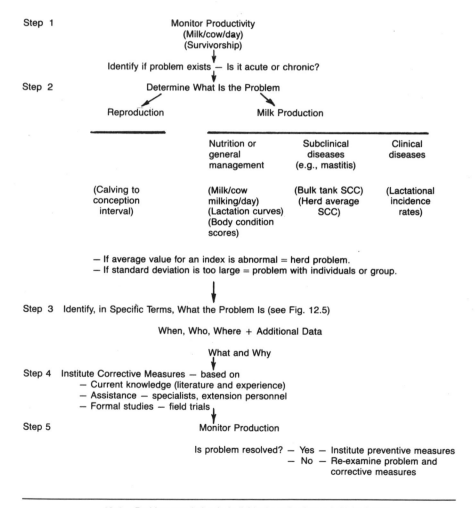

12.4. Problem resolution in individual production unit (dairy herd).

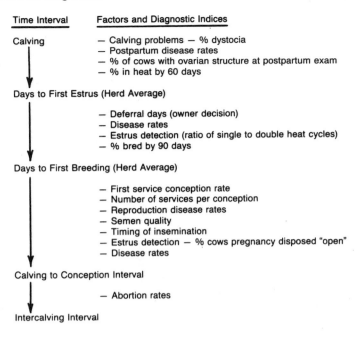

Time Interval	Factors and Diagnostic Indices
Calving	— Calving problems — % dystocia — Postpartum disease rates — % of cows with ovarian structure at postpartum exam — % in heat by 60 days
↓	
Days to First Estrus (Herd Average)	— Deferral days (owner decision) — Disease rates — Estrus detection (ratio of single to double heat cycles) — % bred by 90 days
↓	
Days to First Breeding (Herd Average)	— First service conception rate — Number of services per conception — Reproduction disease rates — Semen quality — Timing of insemination — Estrus detection — % cows pregnancy disposed "open" — Disease rates
↓	
Calving to Conception Interval	— Abortion rates
↓	
Intercalving Interval	

12.5. Use of diagnostic indices (reproduction problem in dairy herd).

The first step in problem resolution is to identify that a problem exists and to define in general terms what the problem is. In this regard, a few production parameters that are both biologically and economically meaningful should be monitored on a regular basis. For a dairy herd, monitoring suitable herd production parameters (such as milk production per unit time and survivorship in adult animals) will indicate when a problem exists. (For calves, growth rates and survivorship would be appropriate parameters to measure.) Milk production per cow per day is probably the most useful overall measure of productivity, biologically and economically, because it incorporates measures of milk production and reproductive performance (Morris 1971). If this is low, one would then proceed to identify whether the major problem lies in reproductive performance, milk production, or both. The temporal pattern of milk/cow/day can easily be monitored by dividing the volume of milk shipped each day by the number of cows in the herd and plotting the result against time. The resultant graph can quickly identify sudden changes in productivity (e.g., reduced milk production), and it can also be used to monitor long-term trends (such as a gradual reduction in productivity due to declining reproductive performance).

Once it is known that a problem exists, the second step is to examine additional parameters to determine what the problem is. For example, the herd average calving-to-conception interval or the percent of the herd pregnant by 120 days are useful parameters for assessing the overall efficiency of a dairy herd's reproductive program. While, the average calving-to-conception interval is perhaps the easier parameter to interpret, determination of which cows to include in the calculation can be difficult. Cows that never conceive will not be included in the calculation, and consequently the parameter may overstate the true efficiency of the breeding program. On the other hand, percent of the herd pregnant by 120 days (or any other agreed upon cut-off point) circumvents this problem and identifies a production deficit quickly. However, it suffers from the drawback that a cow open 200 days has no greater impact on the parameter than a cow open 121 days. Additional parameters worth monitoring in a dairy herd include: milk/cow/day (a measure of nutritional status and other general management factors); bulk tank somatic cell count or the herd geometric mean somatic cell count (indicators of subclinical mastitis); and the lactational incidence rates of the more common clinically evident diseases.

Although changes in any of the parameters described above will eventually result in a change in the overall measure of productivity (i.e., milk/cow/day), there will inevitably be a delay before the change is apparent. Since most of the parameters are readily available, many producers will choose to monitor the more specific parameters on a regular basis. For example, an increase in subclinical mastitis will inevitably result in a reduction in milk/cow/day. However, since many other changes may be taking place in a herd at the same time (e.g., cows drying off and freshening, ration changes, etc.), the reduction in milk/cow/day may not be evident for some time. The bulk tank somatic cell count is a more sensitive indicator of the level of subclinical mastitis and will reflect the change more quickly. Consequently, there is merit in monitoring these more specific parameters to prevent a drop in productivity.

The third step in problem resolution is to determine in very specific terms what the problem is and why it has occurred. An analogous situation in individual animal medicine would be progressing from an observation that a dog has a persistent ocular discharge to a diagnosis of keratoconjunctivitis sica due to inadequate tear production. However, instead of using clinical examinations and diagnostic tests to refine the diagnosis, the veterinarian analyzes herd records and the results of screening tests.

To further define the problem on a herd basis, it is necessary to identify when and where the problem occurs and which animals are affected. In answering these questions, parameters called diagnostic indices (Williamson 1981) are used to assess specific aspects of the production system. As an example, the first service conception rate in a dairy herd is a good indicator of fertility in cows presented for breeding. The herd's average values of these diagnostic indices should be compared to preset targets or goals. In addition, for production units with sufficient animals, it is useful to note the standard deviation of the indices. An abnormal average with an acceptable standard deviation indicates a general herd problem, as, for example, one that would result from inadequate nutrition or a herd-wide management problem. A large standard deviation indicates that individual animals or a subset of the herd constitutes a major part of the problem, and one should identify these abnormal animals and try to determine reasons for their poor performance. A small standard deviation is as important to economic return and ease of management as meeting a stated production average (Blood et al. 1978; Morris 1971).

For herd medicine problems, one of the most important determinations to be made is, When in the production cycle does the problem occur? For a reproductive problem, this question becomes, At what point between calving and eventual conception are events not occurring as expected? To answer this question, the calving-to-conception interval is subdivided and various parameters that assess specific portions of the reproductive program are calculated (Fig. 12.5). For example, if a herd has a prolonged calving-to-conception interval (160 days) but an acceptable average number of days to first breeding (70 days), parameters such as number of services per conception, percentage of cows presented for pregnancy diagnosis that are found to be "open" (a measure of estrus detection in the herd) (Williamson 1981), and incidence rates of cystic ovaries and other reproductive diseases should be examined.

While examining the question, When does the problem occur?, it is also appropriate to examine the temporal distribution of the problem. This may involve determining long-term trends, seasonal variations, and even short-term variations. For example, if a herd has an excessive number of services per conception, it would be appropriate to examine conception rates by day of the week. It is possible that the individuals responsible for inseminations on the weekend are not as skilled as their weekday counterparts. Conception rates may also vary seasonally in response to changes in nutrition and housing.

Determining which animals are involved in a problem requires a criterion by which animals can be classed as "normal" (e.g., 80 days for calving to first breeding or 200,000 cells/ml for a somatic cell count) or "abnormal". Then the percentage of abnormal animals in various groups within the herd can be calculated. It may be informative to compare animals of different age groups, different breeds, high producers versus low producers, etc. For example, determining the prevalence of elevated cell counts in cows in various age groups can be helpful in arriving at a "herd diagnosis" (see Example 1, below).

The question of where the problem is occurring can be answered in a similar manner. The relative frequency with which the problem appears in animals in different pens or barns, or different locations within a barn or a milking string should be determined. This information can then be studied and possible explanations for the pattern such as ventilation problems or inadequate water sources can be sought.

Answering the questions when, who, and where may not completely define the problem at hand and additional data may be required. Once collected, these additional data can be combined with the information about when, who, and where for a detailed specific definition of what the problem is. As an example, a veterinarian may start a problem-solving exercise with the observation that the calving-to-conception interval for a herd is too long and has a large standard deviation. Through the analyses of appropriate records it may be possible to identify that the specific problem relates to very low conception rates in cows bred on Friday, Saturday, and Sunday. The veterinarian and producer would then have to collect additional data or conduct a small trial to determine if the problem relates to cows being bred at the wrong time in their cycle on the weekends (i.e., a problem in estrus detection) or to inappropriate technique on the part of the inseminator.

Once a clear statement has been made as to what the problem is, the number of possible explanations as to why it is occurring will be greatly reduced. In the example above, if it turns out that cows not in heat are being bred on the weekend, the possible explanations might include inability of the person involved to correctly identify the signs of heat, or incorrect recording of cow names and numbers.

This approach to problem solving is not restricted to situations where dramatically serious deficits exist. As the following two examples show, it can be used to help rectify relatively minor or moderate problems to improve the productivity of the herd.

12.2.2.1 PROBLEM RESOLUTION: EXAMPLE 1.   A 90-cow Holstein-Friesian herd in Ontario, Canada had a rolling herd average of 147 BCA units and a daily milk production of 20.7 liters/cow/day. Both production parameters indicated a reasonable level of milk production, but the bulk tank somatic cell count (SSC) had averaged 509,000 cells/ml over the last 6 months. The producer was not particularly concerned, but the veterinarian pointed out that with milk valued at $40/hL, there was a loss in excess of $8000/yr in milk compared to production at a cell count average of 150,000 cells/ml (Dohoo et al. 1984).

To further investigate the problem, the veterinarian classified all the cows as having "elevated SCC" if their most recent individual cow somatic cell count was over 200,000 cells/ml and "normal" if it was less. While investigating when the problem occurred, it was found that the distribution of counts according to the cows' stage of lactation was as follows:

SCC	Stage of Lactation		
	Early	Middle	Late
Elevated	11%	35%	79%
Normal	89%	65%	21%

In general, counts were low early in lactation, suggesting the dry cow therapy program on this farm was adequate and also that the majority of new infections were not occurring around the time of parturition. The dramatic rise in the prevalence of elevated counts throughout the lactation is suggestive of cow-to-cow transmission of a pathogenic agent.

To determine which cows were infected, the cows were classified according to age and cell count status with the following results:

SCC	Age (yr)		
	2	3–5	6 and up
Elevated	25%	55%	75%
Normal	75%	45%	25%

It was quite evident that the prevalence of elevated counts increased with the age of the cows, but since one expects very few elevated counts in first calf heifers, the 25% prevalence observed in this herd was additional cause for concern.

At this point it was concluded that the herd had a high prevalence of infection, with cow-to-cow spread during the lactation being the most likely mechanism of transmission. It was also concluded that most infections were eliminated by the dry cow therapy and that management at the time of calving was adequate since relatively few new infections occurred then.

To further characterize the problem, data about the incidence of clinical mastitis were collected, and composite milk samples from the 75 milking cows were collected for culturing. The incidence of clinical mastitis was 2.7% per month (i.e., 2.7 cases/100 cows/mo), which was deemed acceptable. Of the 31 samples that were culture positive, 26 (84%) yielded *Streptococcus agalactiae*.

The "herd diagnosis" of this problem could now be stated as a high rate of cow-to-cow transmission of *S. agalactiae* during lactation, resulting in a high prevalence of subclinical mastitis with an attendant economic loss in excess of $8000/yr. Resolution of the problem depended on identifying those faults in the milking system and the operator's technique that related either to cow-to-cow transmission of the organism or to increasing the susceptibility of the cows to new infections.

12.2.2.2 PROBLEM RESOLUTION: EXAMPLE 2.   A 200-cow Holstein-Friesian herd in Ontario, Canada had a calving-to-conception interval of 121 days. The dairy farmer, in conjunction with the veterinarian, had set 90 days as the herd objective and, based on an estimated loss of $2.50/cow/extra day open (Dohoo 1982), it was estimated that suboptimal reproductive performance was resulting in a loss of approximately $15,000/yr.

To identify when in the sequence of reproductive events the problem was occurring, the veterinarian examined several diagnostic indices:

Index	Mean	Std. Dev.	Target	Days Lost
Calving to conception (days)	121	52	90	31
First breeding to conception (days)	27	11	30	0
Calving to first breeding (days)	91	37	60	31
Calving to first heat (days)	66	42	45	21
Percent in heat by day 45 postpartum	40%	...	100%	...
Percent bred by day 60 postpartum	19%	...	50%	...

From these data it was apparent that of the 31 days being lost, all of the loss was occurring prior to the first breeding. A proportion of this loss appeared to occur because of the delay between first heat and first breeding, but the greatest loss was due to failure to detect heat early in all cows. The standard deviations for both the calving to first heat and calving to first breeding intervals were too large (in excess of 30% of mean), indicating considerable variability among cows within the herd.

In further investigating the loss of time between first heat and first breeding, it was recognized that since the producer had decided that cows would not be bred prior to 50 days postpartum, not all cows could be bred on their first detected heat. However, of the 210 cows calving, 26 (12.4%) had heats detected on or after day 50, at which time they were not bred. An average of 47 days, about two estrus cycles (called "deferral days"), then elapsed before those cows were again detected in heat and bred. The total days lost by this failure to breed at the first appropriate heat in this small group of cows resulted in an extra 6 days in the calving-to-conception interval when averaged over the whole herd.

Not satisfied with simply identifying one source of inefficiency in the reproductive program, the veterinarian further investigated the problem of deferral days. When the cows were subdivided into heifers and mature cows it was found that 0% and 18.5% of each group, respectively, were deferred. Heifers have a greater persistency of milk production than do cows; consequently a longer calving-to-conception interval in heifers has less detrimental effect on overall productivity. Thus, the veterinarian was concerned that the deferrals were occurring in mature cows instead of in heifers. However, the veterinarian had been continually stressing the importance of early breeding, and when the percentage of cows deferred during the first 6, second 6, and last 4 months of the study period were calculated, the results were 17.0%, 12.8%, and 0%. It appeared that the problem of deferrals had been solved.

The veterinarian then turned to the problem of identifying why cows were not being seen in heat early enough. A number of factors were examined and the results of several were as follows:

Factor	Calving to first heat interval (days)	
	Mean	Standard deviation
Age: 2 years	64	33
3–5 years	62	41
6+ years	68	47
Retained placenta: present	86	48
absent	61	40
Production: above herd average	71	48
below herd average	58	34
Season: summer first year	56	32
winter	77	51
summer second year	61	37

Age did not appear to be a factor in the problem. However, the 26 cows that had retained placentas had a substantially longer interval to first observed heat, suggesting that measures to reduce the incidence of retained placenta might be in order. The problem was also more serious in the higher producing cows, suggesting that the nutrition program in the dry period and early lactation should be reviewed. Finally, the problem appeared to be more serious in the winter. The veterinarian had noticed that the operators were less likely to be around the barn later in the evening during the winter and one possible consequence of this was a reduced level of heat detection.

These analyses were not a complete evaluation of all aspects of the reproduction program on the farm, but they did serve to identify the major problem areas. The problem of deferral days was identified, and with assistance it appeared that the producer had rectified that situation. It was also determined that cows having a retained placenta and cows calving during the winter were more likely to have a prolonged calving-to-first-heat interval. Steps to rectify those problems could be initiated immediately. Finally, the problem of failure to detect heats appeared more serious in high producing cows. A review of the nutritional program along with an evaluation of body condition scores would be required before corrective measures for that problem could be undertaken.

Once the problem area(s) have been identified, corrective action must be taken (step 4, Fig. 12.4). To institute the appropriate directed action, the practitioner's current knowledge may suffice, or the assistance of other personnel may be required. In some cases, the control strategies will not be obvious and further study of the type exemplified in the previous section will be required. Multiphasic screening (biochemical-metabolic profiles) and serologic data can be combined to allow the simultaneous study of the physiologic status and the infection (immune) status of individuals and the herd. Questions such as how many animals to sample, which animals to sample, and how many samples per animal are required for this purpose, remain largely unanswered. Nonetheless, first approximations are possible using the sampling techniques discussed in Chapter 2. The fact that multiphasic screening generally has failed to produce obvious benefits may in part reflect historic limitations with regard to sampling, testing , analysis, and interpretation of results, rather than the true value of the procedure.

If no answer to the problem is obvious, practitioners should be prepared to conduct well-designed, analytic observational studies and/or field trials. It is quite likely that in the future farmers will not demand immediate answers of the veterinarian, but they will demand that the veterinarian know how to find the answers. If the problem is at the herd level, the veterinarian should be able to obtain assistance from personnel at an epidemiologic research unit (10.4). As mentioned, a major reason for the existence of such a unit is to assist in problem solving at the herd level. The latter is very difficult for an individual practitioner to perform because data on many herds (flocks) are required, and the analytic expertise and computer requirements to manipulate and analyze the large volume of data or the ability to conduct multiherd field trials will be beyond the capabilities of most practitioners.

The final stage (step 5, Fig. 12.4) of problem resolution is to monitor the progress of the herd to ensure that the corrective measures have had the desired effect. If production levels fail to increase (or if production is not more efficient), the practitioner should reexamine the diagnostic indices to ensure that the correct problems have been identified. If this is confirmed, the control measures should be reexamined and alternate strategies employed if deemed necessary.

It is highly likely that mistakes will be made as veterinarians enter this new era of health management. Some mistakes are inevitable. The key is that the individual veterinarian, the client, and the veterinary profession must learn from their experiences, so clients get the best current information and advice and the quality of information improves with time. It should be obvious from the preceding discussion that the practitioner of the future is an applied researcher as well as a provider of essential technical services and information. Indeed, the combination of these two activities will likely increase the satisfaction of practitioners and prolong their productive days in practice.

12.3 Sporadic Diseases

Sporadic diseases (4.8.1) occur with low frequency and with no obvious temporal pattern. This definition by no means indicates that a sporadic disease occurs totally at random (i.e., without any pattern), nor does it mean that the disease is of no consequence. In fact, some of the most interesting animal diseases from an epidemiologic point of view belong to the group of sporadic diseases. These include the majority of diseases of general veterinary interest (e.g., chronic, neoplastic, and degenerative disorders; acute noncontagious problems such as traumatic lesions and poisonings; and genetically related problems).

Many sporadic diseases have an unknown or complex multifactorial etiology. An especially interesting group of sporadic diseases are those of comparative relevance to human health problems (e.g., cancer, degenerative diseases, and congenital defects) in relation to their possible environmental determinants. In addition to increased insight into the causes of disease, epidemiologic studies may help practicing veterinarians recognize animals with a high risk of a particular sporadic disease, and thus improve the likelihood of proper diagnosis, treatment, and prevention.

12.3.1 Availability and Validity of Data

A major problem of sporadic disease investigations is obtaining sufficiently accurate epidemiologic data about the disease because of its rare and unpredictable occurrence. Most methods used for retrieval of case data are, by the very nature of the problem, retrospective in their approach. These include surveys of existing records from herds, practices, and laboratories, and the establishment of centralized data banks for such records from one or more institutions to support subsequent retrospective searches for cases of a particular disease. Applications of these and other sources of data will be discussed in more detail later in this section.

The validity of the information on sporadic diseases is of critical importance. Special problems in this regard with studies of sporadic diseases are as follows: (1) often several diagnosticians and institutions contribute cases, and there may be no standardized nomenclature or common diagnostic criteria; (2) definitions of syndromes, particularly those of unknown etiology, tend to change gradually as new diagnostic methods become available, and this increases the problems with retrospective use of case records; (3) only small case series may be available for the study of a rare condition, thus relying heavily on the validity of each recorded event; and (4) biased selection of cases. Because such potential biasing factors are very likely to affect the results of an analytic observational study of a sporadic disease, even though appropriate standard analytic design and analysis are being applied, it is particularly important to utilize the judgment criteria mentioned in 5.5 in any causal interpretation of results.

In case-control and cross-sectional studies (i.e., nonprospective designs) special emphasis needs to be placed on ensuring a proper temporal sequence from exposure to disease. For example, using data from the DHIA system, in a case-control study of mycoplasma mastitis among California dairy herds, an association was found between the occurrence of mycoplasma mastitis and increased culling rates for the same year (Table 12.3). To establish the most likely temporal sequence between these events, culling rates for adjacent years were obtained. Since increased culling coincided with the outbreak, the authors concluded that mastitis was most likely the cause of high culling rates rather than vice versa (in which case high culling rates would have been expected at least for the year preceding the problem) (Thomas et al. 1982).

The application of the remaining criteria for causation may be illustrated from the data found in case-control studies on the relationship between dietary factors and the feline urologic syndrome (FUS). The consistency of findings among different studies in different countries using different scales of characterizing the level of feeding of dry cat foods (DCF) supports causality to be the reason for the observed association between DCF and FUS (Table 12.4). In addition, causality is strengthened by the observed dose-response relationship as well as coherence with other biolo-

Table 12.3. Culling percentages for herds grouped by year of first mycoplasmal mastitis problem

Year first positive for mycoplasma	Number of herds	Culled, 1975 (%)	Culled, 1976 (%)	Culled, 1977 (%)	Mean
1975	5	30.2	25.8	27.8	27.9
1976	8	30.4	37.1	31.3	32.9
1977	11	29.8	29.2	33.5	30.8
Mean for 24 herds		30.1	31.1	31.5	30.9

Source: Thomas et al. 1982, with permission.

Table 12.4. Odds ratios of FUS by level of convenience cat food used in the feeding as reported from recent studies around the world

	Odds ratios	
Level of feeding	Dry cat foods	Canned cat foods
Not normally fed	1	1
Normally fed	4.01**	0.59
Not fed	1	1
Once weekly or less	1.90	0.57
2–6 times weekly	1.69	0.72
Daily	1.73	0.60
Never fed	1	1
Rarely fed	1.70	0.75
Partly fed	8.67***	1.63
Mainly fed	6.11**	1.26
Exclusively fed	. . .	0
Not fed	1	1
Once weekly or less	0.78	0.67
2–6 times weekly	2.33***	0.45**
Daily	3.47***	0.66**
None	1[a] 1[b]	1[a]
<25% of diet	0.60 1.87	0.85
25–50% of diet	0.89 2.50	0.42
51–75% of diet	0.67 2.00	0.25
76–99% of diet	1.71 8.00*	0.36
100% of diet	6.67* 23.33**	1.39
Exclusively or mainly for at least several months	4.73***	. . .
Less than in entry above	1	. . .

Source: Willeberg 1981, with permission.
[a]Based on all FUS cats, initial as well as recurrent episodes.
[b]Based on cats with initial episode of FUS.
Note: Significance, * $= p < 0.05$,   ** $= p < 0.01$,   *** $= p < 0.001$.

gic facts (Willeberg 1981). These examples demonstrate the general benefit from collecting data suitable for establishing a dose-response relationship as the results are much more convincing than merely comparing two levels of a factor (i.e., fed versus not fed, exposed versus not exposed). Also note that the ordering of exposure may be done when the independent variables are ordinal (qualitative) in type, as well as when they are ratio level (quantitative) variables.

Investigating the reasons for lack of consistency in results among different studies may reveal the nature of any bias affecting a study. For example, other issues in FUS are whether castration increases the risk, whether there is a difference in risk among cat breeds, and whether multiple cat households experience more cases than expected from a common risk. Part of the controversy over these issues is due to conflicting evidence between laboratory experiments and epidemiologic studies, and disagreements among published epidemiologic studies (Willeberg 1981). Nonagreement between laboratory experiments and epidemiologic studies of multietiologic sporadic diseases such as FUS may have many explanations. One reason is that multifactorial diseases, such as FUS, often are not suitable for laboratory experiments where changes in only one or a few putative causal factor(s) are investigated at a time. In other words, laboratory studies may not be a relevant model of the spontaneous field situation and the results may not be applicable to the field. Furthermore, to produce a specified minimum number of clinical cases in a laboratory environment, either unrealistically large-scale experiments are required, or extreme exposures not typical of field conditions often must be used to reproduce the disease. The latter feature makes it difficult to extrapolate the laboratory results beyond that setting.

12.3.2 Estimating Frequency

It is difficult to estimate the incidence of a sporadic disease by direct methods such as those discussed in Chapter 2. Therefore indirect methods are often applied, some more appropriate than others. As one example, a retrospective longitudinal study was used to estimate the incidence of the feline urologic syndrome (FUS) in British and U.S. household cat populations. Telephone interviews were conducted with cat owners about episodes of FUS that occurred during the preceding 12-month period. The resulting incidence rate of approximately 0.6% per year agrees well with estimates based on FUS case loads seen in some veterinary practices in England, where the number of cases was related to the estimated cat population at risk in the practice areas after adjusting for possible non-veterinary-attended cases (Table 12.5). (As mentioned throughout this text, caution should be taken not to mistake proportional morbidity rates for incidence rates. It is obviously much easier to calculate the former because data on the total number of cases seen in a practice or a laboratory are more easily available than estimates of the population at risk. Confusion has resulted from published figures of 1–10% of all cats seen in veterinary hospitals being FUS cases, because these figures have been incorrectly termed "incidence of FUS.") As another example of estimating the frequency of sporadic disease, the incidence of LDA in Danish dairy cattle was estimated from an interview survey of veterinarians who provided the number of LDA cases and the average dairy cattle population in their respective practice area over the previous year (Grymer and Hesselholt, 1980) (Table 12.6). Similarly, estimates of the frequency of clinical bovine leukemia in Canada were derived through questioning of selected practitioners as well as routine slaughterhouse data. These data were related to the population at risk to estimate the rate of clinical leukemia (Kellar 1980).

In situations where routine collection of test samples is made for qual-

Table 12.5. Frequency of FUS as reported from recent studies around the world

Rate of cases	Population basis
Annual incidence rates	
34–52 per 10,000	Cats per year at risk in
64 per 10,000	the household cat
60 per 10,000	population
Proportional morbidity rates	
2.1%	All first presentations in the clinic
4.3%	All first presentations in the clinic, excluding nondiagnostic visits
5.7%	All first presentations in the clinics
4.5%	Cat-years at risk[a]
2.8–6.6%[b]	Cat-years at risk[a]
1.6%[c]	All first presentations in the practices, excluding nondiagnostic visits
Min. 0.75%	All cats seen in the clinic
4.5%	All male presentations in the clinic
5.4%	All first presentations in the clinic, excluding nondiagnostic visits

Source: Willeberg 1981, with permission.
[a]Individual cats counted once every year they visited the institution.
[b]Interinstitutional range observed among 13 veterinary colleges.
[c]The value is based on information from only 8 practices.

Table 12.6. Incidence of left abomasal displacement (LDA) in 26 Danish veterinary practices, 1 April 1977 to 31 March 1978

Practice	No. of LDA cases	No. of cows in practice	Incidence of LDA (% per year)
1	32	7,500	0.42
2	9	2,800	0.32
3	5	3,000	0.16
4	18	3,500	0.51
5	12	2,500	0.48
6	11	2,000	0.55
7	8	3,000	0.27
8	14	3,000	0.47
9	8	2,500	0.32
10	57	3,000	1.90
11	4	3,300	0.12
12	15	2,000	0.75
13	20	8,000	0.25
14	4	2,400	0.17
15	28	2,250	1.24
16	11	2,500	0.44
17	6	3,750	0.16
18	13	4,500	0.29
19	52	6,000	0.87
20	29	7,000	0.41
21	20	4,500	0.44
22	8	2,500	0.32
23	7	3,000	0.23
24	14	5,000	0.28
25	20	3,600	0.56
26	9	3,300	0.27
	434	96,400	0.45

Source: Grymer and Hesselholt, 1980, with permission.

ity control (e.g., antibiotic residues in milk and meat) or as part of a routine monitoring program (e.g., of herd prevalence of mastitis), special surveys for sporadic diseases may be carried out inexpensively. For example, in California two state-wide bulk tank surveys were made in 1977–78 to estimate the prevalence of pathogenic mycoplasma in bulk tank milk among dairy herds (Table 12.7).

Because many infections remain subclinical, the prevalence of infection is expected to be much more common than the disease; in fact, the presence of a putative pathogen may not be a good predictor of clinical disease. Similarly, surveys of seroreaction to agents associated with sporadic clinical disorders often show that, although the clinical condition may be sporadic, serological evidence of infection is by no means rare or unpredictable (Table 12.8). For example, clinical disease due to *Histoplasma capsulatum* in the dog is a serious, infrequent, often unpredictable disease, yet infection of dogs with this organism appears to be widespread and usually of little consequence.

Table 12.7. Distribution of herds with bulk tank milk isolations of known myco-plasma pathogens[a]

Number of colonies	Spring survey[b] (2410 herds)		Winter survey (2562 herds)		Combined (4972 herds)	
	No. of positive herds	Positive herd prevalence rate (%)	No. of positive herds	Positive herd prevalence rate (%)	No. of positive herds	Positive herd prevalence rate (%)
1–49	36	1.494	46	1.795	82	1.649
50 +	31	1.286	28	1.093	59	1.187
	67	2.780	74	2.888	141[b]	2.836

Source: Thomas et al. 1981, with permission.

[a]Pathogenic *Mycoplasma* species.

[b]Includes 23 herds with repeat isolations of the same species of *Mycoplasma* in the spring and winter survey, leaving 118 different herds as positive for the combined surveys.

Table 12.8. The prevalence of antibodies against *Coxiella burnetii* (Q-fever) among hospitalized livestock and pets and among stray dogs, University of California, 1973–75

Species	Number tested	Positive		Antibody titers		
		No.	Percent	4	8	>16
Hospitalized animals						
Cattle	28	9	32	3	2	4
Horses	121	31	26	19	10	2
Dogs	724	346	48	213	93	40
Cats	80	7	9	5	1	1
Nonhospitalized						
Dogs (stray)	316	208	66	166	39	3
	1269	601	47	406	145	50

Source: Willeberg et al. 1980, with permission.

The prevalence of sporadic conditions in populations may be more feasible to estimate as part of ongoing disease monitoring systems (e.g., at a slaughterhouse) or from screening a sample of the population, particularly if the condition is chronic. For example, the slaughterhouse data given in Table 12.9 are based on a large sample of animals, and assuming complete and accurate reporting (this is a major assumption), the resulting prevalence estimate should be close to the true population prevalence rate (small sampling variance). This is particularly true if the condition has a low case-fatality rate and does not alter the performance of the animals (i.e., they are not at increased risk of culling or slaughter because they have the disease). Other studies of the prevalence of sporadic diseases performed on very small samples (e.g., a study to estimate the prevalence of systemic lupus erythematosus (SLE) reactions among dogs belonging to people with SLE to investigate if there is an association between SLE in the two species) will have a large sampling error. Because of the large sampling variance, a prevalence estimate of zero is not very meaningful. The data in Table 2.1 can be used to derive upper confidence limits (either 95% or 99%) for the prevalence of disease in these situations. For example, if 1% of a population of 10,000 dogs were randomly selected and none were found to have the disease in question, the anticipated maximum number of cases in that population is 294, giving a 95% upper confidence limit of 2.9%. Despite these calculations, however, one remains rather uncertain of the true prevalence. (For a more detailed discussion of this, see Richards 1982.)

12.3.3 Characterizing the Case Series

Usually, the common characteristics of diseased individuals will be summarized in terms of the age, breed, and sex distribution. However, one must be careful in making inferences about the importance of these demographic factors as determinants of the disease based on the characteristics of diseased animals only. For example, in a descriptive sense it may be true that most cat patients with FUS are domestic shorthair. This, however, only reflects the fact that most household cats are domestic shorthair and it does

Table 12.9. Distribution of mycotoxic porcine nephropathy[a] (MPN) based on data from 10 Danish slaughterhouses in 1968

Sex	Number of MPN cases observed	Number of pigs slaughtered	Prevalence of cases per 10,000 pigs	Ratio: female rate to male rate (relative risk)
Females	248	469,172	5.3	1.4
Males	190	512,360	3.7	1.0
	438	981,532	4.5	. . .

Source: Krogh 1976, with permission.
[a]Kidney damage due to ochratoxin.

not indicate a high risk of FUS for that type of cat.

Similarly, in many case series of canine Cushing's syndrome, there is a predominance of female over male dogs. However, this does not mean that female dogs are at higher risk than males. One reason why the female excess attracts attention may be the fact that in human cases of Cushing's syndrome a true female predominance exists, and thus female excess among a series of canine patients is more likely to be published than a male excess in a canine case series. (This feature has been called a "publication bias.")

12.4   Analytic Observational Studies of Etiology

12.4.1   Case-Control Studies

The best way to make inferences about the etiology of a sporadic disease without accompanying data on the population base from which they originate is to perform a case-control study. This approach is particularly well suited to cope with rare diseases. Case records may be retrieved from institutional files and a control group can be sampled from the same or other sources to represent the population distribution of the factor in question (e.g., age, breed, or sex). Proper statistical comparisons can then be made (e.g., by the Mantel-Haenszel test) contrasting the characteristics of the cases with those of the control series to identify potential risk factors for the disease. Using this method it has been shown that Persian cats are at excess risk of FUS compared to domestic shorthair (Table 12.10) and that male and female dogs have the same risk of canine Cushing's syndrome (Willeberg and Priester 1982). Both these examples are from studies based on the Veterinary Medical Data Program (VMDP), a system specifically designed to support case-control studies. The VMDP may therefore serve to indicate the possibilities and requirements in collecting data to study the epidemiology of sporadic animal diseases.

Table 12.10.   Odds ratio of FUS by breed, Veterinary Medical Data Program, 1964–1973

Breed	Number of cases	Reference population	Odds ratio
Persian	240	3,553	1.4*
Domestic shorthair	2124	46,946	1.0
Siamese	663	15,927	0.8*
Other breeds	1084	23,081	1.0

Source: Willeberg and Priester 1976, with permission.
*Significantly different from 1; $p < 0.001$.
Note: In calculating R and chi-square values, breed risks were adjusted for sex, age, and weight, using the Mantel-Haenszel method.

12.4.1.1 VETERINARY MEDICAL DATA PROGRAM. The Veterinary Medical Data Program (VMDP) was begun by the U.S. National Cancer Institute (NCI) in 1964, at the College of Veterinary Medicine, Michigan State University, to provide a reliable standardized source of data on disease in domestic animals (Priester 1975). A number of veterinary schools in the United States and Canada have participated in this program.

At a collaborating veterinary college, when a patient is discharged or dies, the attending clinician completes a case summary form (or signs a summary form completed by the medical records specialist), including final diagnoses. The case summary, kept with the patient's permanent record file, is used by the medical records specialist to complete a standard VMDP abstract for entry on magnetic tape. The unique identifying number assigned each patient and used whenever that patient returns to the clinic provides a means of subsequently determining how many different patients were seen in each age, breed, sex, or weight subcategory, as well as the diagnostic and/or operative characteristics of each subcategory. In addition, the identifying number makes it possible to assemble a summary of the entire clinical history of an individual by computer, without manually referring to original medical records. (One limitation is that many of the institutions contributing to VMDP are referral institutions, and hence a patient may only be seen for particularly serious diseases because less serious diseases are handled by the client's regular veterinarian.)

Diagnoses and operations entered into VMDP are assigned numeric codes from the Standard Nomenclature of Veterinary Diseases and Operations (1975) and its supplements. The SNVDO codes are based on systematic numbering of (1) all parts of the body, (2) all etiologic agents, and (3) all operative procedures. Combinations are used to code diagnoses and operations. Standard codes for patient information (e.g., age, breed, sex, and weight) are provided on the abstract forms and in the VMDP Users Guide furnished participants.

The summary data on every patient, including diagnoses and operations, are entered on magnetic tape and sent to a central computing facility for storage and analyses. Quarterly tabulations sent to each participating school consist of listings of all cases arranged in numeric sequence according to several classifications such as patient's case number, etiology, or topographic site and summaries of the number of cases in various demographic categories. Each participating school also receives an annual tabulation of its own data, and, if requested, a tabulation made from the combined data submitted by all participants. Combined annual reports for each year from 1968 are kept on file at NCI. From these, one can estimate the total of any diagnosis or operation reported to VMDP. While not useful alone in analytic studies these estimates can be of value as background material or in planning research projects. Consisting of all discharges reported to VMDP since March 1964, the main magnetic tape data bank is available to all VMDP participants and other research groups. If the research will identify a particular school, permission must be sought before publication of results.

With more than 2 million records stored, the VMDP is the largest extant source of data on disease in domestic and pet animals. There have been more than 100 published reports to date based on analyses of these data, on topics as diverse as cancer, congenital heart disease, lead poisoning, endocrine diseases, and the feline urologic syndrome. Currently, the VMDP is being maintained by the College of Veterinary Medicine, Cornell University, Ithaca, New York.

12.4.1.2 OTHER SOURCES OF DATA. All practitioners use their experience and the most recent knowledge when diagnosing and treating cases of sporadic diseases. Yet in some instances, their performance would probably be improved if formal testing of their impressions were periodically carried out based on records from their own or neighboring practices. At one time it was not atypical for practitioners to carry out surveys on their own clients for this purpose; unfortunately, this practice has declined in recent years.

Usually, the relevant information needed to test a particular causal hypothesis is not always in the case records. This is particularly true when investigating specific exposures, although the common attributes (host factors) are often routinely recorded. Thus, it may be necessary to collect supplementary data (e.g., by questionnaires sent to owners of affected animals and owners of a comparison group of control animals). For example, several case-control studies of the role of dietary factors in the feline urologic syndrome (FUS) were carried out using records on FUS cases and selected control cats from clinics. In addition, mailed questionnaires were sent to cat owners inquiring about the composition of the diet.

In a similar manner, data on environmental and managerial factors at the herd level may be collected by personal interview or by questionnaires sent to owners of problem herds identified from routine diagnostic records (e.g., records kept in a practice, laboratory, or slaughterhouse) and to a sample of control herds. For example, in a study of swine enzootic pneumonia, data on barn ventilation were collected by questionnaires, whereas herd size and disease prevalence were estimated from data in the Danish slaughterhouse system. These data are shown in Tables 12.11 and 12.12, and the procedure to calculate the summary odds ratio using the Mantel-Haenszel method is also demonstrated (Willeberg 1980). Note that the crude odds ratio (not adjusted for herd size) is significant, whereas the adjusted odds ratio is not significant (Table 12.12). The relationship of some other factors to enzootic pneumonia prevalence is shown in Table

Table 12.11. Distribution of herds by health status, ventilation system, and herd size in a case-control study of swine enzootic pneumonia

| Herd size | Ventilation system | | | | Total no. of herds (n) |
| | With fan | | Without fan | | |
	Cases (a)	Controls (b)	Cases (c)	Controls (d)	
<200	2	7	4	27	40
200–300	15	30	8	18	71
300–400	13	19	7	10	49
400–500	7	5	2	4	18
>500	54	12	4	1	71
	91	73	25	60	249

Source: Willeberg 1980, with permission.
Cases had $\geq 5\%$ swine enzootic pneumonia (SEP); controls had $<5\%$ SEP.

Table 12.12. Adjustment of odds ratio (data from Table 12.11) by ventilation system for the confounding effect of herd size using the Mantel-Haenszel technique

Herd Size	$\dfrac{a \times d}{n}$	$\dfrac{b \times c}{n}$	$E(a) = \dfrac{(a+b)(a+c)}{n}$	$E(d) = \dfrac{(c+d)(b+d)}{n}$	$V(a) = \dfrac{E(a) \times E(d)}{n-1}$	Odds ratio (OR)
< 200	1.35	0.70	1.35	26.35	0.91	1.93
2–300	3.80	3.38	14.58	17.58	3.66	1.13
3–400	2.65	2.71	13.06	10.06	2.74	0.98
4–500	1.56	0.56	6.00	3.00	1.06	2.80
> 500	0.76	0.68	53.92	0.92	0.71	1.13
	10.12	8.03	88.91	57.91	9.08	2.99 (crude)

Source: Willeberg 1980, with permission.

Notes: Adjusted odds ratio $= \Sigma \dfrac{ad}{n} / \Sigma \dfrac{bc}{n} = \dfrac{10.12}{8.03} = 1.26$

Adjusted $\chi^2 = \dfrac{(|\Sigma \frac{ad}{n} - \Sigma \frac{bc}{n}| - \frac{1}{2})^2}{\Sigma V(a)} = \dfrac{(|10.12 - 8.03| - 0.5)^2}{9.08} = 0.28^{n.s.}$

$^{n.s.}$Non-significantly different from 1, $p > 0.05$.

12.13. As another example of this approach, a practitioner who had several herds with a high frequency of LDA in his district suspected feeding to be a contributory cause. Data on dietary composition were collected from a group of affected herds and from a selected group of nonaffected herds of similar size and production from the same general area. (The herds were matched on herd size, production, and locality.) The results (shown in Table 6.6) supported the idea that rations with low crude-fiber content were associated with increased occurrence of LDA (Grymer et al. 1981). Subsequently, the practitioner was in a much better position to advise on preventive measures against LDA. (Because the information is based on the farmer's own data, acceptance of control programs may be increased over suggested control strategies based on less direct data.)

Table 12.13. Odds ratio analysis of possible determinants of swine enzootic pneumonia (SEP) in Danish herds

	Number of herds		Odds ratio	
Factor/category	Cases ($\leq 5\%$ SEP)	Controls ($> 5\%$ SEP)	Crude	Adjusted for herd size
Herd size				
< 400 pigs slaughtered/yr	49	111	1.0	...
≥ 400 pigs slaughtered/yr	67	22	6.9[b]	...
Ventilation				
No-fan system	25	60	1.0	1.0
Fan system	91	73	3.0[b]	1.3[n.s.,c]
Replacement				
On-farm weaning	12	61	1.0	1.0
Purchase of weaners	104	72	7.3[b]	5.1[b]
Diarrhea				
No infectious diarrhea	56	86	1.0	1.0
Infectious diarrhea	60	47	2.0[a]	1.5[n.s.]
Frequency of other diseases				
$< 3\%$ prevalence at slaughter	55	85	1.0	1.0
$\geq 3\%$ prevalence at slaughter	61	48	2.0[a]	1.9[a]
	116	133	...	...

Source: Willeberg 1980, with permission.
[a]Significantly different from 1, $p < 0.05$.
[b]Significantly different from 1, $p < 0.001$.
[c]As per Table 12.12.
[n.s.]Nonsignificantly different from 1, $p > 0.05$.

Similar examples of this approach are found in studies of factors associated with mastitis (Goodhope and Meek 1980) and factors associated with *Haemophilus pleuropneumoniae* in swine (Rosendal and Mitchell 1983). Although subclinical mastitis is an endemic disease and clinical mastitis is sporadic, the methods used to study their epidemiologies are similar. In the study of pneumonia in swine, questionnaires were sent to registered pork producers in an attempt to estimate the prevalence of the problem as well as to identify risk factors for the syndrome. The low response rate in the swine study (22.5%) and the differential in responses between case and control herds in the mastitis survey (49% versus 81%) indicate the need for caution when interpreting the results of these otherwise well-designed studies.

12.4.2 Cohort Studies

It is rare that data sets suitable for a cohort or longitudinal study of sporadic diseases are available. Although cohort studies have numerous advantages over case-control studies (including the ability to estimate incidence rates among exposed and unexposed individuals), the difficulties in carrying out such studies are numerous. These include the long monitoring period of a large cohort to observe just a few cases, and the necessary tracing of the individuals during follow up makes it an expensive and tedious undertaking. One of the cohort studies concerns testicular tumor development in cryptorchid versus intact dogs (Reif et al. 1979). Many of the problems just mentioned arose in this study. Veterinarians from 22 practices collaborated in the study, and there was a wide variation among practices in the number of cryptorchids identified. This suggested either a difference in the at-risk population or variation in the interest of the practitioners. More than 25% of the dogs initially identified were lost to follow up during the 5-year study; often the owner could not be traced. This loss was particularly great during the first year after diagnosis of the condition or selection for the control cohort. In total, almost 1000 dogs (609 cryptorchids) were monitored and only 14 of these developed testicular neoplasia (Table 12.14). Despite the large effort, this was too few cases to provide valid estimates of breed specific rates. Another example of a cohort study involved a follow up of cats living in households with leukemic cats. The general feline population was used as the nonexposed group for purposes of comparison. In one of the cohorts of exposed cats, over 500 cats were followed for several years; 41 developed leukemia of which 11 (27%) were classified as feline leukemia virus-negative. This percentage of virus-negative leukemic cats was higher than in the general population where the overall rates of leukemia were much lower. Thus, the authors concluded that cats in households with feline leukemia virus excretors were at increased risk of leukemia whether virus was subsequently found in the new leukemia cases or not. This phenomenon of virus-negative leukemic cats is currently explained by the "immunoselection hypothesis" (Essex 1982).

12.4.3 Cross-Sectional and Longitudinal Studies

Longitudinal studies have been applied in a few instances using data bases specifically designed to provide estimates of cancer incidence and

Table 12.14. Age specific rates for testicular neoplasia in cryptorchid dogs from a cohort study comprising 609 cryptorchid and 329 age and breed-matched control dogs, which were monitored for an average of 2 years

Age	Dogs (no.)	Dog-years at risk	Neoplasms (no.)	Age specific rate per 1000 dog-years
2 and under	262	411.3	0	0.00
2–3	153	288.8	0	0.00
4–5	93	199.4	0	0.00
6–7	49	103.0	7	67.96
8–9	31	59.2	4	67.57
10 and over	21	43.3	3	69.28
	609	1105.0	14	12.67

Source: Reif et al. 1979, with permission.

Note: No cases of testicular neoplasia developed among the control dogs during the observation period.

distribution in dogs and cats. One example is the Animal Neoplasm Registry of the Alameda and Contra Costa counties of California (Schneider 1975). In this program, all veterinary practices in a defined geographic area submit data and tissue specimens on all neoplastic conditions to a common pathology laboratory for diagnosis. To establish a reference population, questionnaire surveys (census) of the households in the area are taken repeatedly to estimate the size and characteristics of the population at risk (Schneider 1983).

A somewhat similar situation exists in Denmark, where since 1959 all cattle tumors have been deemed notifiable diseases and must be submitted for histopathology, whether as a biopsy from a clinical case or as tissue samples collected from abattoirs or from necropsies. Statistics are also being prepared on nonenzootic types of leukosis (juvenile, skin, and sporadic adult bovine leukosis). Appropriate population figures from published yearly census reports are used in the conversion of the numerator data to rates. For example, between 1969 and 1980 the incidence rate of sporadic adult leukotic tumors decreased from 4 to 2 per 10^5 cow-years at risk, while the incidence rate of enzootic tumors dropped from 1.5 down to 0.15 per 10^5 cow-years at risk over the same period (Willeberg et al. 1982).

Cross-sectional studies can be conducted on hospitalized animals. Willeberg et al. (1980) carried out a serological survey of Q-fever antibodies among hospitalized animals. This study indicated associations between seroreaction in dogs and their sex (data not shown) and discharge status, respectively (Table 12.15). While sex may be regarded as a contributory factor to seropositive status, the discharge status may possibly be a result of the infection. It is more likely, however, that discharge status and seroreaction are partly determined by a third factor, namely the primary disease for which the dogs were hospitalized. The latter explanation suggests either that dormant Q-fever infections are turned into active ones by various debilitating conditions, or weakened individuals are highly susceptible to a widespread Q-fever agent. This example again illustrates the kind of problems that one may get into in interpretation of results from cross-sectional surveys.

12.5 Ecologic Studies

Ecologic studies typically are investigations involving aggregates of individuals as the unit of analysis when the unit of concern is the individual. The group may be litters, pens, farms, animals in specified geographic areas, etc.

Ecologic studies are performed in situations where it is difficult or impractical to obtain exposure and outcome data on individuals. Also, because they can often be done using existing data sources, they are less

Table 12.15.   Discharge status among hospitalized animals by species and test reaction for *Coxiella burnetii* (Q-fever) antibodies at admission, University of California, Davis, 1973–1975

Species	Serotest result	Discharge status			Mortality (%)
		Alive	Dead	Total	
Dog[a]	Positive	271	74	345	21
	Negative	328	43	371	12
		599	117	716[a]	
	chi-square = 12.71, $p < 0.001$				
Horse	Positive	21	10	31	32
	Negative	70	20	90	22
		91	30	121	
	chi-square = 1.24, $p > 0.20$				
Cat	Positive	6	1	7	14
	Negative	53	20	73	27
		59	21	80	
	chi-square = 0.57, $p > 0.40$				
Cattle	Positive	5	4	9	44
	Negative	15	4	19	21
		20	8	28	
	chi-square = 1.64, $p > 0.20$				

Source: Willeberg et al. 1980, with permission.
[a]Discharge status for 8 dogs was not stated; 1 was seropositive.

time consuming and expensive than prospective studies using the individual as the unit of analysis (Morgenstern 1982). On the other hand, results of ecologic studies are prone to substantial bias, because one must assume that what is true at the group level is true at the individual level since data on individuals are missing. This assumption is frequently incorrect, hence the term for this bias is "ecologic fallacy." In discussing causal associations in 5.6.1, it was stated that if the exposure is measured at a level different than the unit of concern, any causal associations must be indirect in terms of the unit of concern. The current discussion elaborates reasons why the association at the group level may not be valid at the individual level. Certainly whenever ecologic studies are used, the investigators should strive to assess the validity of this assumption, rather than accepting it on faith.

In the Bruce County Beef Health Study, it was noted that groups of cattle fed large amounts of corn silage early in the post-arrival period had higher mortality rates. This association is valid and likely directly causal at the group level. Despite this, it may not be true at the individual level. The missing information is which calves ate corn silage and which died; that is, given that alternate feed (e.g., dry hay) was available, it may have been the calves that ate the alternate feed that died, not those eating the silage. Without firsthand knowledge of what happened in individuals, one must appeal to the fact that the stronger the relationship at the group level, the more likely it is to be true at the individual level.

In another study of dairy cow mortality, a time-series analysis was used to characterize the components of the observed temporal variations in the crude mortality rates (Agger 1983). This technique decomposes the observed variations into various components of time, including an overall linear (secular) trend, a cyclical component, a seasonal component, and an irregular random component. Figure 12.6 shows the cyclical component, and superimposed on this is an economic standard index for the volume of agricultural building investments. A striking correlation between the two curves appears, including a 1–2 year phase difference between a change in the building index and the corresponding change in mortality. Given that most criteria for causation are met, in ecologic terms the covariation may be interpreted as causality between new barn buildings and a resulting higher mortality rate, perhaps due to management problems during the break-in period and the related increased disease occurrence. Although this appears to be a logical and likely explanation of the observed covariation, what happened on individual farms is unknown. In the present example it is not known whether the excess number of cows dying in years following high barn building activity were housed in newly built barns or older barns.

As a final example of an ecologic study, consider the data on canine distemper (CD) and multiple sclerosis (MS) in Table 12.16, (Kurtzke and Priester 1979). The number of CD cases recorded during 1973–1977 in areas of states containing veterinary schools that collaborated in the VMDP were related to two different denominators: (1) the total number of cases in those schools (proportional morbidity rates), and (2) the number of people

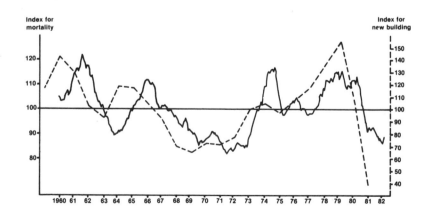

12.6. Comparison of cyclical component (C_t) from time series analysis of monthly crude mortality rate of mature cattle/10,000 cows and heifers that have calved annually from 1960 to 1982 (solid line) with annual volume index for investments in agricultural buildings from 1960 to 1981 (broken line). (Source: Agger 1983, pp. 308–11)

Table 12.16. **Ecologic study of possible association between human cases of multiple sclerosis (MS) and canine distemper (CD) on a state basis. CD cases from VMDP, MS cases from a Veterans Administration study in which matched pairs of MS cases and controls (C) were formed**

Veterinary center	1973–1977 CD cases	Annual number of CD cases per 10^4 dogs treated	Annual number of CD cases per 10^4 human population	MS/C ratio
Michigan	170	48	3.8	1.22
Missouri	204	92	8.6	0.89
Minnesota	85	32	4.4	1.93
Iowa	139	78	9.6	1.09
Indiana	58	39	2.2	0.80
Georgia	244	103	10.2	0.59
California	407	102	9.7	1.22
Ohio	748	157	13.9	1.22
Kansas	185	59	16.2	1.04
Illinois	172	61	3.1	1.03
Colorado	223	74	18.3	1.03
Alabama	172	107	12.2	0.45
	2807	84.1	11.0	. . .
(Total)[a]	(3055)	(81.6)	. . .	(1.00)

Source: Kurtzke and Priester 1979, with permission.
Note: The "risk" of MS by state is expressed as the ratio of MS cases to controls (MS/C). Only states for which VMDP data were available are included. Correlation between MS/C ratio and CD proportion of dogs was $r = -0.22$ and between MS/C ratio and CD proportion on a human population basis was $r = +0.02$, indicating no consistent association of MS with CD.
[a]Second total includes two Canadian centers, plus Texas 1976–1977.

in each area. The list of MS cases was derived from a Veterans Administration study, and for each state the risk of MS was described by the case-to-control ratio (MS/C). There was a weak negative association between the proportional morbidity rate of CD and MS/C ratio ($r = -0.22$) and virtually no association between the number of CD cases per 10^6 humans and the MS/C ratio. The conclusions indicate that there does not appear to be any association between CD and MS; this is consistent with a number of other studies on this subject and supports the lack of a causal relationship.

As mentioned earlier, monitoring disease in animals can be used as an early warning system for humans. At the ecologic level, there is a positive association between bladder cancer occurrence in dogs and the extent of manufacturing in that area; the inference is that chemical pollutants increase the risk of bladder cancer in both dogs and humans (Hayes et al. 1981).

Thus, ecologic studies have a valid role to play in investigating exposure-disease associations; however, they are most useful as indicators of hypotheses that require more detailed evaluation (i.e., where exposure and outcome are measured at the same level in the unit of concern), rather than as final studies on the subject.

References

Agger, J. F. 1983. Production disease and mortality in dairy cows: Analysis of records from disposal plants 1960–82. Proc. 5th Conf. on Prod. Dis. in Farm Animals, Aug. 1983, Uppsala, Sweden.

Blood, D. C. 1979. The veterinarian in planned animal health and production. Can. Vet. J. 20:341–47.

Blood, D. C., R. S. Morris, N. B. Williamson, C. M. Cannon, and R. M. Cannon. 1978. A health programme for commercial dairy herds. I. Objectives and methods. Aust. Vet. J. 54:207–15.

Botterell, E. H. 1976. Maintenance of Animal Health for Food Production. A report for the Ontario Ministry of Agriculture and Food.

Cannon, R. M., R. S. Morris, N. B. Williamson, C. M. Cannon, and D. C. Blood. 1978. A health programme for commercial dairy herds. II. Data processing. Aust. Vet. J. 54:216–30.

Committee on Communicable Diseases Affecting Man. 1976. Procedures to investigate foodborne illness. Int. Assn. Milk, Food, Environ. Sanitarians. Ames, Iowa.

Committee on Communicable Diseases Affecting Man. 1979. Procedures to investigate waterborne illness. Int. Assn. Milk, Food, Environ. Sanitarians. Ames, Iowa.

Davies, G. 1983. Pig health and production recording. U.K. Min. Agric. Fisheries and Food, Booklet 2075.

Dohoo, I. R. 1982. Cost of extended open period in dairy cattle. Can. Vet. J. 23:229–30.

———. 1983. The effects of calving to first service interval on reproductive performance in normal cows and cows with postpartal disease. Can. Vet. J. 24:343–46.

Dohoo, I. R., S. W. Martin, and A. H. Meek. 1984. Disease, production and culling in Holstein-Friesian cows. VI. Effects of management on disease rates. Prev. Vet. Med. 3:15–28.

Erb, H. N., and S. W. Martin. 1980. Interrelationships between production and reproductive diseases in Holstein cows. Data. J. Dairy Sci. 63:1911–17.

Erb, H. N., S. W. Martin, N. Ison, and S. Swaminathan. 1981. Interrelationships between production and reproductive diseases in Holstein cows. Path analysis. J. Dairy Sci. 64:281–89.

Essex, M. E. 1982. Feline leukemia: A naturally occurring cancer of infectious origin. Epidemiol. Rev. 4:189–203.

Esslemont, R. J., A. J. Stephens, and P. R. Ellis. 1981. DAISY: Dairy information system. An aid to record keeping and health management. Proc. Am. Assoc. Bov. Pract. 13:51–60.

Etherington, W. G., W. T. K. Bosu, S. W. Martin, J. F. Cote, P. A. Doig, and K. E. Leslie. 1984a. Reproductive performance in dairy cows following postpartum treatment with GnRH and/or postaglandin: A field trial. Can. J. Comp. Med. 48:245–50.

Etherington, W. G., A. H. Meek, and B. W. Stahlbaum. 1984b. Application of Microcomputers to Facilitate the Collection and Analysis of Health and Production Data on Dairy Farms. Guelph, Canada: Univ. of Guelph.

Goodhope, R. G., and A. H. Meek. 1980. Factors associated with mastitis in Ontario dairy herds: A case-control study. Can. J. Comp. Med. 44:351–57.

Grymer, J., and M. Hesselholt. 1980. Abomasal dislocation—a production disease in intensive dairy herds. Dansk Vet. Tdsskr. 63:852–57.

Grymer, J., M. Hesselholt, and P. Willeberg. 1981. Feed composition and left abomasal displacement in dairy cattle: A case-control study. Nord. Vet. Med. 33:306–9.

Hancock, D. D. 1983. Studies on the epidemiology of mortality and diarrheal morbidity in heifer calves in northeastern Ohio dairy herds. Ph.D. thesis, Ohio State University.

Hanson, R. P., and M. G. Hanson. 1983. Animal Disease Control: Regional Programs. Ames: Iowa State Univ. Press.

Hayes, H. M. Jr., R. Hoover, and R. E. Tarone. 1981. Bladder cancer in pet dogs: A sentinel for environmental cancer? Am. J. Epidemiol. 114:229–33.

Hird, D. W., and R. A. Robinson. 1982. Dairy farm wells in southeastern Minnesota: The relation of water source to milk and milk-fat production. Prev. Vet. Med. 1:37–51.

_____. 1983. Dairy farm wells in southeastern Minnesota: The relation of new water sources (new wells) to milk and milk-fat production. Prev. Vet. Med. 1:97–104.

Hopkins, R. S., R. Olmstead, and G. R. Istre. 1984. Endemic *Campylobacter jejuni* infection in Colorado: Identified risk factors. Am. J. Publ. Health. 74:249–50.

Kellar, J. A. 1980. The economic impact of enzootic bovine leucosis in Canada. Food Prod. Insp. Br. Agric. Canada. Ottawa, Canada.

Krogh, P. 1976. Epidemiology of mycotoxic porcine nephropathy. Nord. Vet. Med. 28:452–58.

Kurtzke, J. F., and W. A. Priester. 1979. Dogs, distemper, and multiple sclerosis in the United States. Acta Neurol. Scand. 60:312–19.

Loew, F. M. 1976. Why are we here? An Emerging Municipal Issue. Proc. 1st Can. Symp. on Pets in Soc. Ottawa, Ont.: Can. Vet. Med. Assoc.

Marcoux, L., M. De Gràce, F. Filiatrault, P. Auger, and L. Jette. 1984. Food poisoning at a Sugar Bush, Quebec. Can Dis. Wkly. Rep. 45:178–80.

Martin, S. W. 1982. Epidemiology: Its role in health maintenance programs. *In* Cost Benefits of Food Animal Health, ed. J. B. Kaneene and E. C. Mather. East Lansing: Michigan State Univ. Press.

Martin, S. W., A. H. Meek, D. G. Davis, J. A. Johnson, and R. A. Curtis. 1982a. Factors associated with mortality and treatment costs in feedlot calves: The Bruce County Beef Project, years 1978, 1979, 1980. Can. J. Comp. Med. 46:341–49.

Martin, S. W., J. D. Holt, and A. H. Meek. 1982b. The effect of risk factors as determined by logistic regression on health of beef feedlot cattle. Proc. 3rd Int. Symp. Vet. Epidemiol. Econ., Sept. 1982, Arlington, Va.

Meek, A. H., W. R. Mitchell, R. A. Curtis, and J. F. Cote. 1975. A proposed information management and disease monitoring system for dairy herds. Can. Vet. J. 16:329–40.

Meek, A. H., S. W. Martin, J. B. Stone, I. McMillan, J. B. Britney, and D. G. Grieve. 1986. The relationship among current management systems, production, disease, and drug usage on Ontario dairy farms. Can. J. Vet. Res. 50:7–14.

Morgenstern, H. 1982. Uses of ecologic analyses in epidemiologic research. Am. J. Publ. Health. 72:1336–44.

Morris, R. S. 1971. Economic aspects of disease control programs for dairy cattle. Aust. Vet. J. 47:358–63.

Morris, R. S., N. B. Williamson, D. C. Blood, R. M. Cannon, and C. M. Cannon. 1978a. A health programme for commercial dairy herds. III. Changes in reproductive performance. Aust. Vet. J. 54:231–46.

Morris, R. S., D. C. Blood, N. B. Williamson, C. M. Cannon, and R. M. Cannon. 1978b. A health programme for commercial dairy herds. IV. Changes in mastitis prevalence. Aust. Vet. J. 54:247–51.

Pepper, T. A., H. W. Boyd, and P. Rosenberg. 1977. Breeding record analysis in pig herds and its veterinary applications. I. Development of a program to monitor reproductive efficiency and weaner production. Vet. Rec. 101:177–80.

Pepper, T. A., and D. J. Taylor. 1977. Breeding record analysis in pig herds and its veterinary applications. II. Experience with a large commercial unit. Vet. Rec. 101:196–99.

Priester, W. A. 1975. Collecting and using veterinary clinical data. In Animal Disease Monitoring, ed. D. G. Ingram, W. R. Mitchell, and S. W. Martin. Springfield, Ill.: C. C. Thomas.

Reif, J. S., T. G. Maguire, R. M. Kenney, and R. S. Brodey. 1979. A cohort study of canine testicular neoplasia. J. Am. Vet. Med. Assoc. 175:719–23.

Richards, M. S. 1982. The detection and measurement of diseases of low prevalence. Proc. 3rd Int. Symp. Vet. Epidemiol. Econ., Sept. 1982, Arlington, Va.

Robertson, J., McD. 1968. Left displacement of the bovine abomasum: Epizootiologic factors. Am. J. Vet. Res. 29:421–34.

Rosendal, S., and W. R. Mitchell. 1983. Epidemiology of *Haemophilus pleuropneumoniae* infection in pigs: A survey of Ontario pork producers, 1981. Can. J. Comp. Med. 47:1–5.

Schneider, R. 1975. A population-based animal tumor registry. In Animal Disease Monitoring, ed. D. G. Ingram, W. R. Mitchell, and S. W. Martin. Springfield, Ill.: C. C. Thomas.

———. 1983. Comparison of age and sex-specific incidence rate patterns of the leukemia complex in the cat and the dog. J. Natl. Cancer Inst. 70:971–77.

Schwabe, C. W. 1984. Veterinary Medicine and Human Health. 3rd ed. Baltimore, Md., Williams & Wilkins.

Schwabe, C. W., H. Riemann, and C. E. Franti. 1977. Epidemiology in Veterinary Practice. Philadelphia, Penn.: Lea & Febiger.

Simensen, E. 1983. An epidemiologic study of calf health and performance in Norwegian dairy herds. Acta Agric. Scand. 33:57–64, 65–94.

Stephens, A. J., R. J. Esslemont, and P. R. Ellis. 1982. DAISY: A dairy herd information system for small computers. In Cost Benefits of Food Animal Health, ed. J. B. Kaneene and E. C. Mather. East Lansing: Michigan State Univ. Press.

Thomas, C. B., P. Willeberg, and D. E. Jasper. 1981. Case-control study of bovine mycoplasmal mastitis in California. Am. J. Vet. Res. 42:511–15.

Thomas, C. B., D. E. Jasper, and P. Willeberg.1982. Clinical bovine mycoplasmal mastitis: An epidemiologic study of factors associated with problem herds. Acta Vet. Scand. 213:53–64.

Thomson, G. W., and I. K. Barker. 1979. Case report: Japanese yew (*Taxus cuspidata*) poisoning in cattle. Can. Vet. J. 19:320–21.

Waltner-Toews, D. 1985. Dairy calf management, morbidity, mortality, and calf related drug use in Ontario Holstein herds. Ph.D. thesis, Univ. of Guelph, Guelph, Canada.

Waltner-Toews, D., S. W. Martin, A. H. Meek, I. McMillan, and C. F. Crouch. 1985. A field trial to evaluate the efficacy of a combined Rotavirus-Coronavirus/*Esherichia coli* vaccine in dairy cattle. Can. J. Comp. Med. 49: 1–9.

Willeberg, P. 1980. The analysis and interpretation of epidemiological data. Proc. 2nd Int. Symp. Vet. Epidemiol. Econ., May 1979, Canberra, Aust.

———. 1981. Epidemiology of the feline urological syndrome. Adv. Vet. Sci. Comp. Med. 25:311–43.

Willeberg, P., and W. A. Priester. 1976. Feline urological syndrome: Associations with some time, space, and individual patient factors. Am. J. Vet. Res. 37:975–78.

———. 1982. Epidemiological aspects of clinical hyper-adrenocorticism in dogs (canine Cushing's syndrome). J. Am. Anim. Hosp. Assoc. 18:717–24.

Willeberg, P., R. Ruppanner, D. E. Behymer, S. Haghighi, J. J. Kaneko, and C. E. Franti. 1980. Environmental exposure to *Coxiella burnetii*: A seroepidemiologic survey among domestic animals. Am. J. Epidemiol. 111:437–43.

Willeberg, P., C. E. Franti, A. Gottschau, J. Flensburg, and R. Hoff-Jorgensen. 1982. A preliminary evaluation of the Danish control program for enzootic bovine leukosis. Proc. 3rd Int. Symp. Vet. Epidemiol. Econ., Sept. 1982, Arlington, Va.

Williamson, N. B. 1981. Reproductive performance and recording systems. Proc. 13th Am. Assoc. Bovine Pract.

Williamson, N. B., R. M. Cannon, D. C. Blood, and R. S. Morris. 1978. A health programme for commercial dairy herds. V. The occurrence of specific disease entities. Aust. Vet. J. 54:252–56.

INDEX

ISBN 0-8138-1856-7

9 780813 818566

Iowa State University Press
2121 South State Avenue
Ames, Iowa 50014

Phone: 800-862-6657
Fax: 515-292-3348